# Practical Fracture Treatment

*To Helen*

*For Churchill Livingstone*

*Publisher:* Mike Parkinson
*Project Editor:* Dilys Jones
*Production Controller:* Debra Barrie
*Sales Promotion Executive:* Duncan Jones

# Practical Fracture Treatment

**Ronald McRae** FRCS (Eng, Glas) AIMBI

With original drawings and illustrations by the author

THIRD EDITION

CHURCHILL LIVINGSTONE
EDINBURGH LONDON MADRID MELBOURNE NEW YORK AND TOKYO 1994

CHURCHILL LIVINGSTONE
Medical Division of Longman Group UK Limited

Distributed in the United States of America by Churchill Livingstone Inc.,
650 Avenue of the Americas, New York, N.Y. 10011, and by associated companies, branches
and representatives throughout the world.

First edition 1981
Second edition 1989
Third edition 1994

ISBN 0-443-04809-6

**British Library Cataloguing in Publication Data**
A catalogue record for this book is available from the British Library.

**Library of Congress Cataloging in Publication Data**
McRae, Ronald.
    Practical fracture treatment/Ronald McRae; with original
drawings and illustrations by the author. — 3rd ed.
        p. cm.
    ISBN 0-443-04809-6
    1. Fractures—Treatment.   I. Title.
    [DNLM: 1. Fracture Fixation—methods.   2. Fracture Fixation–
–methods—atlases.   WE 185 M174p 1994]
RD101.M222   1994
617.1′5—dc20
DNLM/DLC
for Library of Congress                                                        93-7651

The
publisher's
policy is to use
**paper manufactured
from sustainable forests**

Printed in Hong Kong
NPC/01

# Contents

# Preface to the third edition

In this edition I have made changes in most sections to reflect the continuous expansion of the use of internal fixation in the treatment of fractures; at the same time I have tried to preserve where appropriate details of commonly practised methods of conservative management.

To give further assistance in the general assessment of fractures and those who suffer from them, I have included the AO classification of long bone fractures, Tile's classification of pelvic fractures, Gustilo's classification of open fractures, Trauma Scoring, the use of the Mangled Extremity Severity Score, and the Glasgow Coma scale. There is fresh material on a variety of subjects ranging from gunshot wounds to injuries associated with child abuse.

Lastly, I have suggested some guidelines which might be used when it comes to the important matter of communicating by phone and by the written word; the latter is included within a small additional chapter on fracture clinics.

I hope that the reader will find these changes of value.

Gourock, 1993                                                              R. M.

# Preface to the first edition

This book has been written primarily for the medical student, and the introductory section assumes little prior knowledge of the subject. The second part, which deals with particular fractures, is set in places at a more advanced level; it is hoped that the book will thereby continue to prove of value to the student when he moves to his first casualty or registrar post.

In planning this volume, I have paid particular attention to two points. Firstly, the details of each fracture and a good deal of the introductory section have been arranged in a linear sequence. The material has been divided into small packets of text and illustration in order to facilitate comprehension and learning. These packets have been set out in a logical sequence which in most cases is based on the relative importance of the initial decisions which must be made in a case, and the order in which treatment procedures should be carried out. This format is in a few places restrictive, with an imbalance in the amount of information carried by either text or illustration. This must be accepted because of spatial and subject limitations. Generally, however, text and illustration will be found to complement one another. The text, although of necessity brief, is concise and, it is hoped, to the point.

Secondly, fracture treatment has been given in an uncommon amount of practical detail. As there is such a variety of accepted treatments for even the simplest of fractures, this has the danger of attracting the criticism of being controversial and didactic. This is far from my intention, and I have tried to avoid this in several ways. Firstly, as minor fractures and most children's fractures (together forming the bulk of all fractures) are most frequently treated conservatively, the conservative approach I have employed for these injuries should on the whole receive general approval. Secondly, in the more controversial long bone fractures in adults, and in fractures involving joints, I have on the whole pursued a middle course between the extremes of conservative and surgical management. The methods I have singled out for description are those which I consider safest and most reliable in the hands of the comparatively inexperienced. Where alternative methods appear to me to be equally valid I have generally included these. To conceal my own whims I have not always placed these in the order of personal preference. In consequence, I hope that any offence given by the methods described will be restricted to the most extreme quarters.

R. M.

# Acknowledgements

I would like to thank Mrs Mary Kelly for her painstaking care in the preparation of the original typescript, Mr T. H. Norton and Dr Wilson James for their kind help in tracing and allowing me to copy several of the radiographs accompanying the text, and the late Mr James Patrick and my Glasgow colleagues for a number of useful suggestions.

For the second edition, I would like to acknowledge the help of Mr John Bingham, Mr Colin Mainds, and Mr Norton, again, for allowing me to reproduce some of the radiographs which have been added to this work.

# How to use this book

The basic principles of fractures and their treatment are dealt with in the first part of this book. The AO Classification of fractures (pp. 21–22), Trauma Scoring (pp. 35–38) and the Mangled Extremity Severity Score may be noted but do not require detailed study by the undergraduate.

The second part of the book is arranged on a regional basis and may be used as a guide for the handling of specific fractures. Detailed study is not required by the undergraduate, but a superficial reading should consolidate knowledge of the basic principles, and indicate how they are applied in practice.

The following conventions are used in the illustrations and text:

1. Where two sides are shown for comparison, the patient's *right* side is the one affected.
2. Where several conditions are described, and only one illustrated, the first mentioned is the one shown, unless followed by the abbreviation 'Illus.'.
3. In cross references, the number to the left of the comma indicates the page number while that to the right gives the appropriate frame number: e.g. 119, 70 refers to page 119, frame 70.

## Abbreviations

A      = anterior
Illus. = illustrated
L      = lateral or left
M      = medial
N      = normal
P      = posterior
R      = right

# Section A:
# General principles

# 1. Pathology and healing of fractures

**Initial definitions: 1. Fracture:** A fracture is present when there is loss of continuity in the substance of a bone. The term covers all bony disruptions, ranging from one end of the scale when (1) a bone is broken into many fragments (multifragmentary or comminuted fracture) to (2) hair-line and even microscopic fractures at the other. To the layman the word 'fracture' implies a more severe injury than a simple break in the bone, but in the strict medical sense there is no difference between these terms.

**2. Open fractures:** All fractures are either *closed* or *open*. In an open fracture there is a wound in continuity with the fracture, and the potential exists for organisms to enter the fracture site from outside. All open fractures therefore carry the risk of becoming infected. In addition, blood loss from external haemorrhage may be significant. (Note: the term 'compound' is still frequently used to describe a fracture which is open; the term 'simple', to describe a closed fracture, may lead to confusion, and is now largely abandoned.)

**3. Closed fracture:** In a closed fracture the skin is either intact, or if there are any wounds these are superficial or unrelated to the fracture. So long as the skin is intact, there is no risk of infection from outside. (Blood-borne infection of closed fractures is extremely rare.) Any haemorrhage is internal.

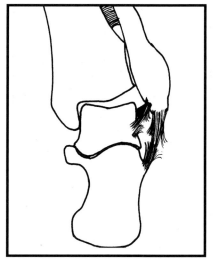

**4. Dislocation:** In a dislocation there is complete loss of congruity between the articulating surfaces of a joint. The bones taking part in the articulation are displaced relative to one another; e.g. in a dislocated shoulder the head of the humerus loses all contact with the glenoid. In the common anterior dislocation the head of the humerus is displaced anteriorly.

**5. Subluxation:** In a subluxation, the articulating surfaces of a joint are no longer congruous, but loss of contact is incomplete. The term is often used to describe the early stages in a condition which may proceed to complete dislocation (e.g. in a joint infection or in rheumatoid arthritis).

**6. Sprain:** A sprain is an incomplete tear of a ligament or complex of ligaments responsible for the stability of a joint; e.g. a sprain of the ankle is a partial tear of the external ligament and is not associated with instability (as distinct from a complete tear). The term sprain is also applied to incomplete tears of muscles and tendons.

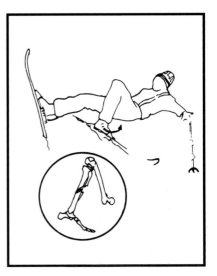

**Causes of fracture:** 7. **Direct violence (a):** Fractures are caused by the application of stresses which exceed the limits of strength of a bone. Violence is the commonest cause. In the case of *direct violence,* a bone may be fractured by being struck by a moving or falling object — e.g. a fracture of the terminal phalanx of a finger by a hammer blow.

8. **Direct violence (b):** A bone may also be fractured if *it* forcibly strikes a resistant object. For example, a fall on the point of the elbow may fracture the olecranon.

9. **Indirect violence:** Very frequently fractures result from indirect violence. A twisting or bending stress is applied to a bone, and this results in its fracture at some distance from the application of the causal force. For example, a rotational stress applied to the foot may cause a spiral fracture of the tibia. Indirect violence is also the commonest cause of dislocation.

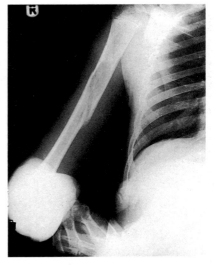

10. **Fatigue fractures:** Stresses, repeated with excessive frequency to a bone, may result in fracture. This mechanism is often compared with fatigue in metals which break after repeated bending beyond their elastic limit. The commonest of these fractures involves the second metatarsal—the march fracture (so called because of its frequency in army recruits).

11. **Pathological fractures (a):** A pathological fracture is one which occurs in an abnormal or diseased bone. If the osseous abnormality reduces the strength of the bone then the force required to produce fracture is reduced, and may even become trivial. For example a secondary tumour deposit may lead to a pathological fracture of the subtrochanteric region of the femur—a common site.

12. **Pathological fractures (b):** Pathological fractures may also occur at the site of simple tumours—e.g. a fracture of the humerus in a child with a simple bone cyst. *The commonest causes of pathological fracture are osteoporosis and osteomalacia.*

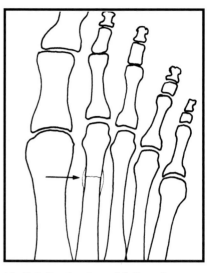

**Fracture patterns and their significance: 13. Hair-line fractures (a):** Hair-line fractures result from minimal trauma, i.e. trauma which is just great enough to produce a fracture but not severe enough to produce any significant displacement of the fragments. Such fractures may be (1) incomplete or (2) complete.

14. **Hair-line fractures (b):** These fractures may be difficult to detect on the radiographs, and where there are reasonable clinical grounds for suspecting a fracture, the rules are quite clear. (1) Additional oblique radiographic projections of the area may be helpful. (2) Do not accept poor quality films. (3) Films repeated after 7–10 days may show the fracture quite clearly (due to decalcification at the fracture site).

15. **Hair-line fractures (c):** *Stress fractures* are generally hair-line in pattern, and are often not diagnosed with certainty until there is a wisp of subperiosteal callus formation, or increased density at the fracture site some 3–6 weeks after the onset of symptoms. Hair-line fractures generally heal rapidly requiring only symptomatic treatment: **but** the scaphoid and femoral neck are notable exceptions.

16. **Hair-line fractures (d):** Radiograph of upper tibia of an athletic adolescent with a 7-week history of persistent leg pain. Previous radiographs were reported as normal. Note the coned view to obtain optimal detail and the incomplete hair-line fracture revealed by bone sclerosis and subperiosteal callus. A crepe bandage support only was prescribed, and the symptoms settled in a further 6 weeks.

17. **Greenstick fractures (a):** Greenstick fractures occur in children, but not all children's fractures are of this type. The less brittle bone of the child tends to buckle on the side opposite the causal force. Tearing of the periosteum and of the surrounding soft tissues is often minimal.

18. **Greenstick fractures (b):** This radiograph illustrates a more severe greenstick fracture of the distal radius and ulna. Note that although there is about 45° of angulation at the fracture site, there is no loss of bony contact in either fracture. The clinical deformity is clearly suggested by the soft-tissue shadow.

**19. Greenstick fractures (c):** Reduction of a greenstick fracture is facilitated by the absence of displacement and by the intact tissues on the concavity of the fracture. Angulation may be corrected by supporting the fracture and applying pressure over the distal fragment (1 and 2). The elastic spring of the periosteum may however lead to recurrence of angulation (3). Particular attention must therefore be taken over plaster fixation and after care.

**20. Greenstick fractures (d):** In the forearm in particular, where angulation inevitably leads to restriction of pronation and supination, some surgeons deliberately overcorrect the initial deformity (1). This tears the periosteum on the other side of the fracture (2). This reduces the risks of secondary angulation (3). Healing in all greenstick fractures is rapid.

**21. Simple transverse fractures (a):** Transverse fractures run either at right angles to the long axis of a bone (1), or with an obliquity of less than 30°. They may be caused by *direct violence,* when the bone fractures directly beneath the causal force (e.g. the ulna fracturing when warding off a blow (a)). They may also result from *indirect violence* when the bone is subjected to bending stresses by remotely applied force (e.g. a fracture of the forearm bones resulting from a fall on the outstretched hand (b)).

**22. Simple transverse fractures (b):** The inherent stability of this type of fracture (illustrated by the model on the right) reduces the risks of shortening and displacement. In the tibia, as a result, weight bearing may be permitted at a comparatively early stage. On the other hand, the area of bony contact is small, requiring very strong union before any external support can be discarded. (NB: The term 'simple' used to describe this and the following fractures means that the fracture runs circumferentially round the bone with the formation of only two main fragments.)

**23. Simple oblique fractures (a):** In an oblique fracture (1) the fracture runs at an oblique angle of 30° or more (O). Such fractures may be caused by (a) direct or (b) indirect violence. In *simple spiral fractures* (2) the line of the fracture curves round the bone in a spiral. Simple spiral fractures result from indirect violence, applied to the bone by twisting (torsional) forces (t).

**24. Simple oblique and spiral fractures (b):** In spiral fractures, union can be rapid (1) as there is often a large area of bone in contact. In both oblique and spiral fractures, unopposed muscle contraction or premature weight bearing readily lead to shortening, displacement and sometimes loss of bony contact (2). [Note: In the AO Classification of Fractures (see later) simple spiral, oblique and transverse fractures are classified as Type A fractures.]

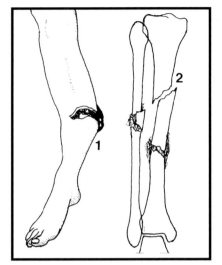

**25. In multifragmentary (comminuted) fractures** there are more than two fragments. *The spiral wedge fracture* (1) is produced by torsional forces (t), and the *bending wedge fracture* (2) by direct (a) or indirect (b) violence. The fragment (B) is often called a butterfly fragment (because of its shape). With greater violence a *fragmented (comminuted) wedge fracture* (3) results. [All these fractures are in Type B in the AO Classification (see later) and their characteristic is that after reduction there is still bony contact between the main fragments (4)].

**26. In multifragmentary complex fractures** (a further division of comminuted fractures) there is no contact between the main fragments after reduction. In *complex spiral fractures* (1) there are two or more spiral elements; in *complex segmental fractures (sometimes called double fractures)* (2) there is at least one quite separate complete bone fragment (S). In *complex irregular fractures* (3) the bone lying between the main elements is split into many irregular fragments. [All these fractures are classified as Type C in the AO Classification.]

**27. Multifragmentary fractures** are generally the result of greater violence than is the case with most simple fractures, and consequently there is an increased risk of damage to neighbouring muscle, blood vessels and skin (1). The fractures tend to be unstable, and delayed union and joint stiffness are common. Segmental fractures are often difficult to reduce by closed methods, and direct exposure may threaten the precarious blood supply to the central segment. Non-union at one level is not uncommon in these fractures (2).

**28. Impacted fractures:** A fracture is impacted when one fragment is driven into the other (1). Cancellous bone is usually involved and union is often rapid. The *stability* of these fractures varies and is more implied than real. Displacement will occur if the fracture is subjected to deforming forces; e.g. without fixation, impacted femoral neck fractures frequently come adrift (2).

**29. Compression (or crush) fractures:** Crush fractures occur in cancellous bone which is compressed beyond the limits of tolerance. Common sites are (1) the vertebral bodies (as a result of flexion injuries) and (2) the heels (following falls from a height). If the deformity is accepted, union is invariably rapid. In the spine, if correction is attempted, recurrence is almost invariable.

**30. Avulsion fractures (a):** An avulsion fracture may be produced by a sudden muscle contraction—the muscle pulling off the portion of bone to which it is attached. Common examples include:
1. Base of fifth metatarsal (peroneus brevis).
2. Tibial tuberosity (quadriceps).
3. Upper pole of patella (quadriceps).
4. Lesser trochanter (iliopsoas).
(These are all AO Type A fractures.)

31. **Avulsion fractures (b):** Avulsion fractures may also result from traction on a ligamentous or capsular attachment: these are often witness of *momentary dislocation;* e.g. (1) an abduction force may avulse the ulnar collateral ligament attachment, with spontaneous reduction. *Late subluxation* (2) is common with this ('gamekeeper's thumb') and other injuries and is especially serious in the case of the spine.

32. **Depressed fracture:** Depressed fractures occur when a sharply localised blow depresses a segment of cortical bone below the level of the surrounding bone. Although common in skull fractures, this pattern is only rarely found in the limbs. There the tibia in the upper third is probably most frequently affected. Healing is rapid; complications are dependent on the site.

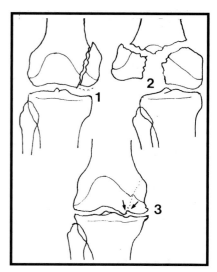

33. **Fractures involving the articular surfaces of a joint.** In *partial articular fractures* (1) part of the joint surface is involved, but the remainder is intact and solidly connected to the rest of the bone. (AO Type B fracture.) In *complete articular fractures* (2) the articular surface is completely disrupted and separated from the shaft. (AO Type C fracture.) When a fracture involves the articular surfaces, any persisting irregularity may cause secondary osteoarthritis (3). Stiffness is a common complication, and this may be minimised by early mobilisation.

34. **Fracture close to a joint:** When a fracture lies close to a joint, stiffness may also be a problem due to tethering of neighbouring muscles and tendons by spread of callus from the healing fracture; e.g. in fractures of the femur close to the knee, the quadriceps may become bound down by the callus, resulting in difficulty with knee flexion.

35. **Fracture–dislocation:** A fracture–dislocation is present when a joint has dislocated and there is in addition a fracture of one of the bony components of the joint. Illustrated is a fracture–dislocation of the shoulder, where there is an anterior dislocation with a fracture of the neck of the humerus. Injuries of this kind may be difficult to reduce and may be unstable. Stiffness and avascular necrosis are two common complications.

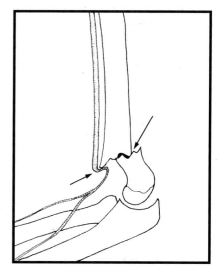

36. **Complicated fractures:** A fracture is described as complicated if there is accompanying damage to major neighbouring structures. The diagram is of a complicated supracondylar fracture of the humerus. (Such an injury might also be described as a supracondylar fracture complicated by damage to the brachial artery.)

**37. Describing the level of a fracture:**
**(a):** *The anatomical divisions* of a long bone
include the epiphysis (E), the epiphyseal plate
(EP), and the diaphysis or shaft (D). Between
the latter two is the metaphysis (M). A fracture
may be described as lying within these
divisions, or involving a distinct anatomical
part; e.g. A = fracture of the tibial diaphysis;
B = fracture of the femoral neck; C = fracture
of the greater trochanter; F = supracondylar
fracture of the femur.

**38. Describing the level of a fracture**
**(b):** For descriptive purposes a bone may be
divided arbitrarily into thirds. In this way
A = fracture of the mid third of the femur;
B = fracture of the femur in the distal third;
C = fracture of the femur at the junction of the
middle and distal thirds.

  The level of a fracture in some cases may be
made quite clear by an eponym; e.g. a Colles
fracture (D) involves the radius, and occurs
within an inch (2.5 cm) of the wrist.

**39. Describing the level of a fracture**
**(c):** *In AO terminology,* long bones are divided
into three unequal segments: *a proximal
segment* (1), a central *diaphyseal segment* (2),
and a *distal segment* (3). The boundaries
between these segments are obtained by
erecting squares (S) which accommodate the
widest part of the bone ends; in the special
case of the femur the diaphysis is described as
commencing at the distal border of the lesser
trochanter.

**40. Describing the deformity:** If there is
no deformity—i.e. if the violence which has
produced the fracture has been insufficient to
cause any movement of the bone ends relative
to one another—then the fracture is said to be
in anatomical position. Similarly, if a perfect
position has been achieved after manipulation
of a fracture, it may be described as being in
anatomical position.

**41. Displacement (i):** Displacement (or
translation) is present if the bone ends have
shifted relative to one another. The direction of
displacement is described in terms of
movement of the distal fragment. For example,
in these fractures of the femoral shaft at the
junction of the middle and distal thirds there is
(1) no displacement, (2) lateral displacement,
(3) posterior displacement, (4) both lateral and
posterior displacement.

**42. Displacement (ii):** Apart from the
direction of displacement, the degree must be
considered. A rough estimate is usually made
of the percentage of the fracture surfaces in
contact; e.g. (1) 50% bony apposition (2) 25%
bony apposition. Good bony apposition
encourages stability and union.

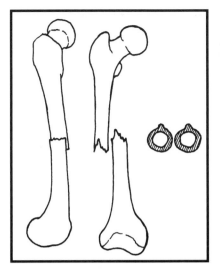

**43. Displacement (iii):** Where none of the fracture surfaces is in contact, the fracture is described as having 'no bony apposition' or being 'completely off-ended'. Off-ended fractures are (1) potentially unstable, (2) liable to progressive shortening, (3) liable to delay or difficulty in union, (4) often hard to reduce, sometimes due to trapping of soft tissue between the bone ends.

**44. Displacement (iv):** (1) Displacement of a spiral or oblique fracture will result in shortening. Displacement of transverse fractures (2) will result in shortening only after loss of bony contact. The amount of shortening may be assessed from the radiographs (if an allowance is made for magnification). Speaking generally, displacement, whilst undesirable, is of much less significance than angulation.

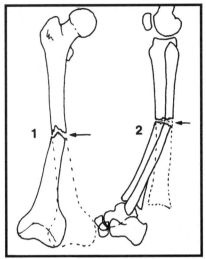

**45. Angulation (i):** The accepted method of describing angulation is in terms of the position of the point of the angle; e.g. (1) fracture of the femur with medial angulation, (2) fracture of the tibia and fibula with posterior angulation. (Both are midshaft fractures.) This method can on occasion give rise to confusion, especially as deformity is described in terms of the distal fragment.

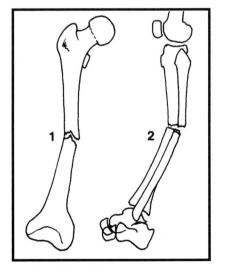

**46. Angulation (ii):** Equally acceptable, and perhaps less liable to error, would be to describe these fractures in the following way: (1) a fracture of the middle third of the femur with the distal fragment tilted laterally, (2) a fracture of the tibia and fibula in the middle thirds, with the distal fragment tilted anteriorly.

**47. Angulation (iii):** Significant angulation must always be corrected for several reasons. Deformity of the limb will be conspicuous (1) and regarded (often correctly) by the patient as a sign of poor treatment. Deformity from displacement (2) is seldom very obvious. In the upper limb, function may be seriously impaired, especially in forearm fractures where pronation/supination may be badly affected (3).

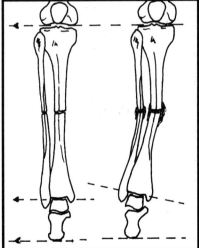

**48. Angulation (iv):** In the lower limb, alteration of the plane of movements of the hip, knee or ankle may lead to abnormal joint stresses, leading to the rapid onset of secondary osteo-arthritis.

49. **Axial rotation (i):** A third type of deformity may be present; this is when one fragment rotates on its long axis, with or without accompanying displacement or angulation. This type of deformity may be overlooked unless precautions are taken and the possibility of its occurrence kept in mind.

50. **Axial rotation (ii):** Radiographs which fail to show both ends of the bone frequently prevent any pronouncement on the presence of axial rotation (1). When both ends of the fractured bone are fully visualised on one film rotation may be obvious (2). The moral is that in any fracture both the joint above and the one below should be included in the examination.

51. **Axial rotation (iii):** Axial rotation may also be detected in the radiographs by noting (1) the position of interlocking fragments (displaced fracture with 90° axial rotation illustrated). If a bone is not perfectly circular in cross-section at the fracture site, differences in the relative diameters of the fragments may be suggestive of axial rotation (2). Axial rotation is of particular importance in forearm fractures.

52. **Open fractures:** *Open* (compound) *fractures* are of two types: those which are open from within out, and others which are open from without in. In fractures which are *open from within out*, the skin is broached by the sharp edge of one of the bone ends. This may occur at the time of the initial injury, or later from unguarded handling of a closed fracture.

53. **Fractures open from within out:** (1) The case may be first seen with bone obviously still penetrating the skin which may be tightly stretched round it. (2) More commonly, the fracture having once broken the skin promptly spontaneously reduces, so that what is seen is a wound at the level of the fracture.

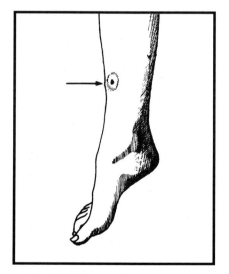

54. **Technically open fracture:** Occasionally the skin damage is minimal, with a small area of early bruising, in the centre of which is a tiny tell-tale bead of blood issuing from a puncture wound; this bead of blood re-appears as soon as it is swabbed. The risks of infection are much less in open-from-within-out fractures than those from without in. This is especially so in the technically open fracture just described.

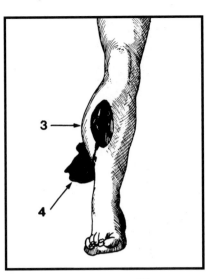

**55. Fractures open from without in (i):** This type of injury is caused by direct violence; the causal force breaks the skin and fractures the underlying bone. Causes include injuries from falling objects (e.g. in the construction industry, mining, rock falls in mountaineering, etc.) and motor vehicle impacts.

**56. Open from without in (ii):** The risks of infection are greater in this type of open fracture as: (1) dirt and fragments of clothing, etc. may be driven into the wound, (2) the skin is often badly damaged; skin may even be lost. In either case, wound healing may be in jeopardy. Difficulty in closure must be anticipated.

**57. Open from without in (iii):** In addition, there may be: (3) damage to surrounding muscle, leading to oedema and further difficulty in wound closure, (4) haemorrhage and shock may be greater than in corresponding within-out fractures. Note also that the fractures are often comminuted—with difficulty in reduction and fixation—and there may be vascular and neurological complications.

## Self test (answers on page 24)

58. Describe the level and pattern of this child's fracture.

59. This is the radiograph of the tibia of a young man who was kicked whilst playing rugby. What is the pattern of fracture? What observations would you make regarding the detection of such a fracture?

60. This is a radiograph of the elbow of an adult injured in a fall. There is obvious clinical deformity. What is the injury?

61. This is a radiograph of the arm of a child severely crushed in a run-over road traffic accident. Describe the injury.

62. What is the pattern of this injury?

63. Describe this fracture. What problems might you anticipate with it?

64. Describe the level and any angulation or displacement that you see in this fracture.

65. Can you detect any abnormality in this AP radiograph of the wrist and forearm of a child?

66. This is the radiograph of a patient who complained of pain in the side of the foot following a sudden inversion injury. Where is the fracture, and what is the pattern of injury?

67. The history in this case is of pain in the back following a fall. What is the pattern of fracture?

68. This radiograph is of the hip of an elderly lady who complained of pain after a fall. What deformity is present? Have you any observations to make regarding any factors contributing to the fracture?

69. What is this pattern of fracture? What is the importance of accurate reduction in this case?

70. What pattern of injury is illustrated in this thumb radiograph? What is its significance?

71. This injury was sustained in a road traffic accident. Describe the pattern of injury and the deformity.

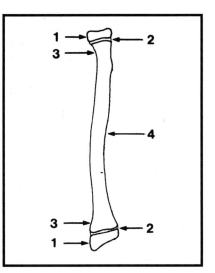

**72. Types of epiphyses:** There are two types of epiphyses: (1) *pressure epiphyses,* which form part of the articulating surfaces of a joint, and (2) *traction epiphyses,* which lie at muscle insertions, are non-articular and do not contribute to the longitudinal growth of the bone.

**73. Traction epiphyses ctd.:** Injuries to the traction epiphyses are nearly always avulsion injuries. The sites commonly affected include: (1) the base of the fifth metatarsal, (2) the tibial tuberosity, (3) the calcaneal epiphysis. Traction injuries are probably the basic cause of Osgood Schlatter's and Sever's disease (2 and 3). Other sites include the lesser trochanter, ischium and the anterior iliac spines.

**74. Pressure epiphyses (a):** Pressure epiphyses are situated at the ends of the long bones and take part in the articulations. The corresponding epiphyseal plates are responsible for longitudinal growth of the bone. (Circumferential growth is controlled by the periosteum.)
*Note:* 1. epiphysis.
　　　 2. epiphyseal plate.
　　　 3. metaphysis.
　　　 4. diaphysis.

**75. Pressure epiphyses (b):** Within the epiphyseal plate (1) is a layer of active cartilage cells (2). The newly formed cells undergo hypertrophy. Calcification and transformation to bone occur near the metaphysis (3). When there is an epiphyseal separation, it occurs at the weakest point, the layer of cell hypertrophy (4). The active region (2) remains with the epiphysis.

**76. Pressure epiphyses (c):** The metaphyseal side of the plate is nourished by vessels from the shaft (M). In the tibia (1) the epiphysis is supplied by extra-articular vessels. Vessels to the femoral head (2) lie close to the joint space and epiphyseal plate (P). There is a variable (up to 25%) contribution from the ligamentum teres. Epiphyseal displacements may lead to avascular necrosis or growth arrest. The head of radius is similarly at risk. C = capsule, A = articular cartilage.

**77. Epiphyseal plate injuries** (Salter and Harris Classification):
Type 1: The whole epiphysis is separated from the shaft.
Type 2: The epiphysis is displaced, carrying with it a small, triangular metaphyseal fragment (the commonest injury).
Type 3: Separation of part of the epiphysis.
Type 4: Separation of part of the epiphysis, with a metaphyseal fragment.
Type 5: Crushing of part or all of the epiphysis.

**78. Type 1 injuries (i):** The epiphysis is separated from the shaft without any accompanying fracture. This may follow trauma in childhood (illustrated is a traumatic displacement of the distal femoral epiphysis) or result from a birth injury. It may occur secondary to a joint infection, rickets or scurvy. Reduction by manipulation is usually easy in traumatic lesions, and the prognosis is good unless the epiphysis lies wholly within the joint.

**79. Type 1 injuries (ii):** An endocrine disturbance is thought to be an important factor in the common forms of slipped upper femoral epiphysis. Avascular necrosis is not uncommon, especially if forcible reduction is attempted after a delay in diagnosis. Growth arrest is seldom a problem (as it occurs in adolescence towards the end of growth, and as most femoral growth is at the distal end).

**80. Type 2 injuries:** The epiphysis displaces, carrying with it a small triangular fragment of the metaphysis (illustrated here in the distal femur). It is caused by trauma and is the commonest of epiphyseal injuries. Its highest incidence is in early adolescence. Growth disturbance is relatively uncommon. Reduction must be early—it becomes difficult after 48 hours by closed methods.

**81. Type 3 injuries:** Part of the epiphysis is separated. Accurate reduction is necessary in this type of injury to restore the smoothness and regularity of the articular surface. The prognosis is generally good unless the severity of the initial displacement has disrupted the blood supply to the fragment. The lower and upper tibial epiphyses are most commonly affected (note separated portion of tibial epiphysis behind lateral malleolus).

**82. Type 4 injuries:** Separation of part of the epiphysis with a metaphyseal fragment. The lateral condyle of the humerus is most commonly affected and must be accurately reduced—open reduction is usually necessary. Failure of reduction leads to bone formation in the gap and marked disturbance of growth.

**83. Type 5 injuries:** Crushing or other damage to the epiphyseal plate. This radiograph of a child who was dragged along the road by a car shows the medial malleolus; part of the epiphyseal plate and the adjacent tibia have been removed by abrasion. (The tibia is also fractured.) The epiphyseal plate may also be crushed in severe abduction and adduction injuries of the ankle.

84. **Growth disturbances (i):** If growth is arrested over part of the epiphyseal plate only, there will be progressive angulatory deformity affecting the axis of movement of the related joint. There will be a little overall shortening. This radiograph shows the tilting of the plane of the ankle joint which occurred in the last case, with deformity of the foot and ankle. In the elbow, injuries of this type may lead to cubitus varus or valgus.

85. **Growth disturbances (ii):** If the whole epiphyseal plate is affected, growth will be arrested, leading to greater shortening of the bone. The final result will depend on the age at which epiphyseal arrest occurred, and the epiphysis involved; obviously the younger the child the greater is the growth loss. Arrest of one epiphysis in paired bones will lead to joint deformity. In the case illustrated, the radial epiphysis on the right has suffered complete growth arrest following a displaced lower radial epiphysis. The ulna has continued to grow at its usual rate; its distal end appears prominent on the dorsum of the wrist, and there is obvious deformity and impairment of function in the wrist. The normal left side is shown for comparison.

86. **Fracture healing:** As a result of the injury, (1) the periosteum may be completely or partly torn, (2) there is disruption of the Haversian systems with death of adjacent bone cells, (3) there may be tearing of muscle, especially on the convex side of the fracture, and damage to neighbouring nerves and blood vessels, (4) the skin may be broached in compound injuries, with risk of ingress of bacteria.

87. **Fracture haematoma (i):** Bleeding occurs from the bone ends, marrow vessels and damaged soft tissues, with the formation of a fracture haematoma which clots. (Closed fracture is illustrated.)

88. **Fracture haematoma (ii):** The fracture haematoma is rapidly vascularised by the ingrowth of blood vessels from the surrounding tissues, and for some weeks there is rapid cellular activity. Fibrovascular tissue replaces the clot, collagen fibres are laid down and mineral salts are deposited.

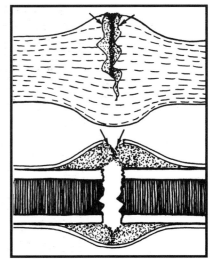

89. **Subperiosteal bone:** New woven bone is formed beneath the periosteum at the ends of the bone. The cells responsible are derived from the periosteum, which becomes stretched over these collars of new bone. If the blood supply is poor, or if it is disturbed by excessive mobility at the fracture site, cartilage may be formed instead and remain until a better blood supply is established.

90. **Primary callus response:** This remains active for *a few weeks only* (1). There is a much less vigorous formation of callus from the medullary cavity (2). Nevertheless, the capacity of the medulla to form new bone remains indefinitely throughout the healing of the fracture.

91. **Bridging external callus (i):** If the periosteum is incompletely torn, and there is no significant loss of bony apposition, the primary callus response may result in establishing external continuity of the fracture ('bridging external callus'). Cells lying in the outer layer of the periosteum itself proliferate to reconstitute the periosteum.

**92. Bridging external callus (ii):** If the gap is more substantial, fibrous tissue formed from the organisation of the fracture haematoma will lie between the advancing collars of subperiosteal new bone. This fibrous tissue may be stimulated to form bone ('tissue induction'), again resulting in bridging callus. The mechanism may be due to a change of electrical potential at the fracture site or to a (hypothetical) wound hormone.

**93. Bridging external callus (iii):** If the bone ends are offset, the primary callus from the subperiosteal region may unite with medullary callus. The net result of the three mechanisms just described is that the fracture becomes rigid, function in the limb returns and the situation is rendered favourable for endosteal bone formation and remodelling.

**94. Endosteal new bone formation (i):** If there is no gap between the bone ends, osteoclasts can tunnel across the fracture line in advance of ingrowing blood vessels and osteoblasts which form new Haversian systems. Dead bone is revascularised and may provide an invaluable scaffolding and local mineral source. This process cannot occur if the fracture is mobile.

**95. Endosteal new bone formation (ii):** The formation of new cortical bone, with re-establishment of continuity between the Haversian systems on either side, cannot occur if fibrous tissue remains occupying the space between the bone ends. If this is present, it must be removed and replaced with woven bone. This is generally achieved by ingrowth of medullary callus which remains active through the healing phase.

**96. Endosteal new bone formation (iii):** Where the bone ends are supported by rigid internal fixation, there is no functional requirement for external bridging callus: as a result external bridging callus may not be seen, or be minimal. Healing of the fracture occurs slowly through the formation of new cortical bone between the bone ends. It is therefore essential that internal fixation devices are retained until this process is complete.

*Remodelling:* After clinical union, new Haversian systems are laid down along the lines of stress. In areas free from stress, bone is removed by osteoclasts. Eventually little trace of external bridging callus will remain. The power to remodel bone in this way is great in children, but not so marked in the adult. In a child, most or all traces of fracture displacement (including even off-ending) will disappear. There is also some power to correct angulation, although this becomes progressively less as the child approaches adolescence. Any axial rotation, however, is likely to remain. In the adult, there is virtually no correction of axial rotation or angulation. It is, therefore, important that axial rotation deformity is always corrected, and that angulation, particularly in adults, should not be accepted.

## 97. **The classification of fractures**

There is no fracture of any bone which has escaped an attempt at classification. Sometimes this has been done on the basis of region and pattern, sometimes through a concept of the stresses to which the bone has been subjected, and usually with an eye on some understanding of the severity of the injury and its prognosis. Unfortunately not everyone has the same ideas regarding the relative importance of the various factors concerned, and as time progresses and knowledge expands the number of classifications that exist has been continuing to grow.

The result is that in nearly every area there is a wealth of classifications, usually with grades, degrees or numbers attached to the originator's name. This bewilders the newcomer, and causes much confusion in those who are attempting to assess the results of various treatments, as the injuries classified by one author may not be easily compared with those described by another. There is too the problem of how to ascribe certain fractures which have been inconsiderate enough to adopt a pattern that does not quite fit within the classification.

No surgeon is able to master the wealth of classifications outside his own specialist area; and for purposes of communication, as far as single injuries are concerned, a fracture is described mainly by its site and pattern, along the lines already detailed. In such circumstances classifications are only mentioned if they have become familiar through long usage, and in some cases classifications of this type may be archaic.

The AO Group have sought a universal classification which is aimed to encompass all fractures, and after many years' work have published full details of their system for the major long bones. This classification (or its general principles) have been adopted in this edition of this book.

## The AO classification of fractures of long bones

The following points should be noted:

1. This is *not* a classification of injuries: it is a classification of fractures.
2. It does not include dislocations, unless they have an associated fracture.
3. It does not differentiate between undisplaced and displaced fractures of the shafts of the long bones (but it does so in the case of certain fractures of the bone ends).
4. It does not give any indication of the relative frequency of particular fractures.
5. The sorting of fractures (beyond the area of the bone involved) depends on the AO Group's assessment of the severity of the fracture; this they define as "the morphological complexity, the difficulty in treatment, and the prognosis". In areas this may reflect a preference for the use of internal fixation rather than conservative methods of treatment.
6. The classification results in an alpha-numeric code which is suitable for computer sorting, and which allows for research purposes (e.g. in assessing the results of any treatment, wherever carried out) the comparison of like with like.
7. Because of the format, it is not descriptive in a verbal sense, and is not suitable for conveying information about the nature of an individual fracture (e.g. over the telephone).

**LOCATION OF THE FRACTURE**    *eg Fracture of the femoral shaft = 32–*

3 TYPES

A = *least severe*

B = *intermediate*

C = *most severe*

*in each Type there are*

3 GROUPS

*In each Group there are*

3 SUB GROUPS

**98. The principles of the AO classification.** 1. The AO classification for long bone fractures may be grasped by likening it to an X-ray storage system, with numbered blocks of filing cabinets: one block for each bone.

Within each block, each filing cabinet (which is also numbered) represents a particular area of each bone: cabinet number 1 stores fractures of the proximal segment, number 2 the diaphysis or shaft, and number 3 the distal segment. In the case of the tibia, there is a fourth cabinet to deal with fractures of the malleoli. (The junction between the segments is determined in the way described on p. 10, Frame 39.) When a fracture bridges the junction between two segments, the segment under which it is classified is determined by the site of the mid-point of the line of the fracture. In practice therefore, a two-digit code determines the **Location** of a fracture: e.g. under 22– would be stored all fractures of the shafts of the radius, or the ulna, or of both these bones.

In *each cabinet* all the radiographs for a single location of fracture are divided into fracture **Types** (represented by the three drawers); the least severe go in drawer A (Type A), those of intermediate severity in B (Type B fractures), and the most severe in C (Type C). Some of the criteria used to differentiate between the three types of fracture have already been indicated (Frames 25, 26, 33) but see Footnote.

Any Type of fracture can be put in one of three **Groups** (represented by folders, and numbered 1–3). The methods of selection are again described later. Within each Group fractures may be further sorted into **Subgroups** (represented by partitions). Each of these **Subgroups** has a numerical representation (.1, .2, .3). [If an even more detailed classification is needed, fractures within each Subgroup can have added **Qualifications.** These can be described by a single number (or two numbers separated by a comma) added in parentheses after the main coding. The first digit in the range 1–6 is used to amplify the description of a fracture's location and its extent, while the second is purely descriptive. The number 7 is reserved to describe partial amputations, 8 for total amputation, and 9 for loss of bone stock.]

As an example of the AO classification, a simple oblique fracture of the proximal part of the femoral shaft would be coded 32–A2.1

3 = THE BONE = the femur
2 = THE SEGMENT = the diaphysis    } THE LOCATION OF THE FRACTURE
– = Separator between Location and Type
A = THE TYPE = A is the least severe type of fracture, with two bone fragments only
2 = THE GROUP = Group 2 includes all oblique fractures
.1 = SUBGROUP = Subgroup .1 includes fractures in the proximal part of the diaphysis where the medullary cavity is wider than in the more central part of the bone.
*Footnote:* the criteria employed in sorting fractures into their appropriate Types, Groups and Subgroups are given in detail in the section on Regional Injuries.

| I | II | IIIA | IIIB | IIIC |

**99. Classification of open fractures (1):**
The classification of Gustilo et al is well established and in common use. It is a practical classification which relates well to the common patterns of injury and their prognosis. Three types are described, with the third being subdivided to allow a more precise grading.

Type I: An open fracture with a wound which is (a) less than 1 cm and (b) clean.

Type II: An open fracture with a wound which is (a) more than 1 cm long and (b) which is not associated with extensive soft tissue damage, avulsions, or flaps.

Type IIIA: An open fracture where there is adequate soft tissue coverage of bone in spite of (a) extensive soft tissue lacerations or flaps or (b) high energy trauma irrespective of the size of the wound.

Type IIIB: An open fracture with extensive soft tissue loss, with periosteal stripping and exposure of bone. Massive contamination is usual.

Type IIIC: An open fracture associated with an arterial injury which requires repair.

**100. Classification of open fractures (2):**
The AO Group use separate classifications for closed and open skin injuries and for injuries to muscle; they employ a separate fourth classification for nerve and vascular injuries. The classification is more complex and is given here for completeness:
Skin lesions in closed fractures (Integuments, Closed):

IC1 = Skin undamaged
IC2 = Contusion of skin
IC3 = Local degloving
IC4 = Extensive (but closed) degloving
IC5 = Skin necrosis resulting from contusion.

Skin lesions in open fractures (Integuments, Open):
IO1 = Skin broken from within out
IO2 = Skin broken from without in, with contused edges but less than 5 cm in length

IO3 = In excess of 5 cm of skin broken, with devitalised edges and local degloving
IO4 = Full thickness contusion, abrasion, skin loss
IO5 = Extensive degloving.

Muscle and tendon injuries in fractures:
MT1 = No muscle injury
MT2 = Local muscle injury, one muscle group only
MT3 = Extensive muscle injury with involvement of more than one group
MT4 = Avulsion or loss of entire muscle groups, tendon lacerations
MT5 = Compartment syndrome; Crush syndrome.

Neurovascular injuries in fractures:
NV1 = No neurovascular injury
NV2 = Isolated nerve injury

NV3 = Isolated vascular injury
NV4 = Combined neural and vascular injury
NV5 = Sub-total or total amputation.

Note that for data storage purposes the above AO soft-tissue classifications are appended to their alpha-numeric fracture classification: e.g. a segmental fracture of the tibia in which there was a small skin wound, no obvious muscle damage, but an associated drop foot would be classified 42–C2/IO2–MT1–NV2: this is *not* a classification for committing to memory!

Note the very approximate correlations between the Gustilo and AO classifications:

Gustilo Type I equivalent to IO1
Gustilo Type II equivalent to IO2
Gustilo Type IIIA equivalent to IO3
Gustilo Type IIIB equivalent to IO4
Gustilo Type IIIC equivalent to IO3–5 + NV2.

58. Transverse fracture of the tibia in the middle third. Simple transverse fracture of the tibia in the middle third (or simple transverse fracture of the tibial diaphysis). There is no significant displacement or angulation, and the fibula is intact. The fracture is of adult pattern and is not a greenstick fracture.

59. Hair-line fracture of the tibial diaphysis (or of the tibia in the lower mid-third). Coned-down views are often helpful; if the initial radiographs appear normal, they should be repeated after an interval if there is continued suspicion that a fracture is present. CAT scans of the suspect area are also often useful.

60. Dislocation of the elbow. The radius and ulna are displaced laterally in relation to the humerus (and also posteriorly, although this is not shown on the single radiograph).

61. This injury cannot be anything but *open* as the right-angled angulation of the greenstick fracture of the radius (at the junction of its middle and lower thirds) indicates. The mottling of the soft-tissue shadows due to air is confirmatory. In addition, there is a greenstick fracture of the ulna in its middle third (note the posterior angulation) and dislocation of the elbow (the ulna appears lateral and the humerus AP). Both fractures are of the diaphysis.

62. Fracture dislocation of the shoulder. The head of the humerus is not congruous with the glenoid. Lateral to it is a large fragment of bone, the avulsed greater tuberosity of the humerus.

63. Segmental (double) fracture of the tibia (complex segmental fracture). The proximal fracture is virtually transverse and in the middle third. The distal fracture is also transverse and situated in the distal third. The fibula is fractured, and the tibia displaced medially. Bony apposition has probably been lost in the proximal fracture. Problems with reduction, fixation and non-union at one level are to be anticipated.

64. Fracture of the radius and ulna in the distal third. In the lateral projection, there is some slight anterior (volar) angulation (posterior (or dorsal) tilting) of the ulna. In the AP view, there is lateral (or radial) displacement of the distal fragments which are virtually off-ended. There is some medial (ulnar) angulation (or the distal fragments are tilted laterally). The radial fracture is oblique with a slight spiral element. The ulnar fracture is transverse.

65. There is a greenstick fracture of the radius. Note the ridging of the radius both medially and laterally just proximal to the epiphysis.

66. Fracture of the base of the fifth metatarsal. This is an avulsion fracture, produced by the peroneus brevis which is inserted into the fifth metatarsal base.

67. The radiograph shows deformity of the body of the first lumbar vertebra which has been reduced in height anteriorly. This is an anterior compression or crush fracture.

68. There is a simple oblique fracture of the proximal femur, running between the lesser and greater trochanters, with a coxa vara deformity (the distal femur is tilted medially). The hip is arthritic, and the disturbance in bone texture in the pelvis and femur is typical of Paget's disease (i.e. this is a pathological fracture).

69. There is a simple oblique fracture of the fibula, which is displaced laterally, accompanied by the talus. The distal end of the fibula is tilted laterally (medial angulation). Unless accurately reduced, this fracture involving a joint is liable to lead to secondary osteo-arthritis.

70. The small fragment of bone detached from the base of the proximal phalanx has been avulsed by the ulnar collateral ligament of the MP joint. It indicates that the thumb has been dislocated, and that there is potential instability at this level.

71. There is a fragmented wedge fracture of the tibial diaphysis. There are four fragments, and the main butterfly fragment of a bending wedge fracture remains in contact and alignment with the main distal fragment. There is a segmental (double) fracture of the fibula. Both fractures are in the middle third. Soft tissue shadows indicate, as might be anticipated, that this is an open fracture. There is lateral angulation (i.e. the distal fragment is tilted medially). During the taking of the AP and lateral radiographs there has been some alteration of position of the fracture: note that in the lateral projection there is considerable *axial rotation* (the foot is lateral, but the upper tibia is almost in the AP plane). Axial rotation is not a feature of the AP projection.

# 2. The diagnosis of fractures and principles of treatment

## 1. History

In taking the history of a patient who may have a fracture, the following points may prove to be helpful, especially when there has been a traumatic incident.

1. What activity was being pursued at the time of the incident (e.g. taking part in a sport, driving a car, working at a height, etc.)?

2. What was the nature of the incident (e.g. a kick, a fall, a twisting injury, etc.)?

3. What was the magnitude of the applied forces? For example if a patient was injured in a fall, it is helpful to know how far he fell, if his fall was broken, the nature of the surface on which he landed, and how he landed; trivial violence may lead one to suspect a pathological fracture: severe violence makes the exclusion of multiple injuries particularly important.

4. What was the point of impact and the direction of the applied forces? In reducing a fracture, one of the principle methods employed is to reduplicate the causal forces in a reverse direction. If a fracture occurs close to the point of impact, additional remotely situated fractures must be excluded.

5. Is there any significance to be attached to the incident itself? For example, if there was a fall, was it precipitated by some underlying medical condition, such as a hypotensive attack, which requires separate investigation?

6. Where is the site of any pain, and what is its severity?

7. Is there loss of functional activity? For example, walking is seldom possible after any fracture of the femur or tibia; inability to weight bear after an accident is of great significance.

**Diagnosis:** In some cases the diagnosis of fracture is unmistakable, e.g. when there is gross deformity of the central portion of a long bone or when the fracture is visible as in certain compound injuries.

*In the majority of other cases, a fracture is suspected from the history and clinical examination, and confirmed by radiography of the region.*

25

2. **Inspection (i):** Begin by inspecting the limb most carefully, comparing one side with the other. Look for any *asymmetry of contour*, suggesting an underlying fracture which has displaced or angled.

3. **Inspection (ii):** Look for any persisting *asymmetry of posture* of the limb: for example, persisting external rotation of the leg is a common feature in disimpacted fractures of the femoral neck.

4. **Inspection (iii):** Look for local bruising of the skin suggesting a *point of impact* which may direct your attention locally or to a more distant level. For example, bruising over the knee from dashboard impact should direct your attention to the underlying patella, and also to the femoral shaft and hip.

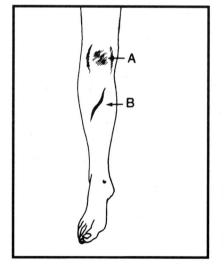

5. **Inspection (iv):** Look for other tell-tale skin damage. For example (A) grazing, with or without ingraining of dirt in the wound, or friction burns, suggests an impact followed by rubbing of the skin against a resistant surface. (B) Lacerations suggest impact against a hard edge, tearing by a bone end, or splitting by compression against a hard surface.

6. **Inspection (v):** Note the presence of: (C) skin stretch marks, (D) band patterning of the skin, suggestive of both stretching and compression of the skin in a run-over injury, (E) pattern bruising, caused by severe compression which leads the skin to be imprinted with the weave marks of overlying clothing. Any of these abnormalities should lead you to suspect the integrity of the underlying bone.

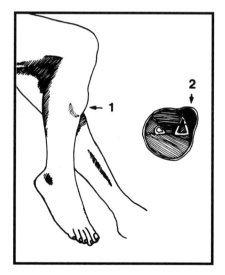

7. **Inspection (vi):** If the patient is seen shortly after the incident, note any localised swelling of the limb (1). Later, swelling tends to become more diffuse. Note the presence of any haematoma (2). A fracture may strip the skin from its local attachment (degloving injury); the skin comes to float on an underlying collection of blood which is continuous with the fracture haematoma.

8. **Tenderness (i):** Look for tenderness over the bone suspected of being fractured. Tenderness is invariably elicited over a fracture (1), but tenderness will also be found over any traumatised area, even though there is no underlying fracture (2). The important distinguishing feature is that in the case of a fracture tenderness will be elicited when the bone is palpated on any aspect (3).

9. **Tenderness (ii):** In eliciting tenderness, once a tender area has been located the part should be palpated at the same level from another direction. For example, in many sprained wrists, tenderness will be elicited in the anatomical snuff-box—but not over the dorsal and palmar aspects of the scaphoid, which are tender if a fracture is present.

10. **Palpation:** The sharp edge of a fracture may be palpable. Note also the presence of localised oedema. This is a particularly useful sign over hair-line and stress fractures. The development of oedema may however take some hours to reach detectable proportions.

12. **Radiographic examination:** In every case of suspected fracture, radiographic examination of the fracture is mandatory. Radiographs of the part will generally give a clear indication of the presence of a fracture and provide a sound basis for planning treatment. In the case where there is some clinical doubt, radiographs will reassure patient and surgeon and avert any later medicolegal criticism.

Radiographers in the United Kingdom receive thorough training in the techniques for the satisfactory visualisation of any suspect area, but it is essential that they in turn are given clear guidance as to the area under suspicion. The request form must be quite specific, otherwise mistakes may occur. At its simplest, the request must state *both the area to be visualised and the bone suspected of being fractured*. It need hardly be stressed that a thorough clinical examination should precede the completion of the radiographic request if repetition and the taking of unnecessary films are to be avoided.

The following table gives some of the commonest errors in requesting (diagnostic errors have been excluded):

11. **Other signs:** If the fracture is mobile, moving the part may produce angulation or crepitus from the bone ends rubbing together. In addition, the patient will experience severe pain from such movement. These signs may be inadvertently observed during routine examination of the patient, but should not be sought unless the patient is unconscious and the diagnosis is in doubt.

13.

| Area suspected of fracture | Typical request | Error | Correct request |
|---|---|---|---|
| Scaphoid | 'X-ray wrist, ? fracture' | Fractures of the scaphoid are difficult to visualise: a minimum of 3 specialised views is required. A fracture may not show on the standard wrist projections | 'X-ray scaphoid, ? fracture' |
| Calcaneus | 'X-ray ankle, ? fracture' 'X-ray foot, ? fracture' | A tangential projection, with or without an additional oblique (along with the usual lateral), is necessary for satisfactory visualisation of the calcaneus. These views are not taken routinely when an X-ray examination of the foot or ankle is called for. | 'X-ray calcaneus, ? fracture' |
| Neck of femur | 'X-ray femur, ? fracture' | Poor centring of the radiographs may render the fracture invisible | 'X-ray hip, ? fracture neck of femur' or 'X-ray to exclude fracture of femoral neck' |
| Tibial table or tibial spines | 'X-ray tibia, ? fracture' | Poor centring may render the fracture invisible, or the area may not be included on the film | 'X-ray upper third tibia to exclude fracture of tibial table' |

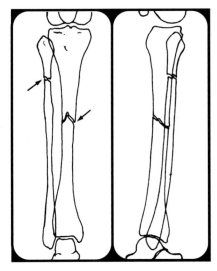

14. **The standard projections:** These are an *anteroposterior (AP) and lateral.* Ideally the beam should be centred over the area of suspected fracture, with visualisation of the proximal *and* distal joints. This is especially important in the paired long bones where, for example, a fracture of the tibia at one level may be accompanied by a fibular fracture at another.

15. **Oblique projections:** In the case of the hand and foot, an oblique projection may be helpful when the lateral gives rise to confusion due to the superimposition of many structures. Such oblique projections may have to be specifically requested when they are not part of an X-ray department's routine.

16. **Localised views:** Where there is marked local tenderness, but routine films are normal, coned-down localised views may give sufficient gain in detail to reveal for example a hair-line fracture: if such films are also negative, the radiographs should be repeated after an interval of 10–14 days if the symptoms are persisting (see also Hair-line Fractures p. 6, 13–16).

17. **Comparison films:** Where there is some difficulty in interpreting the radiographs (for example, in the elbow region in children where the epiphyseal structures are continually changing, or where there is some unexplained shadow, or a congenital abnormality) films of the other side should be taken for direct comparison.

18. **Stress films (i):** Stress films can be of value in certain situations: (a) When a complete tear of a major ligament is suspected, e.g., where the lateral ligament of the ankle is thought to be torn, radiographs of the joint taken with the foot in forced inversion may demonstrate instability of the talus in the ankle mortice. (Local or general anaesthesia may be required in fresh injuries.)

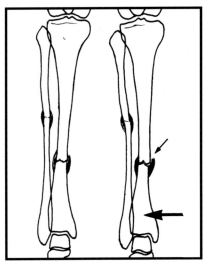

19. **Stress films (ii):** (b) For clarification of doubtful union or possible refracture of a uniting fracture.

There are many other radiological techniques. In particular, computer-assisted tomography and image intensifier screening are often of value in the investigation of spinal injuries. Special techniques are discussed under the appropriate regional sections.

## Pitfalls

A number of fractures are missed with great regularity—sometimes with serious consequences. You should always be on the look-out for the following:

1. An elderly patient who is unable to weight bear after a fall must be examined most carefully. The commonest cause by far is a fracture of the femoral neck, and this must be eliminated in every case. If the femoral neck is intact, look for a fracture of the *pubic rami*. Note that, on the rare occasion, a patient with an impacted fracture of the femoral neck may be able to weight bear, albeit with pain.

2. If a car occupant suffers a fracture of the patella or femur from a dashboard impact, always eliminate the presence of a silent dislocation of the hip.

3. If a patient fractures the calcaneus in a fall, examine the other side most carefully. Bilateral fractures are extremely common, and the less painful side may be missed.

4. If a patient complains of a 'sprained ankle' always examine the foot as well as the ankle. Fractures of the base of the fifth metatarsal frequently result from inversion injuries, and are often overlooked. The mistake of not performing a good clinical examination in these circumstances is compounded by requesting radiographs of the ankle (which do not show the fifth metatarsal bone).

5. In the unconscious patient, injuries of the cervical spine are frequently overlooked. It pays to have routine screening films of the neck, chest and pelvis in the unconscious patient.

6. Impacted fractures of the neck of the humerus are often missed, especially when one view only is taken. Conversely, in children, the epiphyseal line is often wrongly mistaken for fracture.

7. Posterior dislocation of the shoulder may not be diagnosed when it should be at the initial attendance. This is because the humeral head comes to lie directly behind the glenoid, and is not detected if only a single AP projection is taken. If there is a strong suspicion of injury, and especially if there is deformity of the shoulder, a second projection is *essential* if no abnormality is noted on the AP film.

8. Apparently isolated fractures of either the radius or ulna should be diagnosed with caution. The Monteggia and Galeazzi fracture–dislocations are still frequently missed. In the same way, it is unwise to diagnose an isolated fracture of the tibia until the whole of the fibula has been visualised; fracture of the tibia close to the ankle is, for example, often accompanied by fracture of the fibular neck.

9. At the wrist, greenstick fractures of the radius in children are often overlooked due to lack of care in studying the radiographs.

10. In adults, fractures of the radial styloid or Bennett's fracture may be missed or treated as suspected fractures of the scaphoid. Complete tears of ulnar collateral ligament of the MP joint of the thumb are frequently overlooked, sometimes with severe resultant functional disability.

## The treatment of fractures

**Primary aims:** The primary aims of fracture treatment are:
1. The attainment of sound bony union without deformity.
2. The restoration of function, so that the patient is able to resume his former occupation and pursue any athletic or social activity he wishes.

To this might be added 'as quickly as possible' and 'without risk of any complications, whether early or late'. These aims cannot always be achieved, and in some situations are mutually exclusive. For example, internal fixation of some fractures may give rapid restoration of function, but at the expense of occasional infection. The great variations that exist in fracture treatment are largely due to differences in interpretation of these factors and their relevance in the case under consideration.

**Priorities of treatment/multiple injuries:** If a fracture is a patient's sole injury, it is usually possible to proceed with its treatment without undue delay (although unfitness for anaesthesia may sometimes upset this ideal). If, however, a fracture is complicated by damage to other structures, or involvement of other systems, then treatment of the fracture usually takes second place. Immediate action must be taken to correct any life-endangering situation which may be present or anticipated. Therefore, when the patient is first seen, a rapid overall examination must be made to detect any condition which merits priority in treatment. In cases of multiple injury, especially when the patient is unconscious, routine screening films of the skull, cervical spine, chest and pelvis should be carried out.

The following situations may require consideration:

**1. Respiratory obstruction or impairment.** (i) Any blood, mucus or vomit must be removed from the upper respiratory passages by suction or swabbing. Dentures should be looked for and extracted. In the more minor situations, respiratory obstruction may be avoided by support of the jaw, a simple airway, and turning the patient on his side.

An endotracheal tube may have to be passed in a number of situations: (a) in the unconscious patient with an absent gag reflex; (b) where inhalation of mucus or vomit has already taken place (or is suspected), for clearing of the respiratory passages under vision; (c) for the more effective management of cases where there is respiratory difficulty or evidence of hypoxia – e.g in cases of flail chest. Where there is need for intubation in a patient when a cervical spine injury is suspected, the procedure should be carried out with great care, avoiding excessive cervical spine extension; naso-tracheal intubation should be used.

After intubation it is usually wise to assess the arterial blood gas levels so that if these remain impaired the appropriate steps may be taken (e.g. reviewing the diagnosis).

(ii) An open chest wound must be immediately covered to reduce the risks of tension pneumothorax. A vaseline gauze dressing, covered with a swab, and firmly secured to the skin with broad adhesive tape is usually quite adequate in the emergency situation.

(iii) If there is evidence of a tension pneumothorax (hyper-resonance and decreased breath sounds on the affected side, or tracheal shift to the other), or of pneumothorax or haemothorax, the appropriate chest cavities should be drained by intercostal catheters connected to water seal drains. If the diagnosis is in doubt, the chest should be tapped in the fifth interspace in the mid-axillary line.

(iv)  If there is evidence of paradoxical respiration due to flail rib segments, blood gas levels should be estimated; slight impairment of respiratory function may be managed by giving oxygen by inhalation and analgesics with caution. When the blood gas levels are seriously disturbed, and especially in the presence of a concurrent head injury, some form of assisted respiration is usually the best method of management.

**2.  Haemorrhage and shock.** (i) External haemorrhage may be severe and if so must be brought under rapid control. Local padding or packing with firm bandaging is usually adequate, but in the uncommon situations where this fails a tourniquet may be required. This must be adequately applied; too little pressure will increase the blood loss by preventing venous return, and too great a pressure will endanger underlying nerves. A pneumatic tourniquet should always be applied in preference to any other type.

(ii)  Internal haemorrhage: There may be significant internal haemorrhage from the extravasation of blood into the soft tissues in the area of a fracture. This is especially the case in fractures of the pelvis and femur and where there are multiple fractures. Serious blood loss may also occur in chest injuries where there may be rapid bleeding into the chest cavities and the formation of a haemothorax. In the abdomen, there may also be serious loss from rupture of the spleen and liver, and from mesenteric tears. Where there is major intra-abdominal haemorrhage, urgent exploration may be required.

(iii) Oligaemic shock: In any significant injury the pulse and blood pressure should be charted at 15-minute intervals, a sample of blood taken for grouping and cross-matching, and a good intravenous line set up. An attempt should be made to work out how much blood the patient is likely to have lost and the amount and rapidity of future losses. Great accuracy cannot be expected, but it is important to have a clear idea of the replacement likely to be required and to strive to remain in control of the situation. Oligaemic shock should not be allowed to occur; it should be anticipated and prevented, but if present it must be properly and adequately treated. Remember that shock may be well compensated in the initial stage, and serious blood loss may occur before there is any major disturbance of the pulse rate or blood pressure; in the young especially, these signs of shock may not just indicate the patient is suffering from shock, but that he is dying of it. If the estimated total loss is a litre or less (in an adult) replacement should not be required, and plasma or a plasma expander held in reserve. If the estimated loss is 2 litres, 1–1½ litres may be replaced in the form of plasma and/or a plasma expander; 1 litre of cross-matched blood may be held in reserve. If the losses are much in excess of 2 litres, whole blood will be required, but a decision that has frequently to be made is whether the patient can wait until full cross-matching can be carried out. In many cases, if blood loss is slow and controlled, and there has been a good response to initial infusions of plasma or a plasma expander, the patient's condition may be maintained by the administration of up to 2 litres of plasma—during the waiting period. In other cases, where for example the patient arrives exsanguinated, it may be essential to resuscitate using substantial quantities of unmatched group O Rh–ve blood. Where a large replacement is required, all blood should be warmed. Every 3 litres of blood should be followed with a litre of fresh frozen plasma. After 5 litres of blood, platelets should be given.

The following figures have been suggested in estimating blood losses:

| | |
|---|---|
| Closed fracture of the femoral shaft | ½–1 litre |
| Open ring fractures of the pelvis | 2–3 litres |
| Intra-abdominal haemorrhage | 2–3 litres |
| Haemothorax | 1–2 litres |

To this must be added the volume of any external haemorrhage. The total loss from two or more injuries is less than the sum of the individual losses. The effectiveness and balance of the replacement may be gauged (a) by the level and stability of the pulse and blood pressure, (b) by inserting a catheter and measuring the urinary output (normal value for a 70 kg man = 3 ml or more every 5 minutes), (c) by serial estimations of the haematocrit which should be maintained at about 30%.

**3. Head injury:** (i) Where there is a head injury the following procedures should be followed:

(a) The unconscious patient should be intubated to minimise the risks of cerebral hypoxia.

(b) A complete neurological examination must be carried out and the results charted, using a suitable set of protocols (such as the Glasgow Coma Scale, see p. 34); the examination should be repeated at regular intervals. Of particular significance is (1) a history of a post-traumatic lucid interval; (2) a history of progressive deterioration in the level of consciousness; (3) focal neurological signs; (4) a rising blood pressure and falling pulse rate.

(c) Where there is evidence of increased intracranial pressure further investigation with a CAT scan should be carried out. If an extradural haematoma is discovered its immediate evacuation should be undertaken. If a subdural haematoma is found this should be also promptly removed. If there is evidence of diffuse cerebral oedema, surgery is contraindicated, and an infusion of a hyperosmolar solution of Mannitol may be commenced. Where appropriate (and in a specialist unit), monitoring of the intracranial pressure may be carried out using a catheter inserted into the lateral ventricle.

As far as the the treatment of accompanying fractures is concerned, the following points should be noted: Where there is a head injury present which requires urgent investigative procedures or operative intervention (for example an extradural haemorrhage with deterioration in the level of consciousness) this will take priority over the local treatment of most fractures. A combined procedure may often be planned with advantage but certainly in all cases some estimate should be made as to when definitive treatment of the fracture is likely to be possible. Depending on that interval there is the choice of a variety of initial procedures which may include the application of sterile dressings or light packing of open wounds, supporting an injured limb with sandbags or an inflatable splint in such a position that the distal circulation is maintained, or the use of light temporary plaster splintage.

**Glasgow Coma Scale**

A patient is defined as being comatose if he does not open his eyes, if he does not obey commands, and if he does not utter recognisable words. The severity of the coma may be assessed by assigning a value to the eye, motor and verbal responses, and summing these. By repeating the examinations at regular intervals progress may be monitored, and any deterioration (suggesting intracranial complications) recognised at an early stage.

| *Variable* | *Score* |
|---|---|
| **Eye-opening** (E) | |
| Spontaneous | 4 |
| To speech | 3 |
| To pain | 2 |
| Nil | 1 |
| **Best motor response** (M) | |
| Obeys | 6 |
| Localises | 5 |
| Withdraws | 4 |
| Abnormal flexion | 3 |
| Extensor response | 2 |
| Nil | 1 |
| **Verbal response** | |
| Oriented | 5 |
| Confused conversation | 4 |
| Inappropriate words | 3 |
| Incomprehensible sounds | 2 |
| Nil | 1 |

The coma score = E+M+V, with a value of 3 being the worst possible response, and 15 the best. A value of less than 7 indicates severe coma, 8–12 moderate, and 13–14 mild. Severe injuries are infrequent, and most patients who develop haematomas requiring surgery are classified as moderate or minor on admission.

(ii)  Where there is a head injury in which the immediate prognosis is hopeless any temporary splintage of the fracture should be retained but no fresh treatment planned.

(iii)  Where no active neurosurgical treatment is contemplated and the prognosis regarded as very poor but not absolutely hopeless, it is usually possible to devise some simple measures to give reasonable support to the injured part but at the same time permitting more definitive treatment in the near future should unexpected improvement occur.

**4.  Cardiac tamponade: intrathoracic rupture of the aorta**. Prompt drainage of an intrapericardial haematoma may be a life-saving measure. Aortic rupture may not be immediately fatal and be detected by the characteristic squaring-off of the mediastinal shadow on radiographs of the chest. Arrangements should be made without delay for exploration; as by-pass facilities will be required, in some cases this will require transfer of the patient to a specialist unit. Thoracotomy may also be indicated where there is a tracheal, bronchial or oesophageal injury, or a penetrating injury to the mediastinum.

**5.  Visceral complications**. Injury to the solid abdominal organs (especially the liver, spleen and kidneys) may give rise to severe intra-abdominal haemorrhage. Haemorrhage may also follow mesenteric tears and ruptures of the stomach and intestine with which the problems of perforation are also associated. Suspected intra-abdominal injuries may be investigated by (a) peritoneal lavage, where the presence of blood, bile or digestive contents may be diagnostic; (b) CAT scans, which are generally of much greater diagnostic value than plain recumbent abdominal radiographs; (c) in the case of the urinary tract, examination of the urine for blood; an intravenous pyelogram and cystogram, and in certain pelvic fractures a urethrogram may also be employed (see Complications of Pelvic Fractures, p. 249). Abdominal exploration takes priority over fracture treatment (see also Complications of Fractures, p. 88).

## Evaluation of patients with multiple injuries

**Trauma scoring; Hospital Trauma Index; Injury Severity Score:**
Several systems have been developed in an attempt to assess the severity of injuries. These may be used as an alert for the need for prompt and expert treatment; they may give an indication of the prognosis; and over a period they may be used statistically to evaluate the performance of a team, unit or hospital, or to draw attention to some injury pattern where treatment efforts might be profitably concentrated.

The two main systems in use are the Abbreviated Injury Scale (AIS), and the Hospital Trauma Index (HTI). Both classifications are largely comparable, and for normal working purposes grade injuries into five degrees of severity:

0 = None
1 = Minor
2 = Moderate
3 = Major, but not life-threatening
4 = Severe, life-threatening, but survival probable
5 = Critical, survival uncertain.

*Where the injury is isolated* (i.e. the case is not one of multiple injuries), there is no problem and the grade into which the injury falls is used as required.

*Where there are multiple injuries* the addition of the values obtained from the AIS or HTI tables does not give an accurate indication of severity, being overly pessimistic regarding outcome. It has been found, however, that if the grade figures are manipulated, a figure is reached which can be used with some measure of accuracy as a prognostic indicator in cases of multiple injury.

In practice, the patient's three worst injuries are assessed and the relevant grade numbers are each squared before being added together. If several injuries lie within the same area, only the worst is selected. The break point for the resultant sum is in the area of 50. The following points may be noted:
- Score < 10: death rare in any patient under the age of 50.
- Score 10–20: mortality 4–30%, depending on age.
- Score > 50: Only rare survival, and only in exceptional circumstances and with prompt treatment by specialised staff. In this group nearly all the deaths occur within the first week, and half within the first hour.

In all groups the mortality rate rises with age; for example when the score lies between 10 and 19, the mortality rate in the 70+year age group is more than 8 times the rate for those under 50 years. The effects of age are somewhat paradoxically most noticeable when the Injury Severity Scores are comparatively low.

- Score 10–15: The response to treatment of cases within this band does most to throw light on the evaluation of the standard of medical care offered by any team or department. Cases within this group are sufficiently ill to be adversely affected by poor care; but they are not so ill that no matter how expert the treatment they cannot survive.

**Summary of Hospital Trauma Index:** Six areas must be considered when using this method of assessment: Respiratory, Cardiovascular, Nervous system, Abdominal, Extremities, Skin and Subcutaneous. A seventh area of Complications can be included for assessments which are made at a late stage.

## Respiratory

| | | |
|---|---|---|
| 1 | (minor) | Chest discomfort—minimal findings |
| 2 | (moderate) | Simple rib or sternal fracture, chest wall contusion with pleuritic pain |
| 3 | (major) | Multiple rib or first rib fracture, haemothorax, pneumothorax |
| 4 | (severe) | Open chest wound, flail chest, tension pneumothorax with normal BP, simple laceration of diaphragm |
| 5 | (critical) | Acute cyanotic respiratory failure, aspiration, tension pneumothorax with lowered BP, complicated laceration of diaphragm |

## Cardiovascular

| | | |
|---|---|---|
| 1 | (minor) | Less than 500 ml blood loss (less than 10% blood volume) with no change in perfusion. |
| 2 | (moderate) | Blood loss of 500–1000 ml (10–20% blood volume), decreased skin perfusion but normal urinary output, myocardial contusion with normal BP |
| 3 | (major) | Blood loss of 1000–1500 ml (20–30% blood volume), decreased skin perfusion, slight decrease in urinary output, tamponade, BP 80 mmHg |
| 4 | (severe) | Blood loss 1500–2000 ml (30–40% blood volume), decreased skin perfusion, urinary output less than 10 ml per hour, tamponade, conscious, BP less than 80 mmHg |
| 5 | (critical) | Blood loss in excess of 2000 ml (40–50% loss of blood volume), restless, coma, cardiac contusion or arrythmia, BP unrecordable. |

## Nervous system

| | | |
|---|---|---|
| 1 | (minor) | Head injury with or without scalp laceration, but no loss of consciousness or skull fracture |
| 2 | (moderate) | Head injury with unconsciousness of under 15 minutes, skull fracture, cervical pain with minimal findings, one facial fracture |
| 3 | (major) | Head injury with coma of more than 15 minutes, depressed skull fracture, cervical spine fracture or dislocation with positive neurological findings, multiple facial fractures |

4  (severe)  Head injury with coma in excess of 1 hour or with positive neurological findings, cervical spine fracture or dislocation with paraplegia

5  (critical)  Head injury with coma and no response to stimuli up to 24 hours, cervical spine fracture or dislocation with quadriplegia

### Abdominal

1  (minor)  Mild abdominal wall, flank or back pain with tenderness but no peritoneal signs

2  (moderate)  Acute flank, back or abdominal discomfort and tenderness, fracture of a seventh to twelfth rib.

3  (major)  Isolated injury to liver (minor), small bowel, spleen, kidney, body of pancreas, mesentery, ureter, urethra, fractures of ribs 7–12.

4  (severe)  Two major injuries: of rupture of the liver, bladder, head of pancreas, duodenum, colon, (large) of mesentery.

5  (critical)  Two severe injuries: crushing of liver; major vascular, including thoracic or abdominal aorta, vena cava, iliacs, hepatic veins.

### Extremities

1  (minor)  Minor sprain or fracture not involving a long bone

2  (moderate)  Closed fracture of humerus, clavicle, radius, ulna, tibia, fibula, involvement of a single nerve

3  (major)  Multiple moderate fractures, open moderate, closed femur, stable pelvis, major dislocation, major nerve injury.

4  (severe)  Two major long bone fractures, open fracture of femur, crushing or amputation of limb, unstable pelvic fracture

5  (critical)  Two severe or multiple major fractures

### Skin and subcutaneous

1  (minor)  Less than 5% burns, abrasions, contusions, lacerations

2  (moderate)  Burns of 5–15%, extensive contusions, avulsions 8–15 cm, lacerations totalling 30 cm in length

3  (major)  Burns of 15–30%, avulsions of 30 cm

4  (severe)  Burns of 30–45%, avulsion of leg or arm

5  (critical)  Burn of 45–60%

### Complications

1  (minor)  Minor wound infection, atelectasis, cystitis, superficial thrombo-phlebitis, temperature of >38.5°C

2  (moderate)  Major wound infection, atelectasis, pyelonephritis, septic or deep thrombo-phlebitis, temperature of >38.5°C

3  (major)  Intraperitoneal abscess, pneumonia, anuria or oliguria with raised serum urea, jaundice, less than 6 units of gastrointestinal (GI) haemorrhage, respiratory distress syndrome for less than 1 day

4  (severe)  septicaemia, empyema, peritonitis, pulmonary embolism with normal BP, renal failure with dialysis of less than 1 week, more than 6 units of GI haemorrhage, less than 3 days of respiratory distress syndrome

4 (critical) Septicaemia with fall in BP, pulmonary embolism with fall in BP, renal failure for 7–40 days, GI haemorrhage of more than 12 units, respiratory arrest, more than 3 days of respiratory distress syndrome on ventilator.

*Example:* A man aged 30 years has been admitted after being injured in a gas explosion. He was rendered unconscious for about half an hour, but skull films show no fracture and there is no sign of any intracranial damage. He has 35% superficial burns of the face, chest and abdomen. Radiographs of the chest have confirmed multiple rib fractures with a one-sided pneumothorax, but there is no immediate respiratory difficulty. He has also sustained a closed fracture of the left tibia.

Injury Severity Score:

| | | |
|---|---|---|
| Nervous system | 3 | square =  9 |
| Skin | 4 | square = 16 |
| Respiratory | 3 | square =  9 |
| Extremities | 2 | square =  4. |

Only the three most severe injuries are summed, so that the Injury Severity Score would be 34. Age in this case is not a further disadvantage, but nevertheless he will require prompt, expert treatment; with this his chances of survival are good. In treating him priority would be given to the management of his chest injury (e.g. by confirming the presence of a good airway, administering oxygen, inserting a chest drain, and estimating the blood gases) and by prevention or treatment of oligaemic shock (e.g. by removal of blood for grouping, cross-matching, assessment of haemoglobin and haematocrit; and by the establishment of a good intravenous line, with monitoring of a pulse, blood pressure, and urinary output (after insertion of a catheter)). The tibial fracture should be splinted at an early stage to help relieve pain and reduce local haemorrhage. The progress of the head and chest injuries will require careful monitoring and the fluid replacement programme carefully carried out. The large area that has been burned will in itself demand heavy and appropriate fluid replacement.

Once the emergency procedures have been instituted and the immediate situation brought under control, thought can be given to how to deal with the burns and the limb injury; this will be dictated by the exact nature of both these injuries.

**Treatment of the fracture itself:** The initial stages are clear:

(a)  Undue movement at the fracture site should be prevented by the use of temporary splintage till radiographic and any other examination is complete. This will reduce pain and haemorrhage and minimise the chances of a closed fracture becoming open. In the case of the lower limb, support with pillows and sandbags may be adequate. In both the upper and the lower limbs inflatable splints are invaluable.

(b)  If the deformity is so great that the skin overlying a fracture or dislocation is seriously endangering the viability of the overlying skin, it is usually advisable to do something to correct this; in many cases gentle repositioning of the distal part of the limb is sufficient; the use of Entonox may be required.

(c)     If the fracture is an open one, a bacteriological swab should be taken and the wound covered with sterile dressings. Antibiotic therapy should be commenced immediately; the choice of therapy is dependent on the current status of bacterial flora in wound infections occurring in the particular local situation.

(d)  The fracture should be fully assessed by clinical and radiological examination: the site, pattern, displacement and angulation should be noted. Involvement of the skin, and damage to related structures such as important nerves or blood vessels should be assessed.

With this information the following key decisions must be made:
1.  Does the fracture require reduction?
2.  If reduction is required, how is it planned to carry this out?
3.  What support is required till union occurs?
4.  If the fracture is open, how will this influence treatment?
5.  Does the patient require admission to hospital?
Some observations about these decisions will be made in sequence.

**1.  Does the fracture require reduction?** It is obvious that an undisplaced fracture does not require reduction, but unfortunately one still sees fractures in anatomical position subjected to manipulation, although only rarely are they displaced as a result of this.

If a fracture is only slightly displaced, reduction may nevertheless be highly desirable, as for example in fractures involving the ankle joint, where even slight persisting deformity may lead to the development of osteo-arthritis. In other situations, some displacement may often be accepted, depending on: (a) the site involved, (b) where good remodelling may be anticipated (especially in children), (c) if the patient is very old, when the risks of anaesthesia, etc., may be considered to outweigh a problematical improvement.

If the fracture is appreciably angled or rotated, reduction is generally essential for cosmetic and functional reasons (but see under appropriate fractures).

**2.  If the fracture requires reduction, how is it planned to carry this out?** (a) The commonest method is by the application of traction, followed by manipulation of the fracture, under general anaesthesia. General anaesthesia has most to offer in terms of muscle relaxation, duration and overall versatility, but for minor procedures regional anaesthesia and intravenous diazepam are popular and useful measures, with the advantage that waiting time may be reduced.

(b)  Continuous traction is used to achieve a reduction in fractures of the femur and fracture dislocations of the cervical spine. It is used less commonly for a number of other fractures.

(c)  Open reduction of the fracture is carried out: (i) as an obvious part of the treatment of an open fracture—i.e. debridement of the wound exposes the fracture which may be reduced under vision, (ii) where conservative methods have failed to give a satisfactory reduction, (iii) where it is considered that the best method of supporting the fracture involves internal fixation, and exposure of the fracture is a necessary part of that procedure.

**3.  What support is required until union of the fracture occurs?** *(a) Non-rigid methods of support:* Arm slings, bandages and adhesive strapping may be used, and serve some of the following purposes.

(i)  Firm support, in the form for example of crepe bandaging or circular woven bandaging, may help to limit swelling and oedema, and restrict the spread of haematoma.

(ii) Slings are often employed for elevation purposes, especially to limit gravitational swelling of the hand and fingers in upper limb injuries.

(iii) Pain may be relieved by the restriction of movement.

(iv) By restriction of limb movement, forces acting on the bone ends may be reduced to a level at which relative movement is unlikely, or insufficient to interfere with healing. This applies particularly to impacted fractures.

*(b) Continuous traction:* Traction may be maintained for several weeks, while holding a fracture in reduction. Fractures of the femoral shaft are frequently treated by this method. Traction may be effected through the skin (skin traction) by, for example, adhesive strapping, or through bone (skeletal traction) by, for example, a Steinman pin.

*(c) Plaster fixation:* Plaster of Paris, generally in the form of plaster-impregnated bandages, is the commonest method of supporting a fracture. The plaster is carefully moulded to fit the contours of the limb, and the quick-setting properties of the plaster allow the limb to be held without undue strain in the correct position until setting has occurred. For a plaster to achieve its purpose, care must be taken over its application and subsequent supervision. A disadvantage of plaster splints is that they soften if they are allowed to become wet. There are a number of plaster substitutes now available to overcome this problem, but none as yet combine the unique properties of plaster with moderate cost.

*(d) Internal fixation:* Internal fixation is indicated: (i) Where a fracture cannot be reduced by closed methods (e.g. a fracture of the tibia with soft tissue between the bone ends or many fractures of the forearm bones);

(ii) Where a reduction can be achieved but it cannot be satisfactorily held by closed methods (e.g. fractures of the femoral neck);

(iii) Where a higher quality of reduction and fixation is required than can be obtained by closed methods (e.g. some fractures involving articular surfaces).

(iv) In the case of multiple injuries involving the lower extremities, the risks of respiratory distress syndrome, fat embolism and other serious post-injury complications are considerably reduced by early operative stabilisation of lower extremity (especially femoral) fractures. (Respiratory function is improved when the patient can sit up, reducing abdominal pressure on the diaphragm with its risks of atelectasis; and less analgesia is required for fracture pain, with less respiratory depression resulting.) The present tendency in dealing with the multiply injured patient is to stabilise (with internal or external fixation) all major lower limb fractures as soon as the patient's general condition will allow, and preferably as part of the initial treatment on the day the injuries are sustained.

In addition, there is a controversial area where the risks of internal fixation in a particular set of circumstances are outweighed, in the experience and opinion of the surgeon in charge, by the advantages.
Some of the factors involved may include:

(i) The possibility of achieving and maintaining a high quality reduction.

(ii) Earlier mobilisation of joints, with less risk of permanent stiffness, disuse osteoporosis, etc.

(iii) Earlier discharge from hospital, and earlier return to full function (including work, athletic activities, etc.).

Some of the disadvantages of internal fixation are:

(i) The possibility of introducing infection. The consequences may be serious (e.g. chronic bone infection with non-union, which may sometimes necessitate amputation).

(ii) Internal fixation techniques require a degree of mechanical aptitude and experience on the part of the surgeon if the occasional serious failure is to be avoided.

(iii) To cover a wide range of fracture situations, a fairly formidable number of instruments and fixation devices will be required.

(iv) As on the whole the time under anaesthesia is much longer than when conservative measures are employed, the patient's general condition and health is of greater concern: the services of an expert anaesthetist are more frequently required.

The methods of achieving internal fixation include the use of a wide range of devices (screws, nails, plates, etc.).

*(e) External skeletal fixation:* With this method the bone fragments are held in alignment with pins inserted percutaneously. Two common methods of placing the pins are used; in one, each pin is passed through the skin and a bone fragment, and exits through the skin on the other side. More commonly, a cantilever system is used, with rigid pins each of which is screwed into a bone fragment and protruding from one side of the limb only. One to six pins are fixed in each bone fragment. The fracture is reduced with the pins in situ (at open operation, or by using an image intensifier). The pins are then held in proper relation to one another by a rigid external support. The ends of the pins are connected together with a rigid system of mechanical clamps; in emergency situations plaster bandages may be used for this purpose.

Such systems are of particular value in the management of open fractures where the state of the skin and other factors may make the use of internal fixation devices undesirable. Cantilever (one-sided) systems give the best access for the dressing of open wounds.

The use of external fixators is sometimes followed, even in the case of closed fractures, by pin track infections. The quality of the fixation is also dependent on the pins remaining tight in the bone, and there is some risk of non-union.

*(f) Cast bracing:* Cast-bracing techniques are sometimes employed some weeks after the initial conservative management of a fracture. The method is used particularly in the treatment of fractures of the femur and tibia. In the case of fractures of the femur, one method employs two supports—one for the thigh and one for the leg below the knee—linked together by hinges at the side of the knee. Sufficient fixation may be achieved thereby to allow early ambulation.

**4. If the fracture is open, how will this influence treatment?** The following points will require separate consideration:

(a) As debridement of the wound will almost certainly by needed, general anaesthesia and theatre facilities are essential.

(b) In every case, potential difficulty in skin closure and cover of the fracture must be anticipated, and at least one possible line of treatment worked out prior to the patient being taken to theatre.

(c) If the wound is badly soiled, and the skin damage substantial, the use of large implants is discouraged. The wider stripping of the tissues required for the insertion of some internal fixation devices may disseminate any infecting organisms and cause further (albeit local) tissue damage. The presence of inert material in the tissues may act as a nidus for infection, so that it is difficult for any local infection to be overcome. The bulk of an internal fixation device may make wound closure more difficult, and subsequent swelling is more likely to lead to sloughing of devitalised skin over any prosthesis. If intramedullary nailing is to be employed, reaming of the medullary canal should be avoided.

If wound contamination is judged to be slight, and if good cover of the fracture can be obtained, internal fixation of the fracture is often carried out where it is felt to contribute to the chances of union and a successful outcome. Where there is much tissue damage, and the risks of infection are high, the use of an external fixator should be considered.

(d) Open fractures are usually associated with greater damage to surrounding soft tissues than is found in closed fractures. Postoperative swelling is invariable, is often severe, and may lead to circulatory impairment in the limb. Special precautions must be taken over the type of splintage used, and the limb must be elevated. Admission for observation of the patient and of the limb circulation is almost invariably required. In some cases there is serious elevation of pressure within the closed fascial compartments of the limb: this may be suspected on clinical grounds and be confirmed by manometry (when the intra-compartmental pressure exceeds 30 mmHg). It is treated by surgical decompression. In the case of the tibial compartments, this is done preferably by splitting the roofs of all the compartments and not just of the one that is principally involved.

(e) As a rule, open fractures are associated with greater violence, more initial deformity and more direct soft-tissue damage. Neurological and vascular damage is more common, and should be looked for; if found, then the appropriate additional treatment will be required.

(f) The majority of open fractures have microbial contamination which may be of both gram-negative and gram-positive organisms. The risk of the development of infection is closely related to the degree of soft tissue injury. There are special risks from organisms acquired from farmyards, fresh water contamination, and hospital environments (e.g. *Clostridium perfringens*, *Pseudomonas aeruginosa*, penicillin-resistant staphylococci). It is considered that the duration of antibiotic courses should be short to reduce the risks of the emergence of resistant strains. Swabs should be taken from wounds on admission.

Gustilo et al recommend the following: For Type I fractures, a single dose of 2.0 g of cephalosporin on admission followed by 1.0 g every 6–8 h for 48–72 h; for Type II or Type III injuries, gram-negative and gram-positive prophylaxis is necessary; as well as cephalosporin in the previously recommended dosage, the patient should be given aminoglycosides (tobramycin), 1.5 mg per kg body weight on admission, and 3.0–5.0 mg per kg body weight daily thereafter in divided doses. This must be adjusted if there is renal insufficiency. If there is risk of clostridial infection, 10 million units of penicillin should also be given. If any secondary procedure (e.g. internal fixation, delayed wound closure) is being performed, the antibiotic courses should be repeated.

Attention should also be paid to tetanus prophylaxis.

If wound contamination is judged to be slight, antibiotics may or may not be given, depending to some extent on the assessment of the particular circumstances of the case and of unit policy. (See Chapter 4 for details of local treatment.)

(g)  In the most severe open injuries, where there is perhaps much comminution of bone, extensive crushing of muscle, gross wound contamination and neurological damage, primary amputation may have to be considered.

The decision to amputate is not an easy one to make, especially in a climate where success in the re-attachment of severed limbs is not unusual. Nevertheless it must be borne in mind that even with the most sophisticated techniques, requiring perhaps many operations spread over months or years, there may be ultimate failure; when amputation is then carried out, and an artificial limb fitted, the rapidity of his rehabilitation may tempt the previously demoralised patient to wish that the decision to amputate had been made at the beginning.

Such an irrevocable line of treatment should not of course be suggested to a patient without the backing of a second, independent, senior opinion. In coming to a decision it may be helpful to consider the **Mangled Extremity Severity Score** (Johansen et al). This scheme has been: devised to give a quantitative assessment of the severity of injury to a limb, and to offer a guide in making the difficult decision as to whether it is worth striving to save a limb or to minimise losses and advise a primary amputation.

In applying the scheme, four factors are considered and the scores for each are added together to obtain a total. A score of 7 or more is considered a highly reliable guide to the need for amputation. (In a large series no false positives were found, i.e. in no case where the score was 7 or more was there ultimate survival of the limb.) On the other hand as might be expected a score of less than 7 does not necessarily guarantee that amputation may not eventually be required.

The scoring emphasises the great importance of the early restoration of good tissue perfusion.

The four factors and their scoring:

**1.  The skeletal/soft-tissue injury:**

- Low energy injury (stab wound; closed fracture; low velocity gunshot wound)                                                                                   1
- Medium energy injury (open fracture; multiple fractures, dislocation)                                                                                         2
- High energy injury (shotgun wound; high velocity gunshot wound; crush injury)                                                                                 3
- Very high energy injury (as above, but with gross contamination, soft tissue avulsion)                                                                        4

## 2.  Limb ischaemia
- Pulse reduced or absent, normal perfusion:

    less than 6 hours                                                        1

    more than 6 hours                                                       2
- Pulseless; paraesthesiae; reduced capillary refill:

    less than 6 hours                                                        2

    more than 6 hours                                                       4
- Cool, paralysed, insensate limb:

    less than 6 hours                                                        3

    more than 6 hours                                                       6

## 3.  Shock
- BP more than 90 mm                                                       0
- Transient hypotension                                                    1
- Persistent hypotension                                                   2

## 4.  Age
- <30 years                                                                0
- 30–50 years                                                              1
- >50 years                                                                2

For example:

(a)  A man aged 25 years involved in a road traffic accident 3 h previously is found to have an open fracture of the tibia, with reduced tissue perfusion and absent distal pulses; he is normotensive. The Mangled Extremity Severity Score would be 4 (age score = 0, open tibial fracture = 2; circulatory impairment = 2; shock = 0), so that other things being equal, primary amputation would not be considered, but an aggressive attempt to save the limb should be made (e.g. by fixation of the fracture and arterial reconstruction).

(b) A man of 60 is brought in with a gunshot fracture of the femur sustained 8 h previously. The limb is cold and paralysed, and the sensation absent. There is transient hypotension. The Mangled Extremity Severity Score would be 12 (age = 2; gunshot wound = 3; ischaemia = 6; shock = 1) and primary amputation would be advised.

**5.  Does the patient require admission to hospital?** In most cases the decision is an easy one, being related to the seriousness of the injury, the nature of the treatment and the need for continuous observation. The main criteria for admission very frequently overlap, and include the following:

*(a) Admission dictated by treatment:* Admission may be dictated by problems associated with anaesthesia—undue delay before anaesthesia, a prolonged anaesthetic, or where the anaesthetic is administered very late at night and recovery would be occurring at an inconvenient time in the early morning.

Admission will also obviously be required if the patient is being treated by continuous traction, partly because of the continuous use of special equipment, and partly because of the expert supervision required.

Most commonly, admission will be required when as a result of his injury the patient must be confined to bed.

*(b) Admission for observation:* Where there is appreciable risk of complications developing, admission may be required for continuous observation. This is obvious in the case of associated head injury, abdominal injury, or in the case of general multiple trauma.

Of particular relevance is admission for observation of the circulation in an injured limb. The majority of tibial fractures in adults, and ideally all supracondylar fractures in children should be admitted for elevation of the limb and observation of the circulation.

After open injuries (with the possible exceptions of fingers and toes) admission is advisable so that any developing infection can be detected and dealt with as early as possible.

*(c) Admission for general nursing care:* Many fracture cases may or may not require special treatment, but are nevertheless completely dependent on good nursing care. This applies particularly to fractures of the pelvis and spine where the patient is confined to bed. It also applies to other less obvious situations, such as the patient with fractures of both arms, who may be rendered virtually helpless with two comparatively minor injuries.

*(d) Admission for mobilisation:* Admission may be required for a period until the patient adapts to the limitations of his fracture and his splintage: for example, until a patient becomes sufficiently adept in the use of his crutches that he can manage in his own home.

*(e) Admission for social reasons:* Many elderly and infirm people, living alone or with equally affected relatives, may just be able to cope with life prior to injury. Even a minor fracture may render them unable to return to their normal environment. Admission is a necessity if no other help is available, and of course treatment is aimed at getting them fit to return home. Opportunity may be taken of their admission to investigate and treat any concurrent physical problem. If recovery is poor, assistance from hospital and domiciliary occupational therapists, social workers or geriatricians may be required.

*(f) Admission in the case of suspected child abuse:* where there is the possibility of non-accidental physical injury ('battered baby' syndrome), a child returned to the home environment may be put at risk of further injury which might be life-threatening, and admission is mandatory under such circumstances.

The possibility of child abuse should always be kept in mind, especially in dealing with injuries sustained by children under the age of 3 years (80% of cases lie within this age group). The other factors which might alert you include the following:

1. The presence of a fracture with no history of injury, or a vague history which is not in keeping with the nature or the extent of the injury.
2. The presence of multiple fractures or other injuries, especially when these are at different stages of healing, indicating that they have occurred as the result of separate incidents.
3. The presence of multiple soft tissue injuries, including swellings, bruises, burns, welts, lacerations and scars. There may be hand infections secondary to local burns: again, the appearance of these having occurred with a time interval between them is of importance.
4. If there is a head injury, radiographs of the skull may show evidence of fracture or widening of sutures, possibly from raised intracranial pressure secondary to cerebral oedema or subdural haematoma (which is found in about 25% of child abuse victims).
5. Evidence of failure to thrive, growth retardation, fever, anaemia or seizures.
   The commonest fractures that are found, in order of frequency, are of the

ribs, humerus, femur, tibia and skull, and in the average case 3–4 fractures are present. In the case of the long bones, the shafts are now recognised as being most commonly involved: in the older lesions there may be gross deformity and exuberant callus (due to lack of fixation). The presence of multiple lesions in varying states of healing is pathognomonic.

In the metaphyseal region the fractures may be impacted with copious new bone formation; there may be buckling of the bone without much in the way of new bone formation; or there may be irregular deformity with new bone appearing in layers as a result of repeated trauma. In some cases there is periosteal avulsion with marked local tenderness; this may not be detected on the initial films, but may show up if the radiographs are repeated after 10 days (with the formation of subperiosteal new bone).

Injuries to the epiphyses and the growth plates are very uncommon in cases of child abuse (whereas this pattern of injury is seen frequently in other forms of trauma).

Apart from admission and the carrying out of treatment appropriate to the fractures or other injuries, further investigations should usually include the following:

1. Review of the records of previous admissions.
2. Observations of the child's weight and height.
3. Obtaining an X-ray skeletal survey, including the skull.
4. Obtaining clinical photographs.
5. Most importantly, informing the Social Services so that the child's home background can be looked into, and the appropriate action taken to safeguard the child should the diagnosis of child abuse seem likely.

# 3. Closed reduction and fixation of fractures

1. **Closed reduction of fractures: Basic techniques (1):** The direction and magnitude of the causal force (1) and the deformity (2) are related, and may be worked out from the history, the appearance of the limb and the radiographs. Any force required to correct the displacement of a fracture is applied in the opposite direction (3).

2. **Basic techniques (2):** The first step in most closed reductions is to apply traction—generally in the line of the limb (1). Traction will lead to the disimpaction of most fractures (2) and this may occur almost immediately in the relaxed patient under general anaesthesia. Traction will also lead to reduction of shortening (3), and in most cases to reduction of the deformity (4).

3. **Basic techniques (3):** Any residual angulation following the application of traction may be corrected by using the heel of the hand under the fracture (1) and applying pressure distally with the other (2).

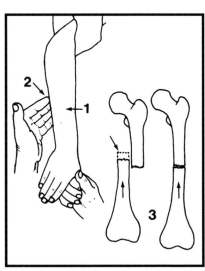

6. **Basic techniques (6):** After reduction of the fracture it must be prevented from redisplacing until it has united. The methods include the following:
Plaster fixation (p. 49–53).
Skin and skeletal traction (for examples, see p. 274–275).
Thomas splint (see p. 276–280).
Cast bracing (see p. 281, 310).
Rigid external fixation (see p. 313).

4. **Basic techniques (4):** In some fractures there may be difficulty in reduction due to prominent bony spikes or soft tissue interposition. Reduction may sometimes be achieved by initially increasing the angulation prior to manipulation. This method of unlocking the fragments must be pursued with care to avoid damage to surrounding vessels and nerves.

5. **Basic techniques (5):** The effectiveness of reduction may be assessed by noting the appearance of the limb (1), by palpation, especially in long bone fractures (2), by absence of telescoping (i.e. axial compression along the line of the limb does not lead to further shortening) (3), and by check radiographs.

7. **Protection of the skin: Stockingette:**
A layer of stockingette is usually applied next to the skin (1). This has several functions: it helps prevent the limb hairs becoming caught in the plaster, it facilitates the conduction of perspiration from the limb, it removes any roughness caused by the ends of the plaster and it may aid in the subsequent removal of the plaster. After the plaster has been applied, the stockingette is turned back (2).

8. **Stockingette** *ctd:* After the stockingette has been reflected, excess is removed, leaving 3–4 cm only at each end (3). The loose edge of stockingette is then secured with a turn or two of a plaster bandage (if a complete plaster is being applied) or with the encircling gauze bandage in the case of a slab.

9. **Wool roll:** A layer of wool should be used to protect bony prominences (e.g. the distal ulna). In complete plasters, where swelling is anticipated, several layers of wool may be applied over the length of the limb; the initial layer of stockingette may be omitted. Wool roll is also advisable where an electric saw is used for plaster removal.

10. **Felt:** Where friction is likely to occur over bony prominences, protection may be given with felt strips or felt cut-outs, fashioned to isolate the area to be relieved (e.g. the vertebral and iliac spines, the pubis and manubrium in plaster jackets). Adhesive felt should not be applied directly to the skin if skin eruptions are to be avoided.

11. **Plaster slabs (1):** These consist of several layers of plaster bandage and may be used for the treatment of minor injuries or where potentially serious swelling may be anticipated in a fracture. In their application, slabs are cut to length (1), and trimmed as required (2) to fit the limb before being applied (3). Slabs may also be used as foundations or reinforcements of complete plasters.

12. **Plaster slabs (2):** If a slab dispenser is available, measure the length of slab required and cut to length. A single slab of six layers of bandage will usually suffice for a child. In a large adult, two slab thicknesses may be necessary. In a small adult, one slab thickness may be adequate with local reinforcement.

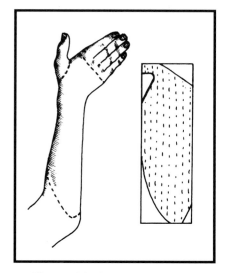

13. **Plaster slabs (3):** Alternatively, manufacture a slab by repeated folding of a plaster bandage, using say 8–10 thicknesses in an adult and six in a child as described (1). Turn in the end of the bandage (2) so that when the slab is dipped the upper layer does not fall out of alignment.

14. **Plaster slabs (4):** Ideally the slab should be trimmed with plaster scissors so that it will fit the limb without being folded over. For example, a slab for an undisplaced greenstick fracture of the distal radius should stretch from the metacarpal heads to the olecranon. It may be measured (1) and trimmed as shown, with a tongue (2) to lie between the thumb and index.

15. **Plaster slabs (5):** In a Colles fracture where the hand should be placed in a position of ulnar deviation, the slab should be trimmed to accommodate this position, a stage that is often omitted in error. The preceding two plaster slabs are examples of dorsal slabs.

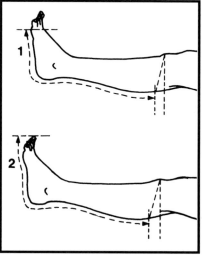

16. **Plaster slabs (6):** An anterior slab may be used as a foundation for a scaphoid plaster, or to treat an injury in which the wrist is held in dorsiflexion (measuring from a point just distal to the elbow crease with the elbow at 90°, to the proximal skin crease in the palm). The proximal end is rounded (1) while the distal lateral corner is trimmed for the thenar mass (2).

17. **Plaster slabs (7):** For the ankle (1) a plain untrimmed slab may be used, measuring from the metatarsal heads to the upper calf, 3–4 cm distal to a point behind the tibial tubercle.

For the foot (2) where the toes require support, choose the tips of the toes as the distal point.

18. **Plaster slabs (8):** Owing to the abrupt change in direction of the slab at the ankle, the slab requires cutting on both sides so that it may be smoothed down with local overlapping.

19. **Plaster slabs (9):** The same technique of side cutting is required for long arm plaster slabs (1). These are measured as indicated from the upper arm to the metacarpal heads, with a cut-out at the thumb as in a Colles plaster slab (2).

20. **Plaster slabs (10):** Wetting the slab: hold it carefully at both ends, immerse completely in tepid water, lift out and momentarily bunch up at an angle to expel excess water. Plaster-setting time is decreased by both hot and soft water.

21. **Plaster slabs (11):** Now consolidate the layers of the slab. If a plaster table is available, quickly place the slab on the surface and, with one movement with the heels of the hands, press the layers firmly together. (Retained air reduces the ultimate strength of the plaster and leads to cracking or separation of the layers).

22. **Plaster slabs (12):** Alternatively, consolidate the layers by holding the plaster at one end and pulling between two adducted fingers (1). Repeat the procedure from the other edge (2).

23. **Plaster slabs (13):** Carefully position the slab on the limb and smooth out with the hands so that the slab fits closely to the contours of the limb without rucking or the formation of sore-making ridges on its inferior surface.

24. **Plaster slabs (14):** At this stage any weak spots should be reinforced. Where there is a right-angled bend in a plaster—for example at the elbow or the ankle—two small slabs made from 10 cm (4″) plaster bandages may be used as triangular reinforcements at either site. A similar small slab may be used to reinforce the back of the wrist.

**25. Plaster slabs (15):** In the case of a long leg plaster slab, additional strengthening at the thigh and knee is always necessary, and this may be achieved by the use of two additional (15 cm) (6″) slabs.

**26. Plaster slabs (16):** Where even greater strength is required, the plaster may be girdered. For example, for the wrist, make a small slab of six thicknesses of 10 cm (4″) bandage and pinch up in the centre (1). Dip the reinforcement, apply, and smooth down to form a T-girder over the dorsum (2).

**27. Plaster slabs (17):** Girdering may also be achieved without a separate onlay. The basic plaster slab is pinched up locally after being applied to the limb. Care must be taken to avoid undue ridging of the interior surface.

**28. Bandaging (1):** Bandages used to secure plaster slabs should be of open weave (cotton or muslin) and be thoroughly wetted. This is to avoid tightening from shrinkage after coming in contact with the slab. Secure the end of the bandage between the thumb and fingers, and squeeze several times under water.

**29. Bandaging (2):** Apply to the limb firmly, but without too much pressure (1). Do not use reverse turns, which tend to produce local constrictions. The ends of the underlying stockingette may be turned back and secured with the last few turns of the bandage (2). On completion, secure the bandage with a small piece of wetted plaster bandage.

**30. Complete POP technique:** (1) The skin should be protected as previously described, using where applicable stockingette, wool roll and felt. (2) The following sizes of plaster bandage are recommended for normal application:

| | |
|---|---|
| Upper arm and forearm | 15 cm (6″) |
| Wrist | 10 cm (4″) |
| Thumb and fingers | 7.5 cm (3″) |
| Trunk and hip | 20 cm (8″) |
| Thigh and leg | 20 cm (8″) |
| Ankle and foot | 15 cm (6″) |

**31. Plaster bandage wetting (1):** Plaster bandages should be dipped in tepid water. Secure the end of the bandage with one hand to prevent the end becoming lost in the mass of wet bandage. Hold the bandage lightly with the other without compression. Immerse at an angle of 45°, and keep under water until bubbles stop rising.

**32. Plaster bandage wetting (2):** Remove excess water by gently compressing in an axial direction and twisting slightly. Alternatively, pull the bandage through the encircled thumb and index while lightly gripping the bandage.

**33. Plaster bandage application (1):** Most moulding of the plaster will be required at the wrist in upper limb plasters, and at the ankle in lower limb plasters. It is often useful to apply the more proximal parts first, so that moulding can be more profitably carried out against a set or nearly set cuff of plaster on the forearm or calf (i.e. start a forearm plaster at the elbow, and a below knee plaster at the tibial tubercle).

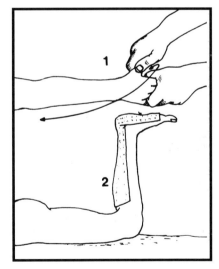

**34. Plaster bandage application (2):** Roll each bandage without stretching if there is no wool beneath; if there is a layer of wool, and no swelling is anticipated, a little even pressure may be applied to compress the wool to half thickness. Plain tucks may be used distally to ensure a smooth fit, but figure-of-eight or reverse turns should not be used if local constriction is to be avoided.

**35. Plaster bandage application (3):** After the application of each bandage smooth the layers down to exclude any trapped air and consolidate the plaster. A second and if necessary a third bandage may be applied to complete the proximal portion. Each bandage should extend 2–3 cm distal to the previous, and be well smoothed down. The distal part may then be completed, and the hand or foot portion moulded before setting is complete.

**36. Plaster bandage application (4):** Where possible the assistant should hold the limb in such a way that the surgeon has a clear run while applying the plaster (1). Where support must be given to a part included in the plaster, the flats of the hands should be used, and the hands eased proximally and distally to avoid local indentation. Where slabs are used, try to let gravity assist rather than hinder (2).

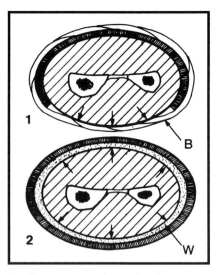

37. **Removal of rings (1):** Wherever possible rings should be removed in case finger swelling leads to distal gangrene. A tight ring can generally be coaxed from a finger if it is well coated with olive oil or a similar lubricant. If this fails, the finger may sometimes be sufficiently compressed by binding it with, for example, macrame twine to allow removal as shown.

38. **Removal of rings (2):** Otherwise a ring may be cut with a ring cutter (1) or a saw cut may be made with a fine tooth hack-saw on to a spatula (2) to spring the ring. Ring removal is nevertheless sometimes obsessively pursued. If significant swelling is unlikely, the ring loose below the knuckle, the patient intelligent and the potential danger is indicated, it may be retained with acceptable safety.

39. **Plaster precautions (1):** After an acute injury, if much swelling is anticipated (1) use a plaster slab in preference to a complete plaster. The retaining bandages have more 'give' than plaster, and are more readily cut in an emergency. (2) If a slab does not give sufficient support, then allow for swelling with a generous layer of wool beneath the plaster. (W = wool; B = bandage.)

40. **Plaster precautions (2):** Consider splitting any complete plaster. This should be done *routinely* after any operative procedure when swelling may be considerable (from tourniquet release, postoperative oedema, etc.). Use a sharp knife and cut down through the plaster to the underlying wool. (The wool protects the skin.) This should be done immediately after application of the plaster before it has had time to dry out.

41. **Plaster precautions (3):** Be sure the plaster has been *completely* divided down to the wool along its whole length (1). (Any remaining strands will act dangerously as constricting bands.) You should be able to see the wool quite clearly. The plaster edges should spring apart by 5–10 mm or they may be eased apart by the handle of the knife, thereby dynamically relieving any underlying pressure (2).

42. **Elevation (1):** Wherever possible, the injured limb should be elevated. In the case of the hand and forearm in a patient who has been admitted, the limb may be secured in stockingette (or in a roller towel using safety pins) attached to a drip stand at the side of the bed. Elevation should be maintained at least until swelling is beginning to resolve.

43. **Elevation (2):** In the case of the ambulant patient a sling may be used, provided the arm is kept high enough (1). If the sling is too slack the arm will hang down, encouraging oedema (2).

44. **Elevation (3):** In the case of the lower limb, the leg may be elevated on pillows (1). The end of the bed may be raised on an A-frame or on chairs (2). The ambulant patient should be advised to keep the foot as high as possible on a couch or chair whenever he is at rest.

45. **Exercise:** Those parts free of plaster should be exercised as frequently as possible: for example, the fingers in a Colles fracture (and later the elbow and shoulder). The patient should be shown how she should curl the fingers into full flexion and then fully extend them. She should be given clear instructions as to how frequently she should perform these exercises (e.g. for 5 minutes every waking hour).

**Instructions for Patients in Plaster of Paris Splints**

A. (1) If fingers or toes become swollen blue, painful or stiff, raise limb.

(2) If no improvement in half an hour call in Doctor or return to hospital immediately.

B. (1) Exercise all joints not included in plaster—especially fingers and toes

(2) If you have been fitted with a walking plaster walk in it.

(3) If plaster becomes loose or cracked—report to hospital as soon as possible.

46. The patient who is being allowed home must be given clear warnings to return should the circulation appear in any way to be impaired. Inform the patient or, where appropriate, a relative who will be looking after the patient. It is also useful to reinforce this by pasting an instruction label (such as the one illustrated) directly to the plaster.

47. **After care of patients in plaster:** Note the following: (i) *Is there swelling?* Swelling of the fingers or toes is common in patients being treated in plaster, but the patient must be examined carefully for other signs which might suggest that circulatory impairment is the cause, rather than the local response to trauma. If there is no evidence of circulatory impairment, the limb should be elevated and movements encouraged.

48. (ii) *Is there discoloration of the toes or fingers?* Compare one side with the other; bluish discoloration, especially in conjunction with oedematous swelling distally, suggests that swelling of the limb within the plaster has reached such a level as to impair the venous return, and appropriate action must be taken.

49. (iii) *Is there any evidence of arterial obstruction?* Note the five Ps: intense **pain, paralysis** of finger or toe flexors, **paraesthesiae** in fingers or toes, **pallor** of the skin with disturbed capillary return, and **'perishing cold'** feel of the fingers and toes. Arterial obstruction requires *immediate, positive action.*

50. **Treatment of suspected circulatory impairment (1):** (a) Elevate the limb (1). (b) In the case of a plaster slab, cut through the encircling bandages and underlying wool (2) until the *skin is fully exposed,* and ease back the edges of the plaster shell until it is apparent that it is not constricting the limb in any way.

51. **Treatment (2):** Where the plaster is a complete one, split the plaster throughout its entire length. *Ease* back the edges of the cast to free the limb on each side of the midline. *Divide* all the overlying wool and stockingette and turn it back till skin is exposed. The same applies to any dressing swabs hardened with blood clot.

52. **Treatment (3):** If the circulation has been restored, gently pack wool between the cut edges of the plaster (1) and firmly apply an encircling crepe bandage (2). If this is not done, there is risk of extensive skin ('plaster') blistering locally. If the circulation is not restored, re-appraise the position of the fracture and suspect major vessel involvement. *On no account adopt an expectant and procrastinating policy.*

53. (iv) *Can the plaster be completed?* If the plaster consists of a back-slab or shell, completion depends on your assessment of the present swelling, and your prediction of any further swelling. Most plasters may be completed after 48 hours; but if swelling is very marked completion should be delayed for a further 2 days, or until it is showing signs of subsiding.

54. (v) *Is the plaster intact?* Look for evidence of cracking, especially in the region of the joints (1). In arm plasters, look for anterior softening (2) and softening in the palm (3). In the leg, look for softening of the sole piece (4), the heel (5) and calf (6). Any weak areas should be reinforced by the application of more plaster locally.

55. (vi) *Is the plaster causing restriction of movement?* Look especially for encroachment of the palm piece on the ulnar side of the hand, restricting MP joint flexion (1). In forearm plasters, look also for restriction of elbow movements. In below-knee plasters, note if the plaster is digging in when the knee is flexed (2). Trim the plaster as appropriate (3).

56. (vii) *Is the plaster too short?* Note especially the Colles-type plaster with inadequate grip of the forearm (1); note the below-knee plaster which does not reach the tibial tuberosity (2) and which, apart from affording unsatisfactory support of an ankle fracture, will inevitably cause friction against the shin. Extend the defective plasters where appropriate (3).

57. (viii) *Has the plaster become too loose?* A plaster may become loose as a result of the subsidence of limb swelling and from muscle wasting. If a plaster is slack, then the support afforded to the underlying fracture may become inadequate. Assess looseness by attempting to move the plaster proximally and distally, while noting its excursion in each direction.

58. *Has the plaster become too loose? ctd.:* In the leg, grasp the plaster and pull it distally; note how far the toes disappear into the plaster. If a plaster is loose, it should be changed unless (a) union is nearing completion and risks of slipping are minimal or (b) a good position is held and the risks of slipping while the plaster is being changed are thought to be greater than the risks of slipping in a loose plaster.

59. (ix) *Is the patient complaining of localised pain?* Localised pain, especially over a bony prominence, may indicate inadequate local padding, local pressure and pressure sore formation. In a child it may sometimes suggest a foreign body pushed in under the plaster. In all cases, the affected area should be inspected by cutting a window in the plaster and replacing it after examination.

60. **How to remove a plaster: plaster slabs:** Plaster shells or slabs are easily removed by cutting the encircling open weave bandages which hold them in position. Care must be taken to avoid nicking the skin, and Bohler scissors are helpful in this respect.

61. **Removing complete plasters: Using shears (1):** The heel of the shears must lie between the plaster and the limb. Subcutaneous bony prominences such as the shaft of the ulna (1) should be avoided to lessen the risks of skin damage and pain. Instead, the route of the shears should be planned to lie over compressible soft-tissue masses (2).

62. **Using shears (2):** If possible, avoid cutting over a concavity. If the wrist is in moderate palmar flexion as in a Colles plaster, the plaster should be removed by a dorsal cut (1). In a scaphoid plaster, the dorsal route should be avoided (2) and the plaster removed anteriorly.

63. **Using shears (3):** Where there is the right-angled bend of the ankle to negotiate, it is often helpful to make two vertical cuts down through the sole piece (1) and turn it down (2). This then gives access for the shears to make a vertical cut behind the lateral malleolus (3) and then skirt forwards over the peronei (4). The remaining plaster may then be sprung open.

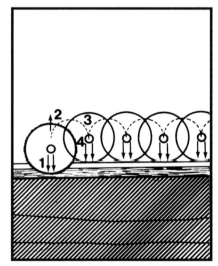

64. **Using shears (4):** Keep the lower handle (L) parallel to the plaster, or even a little depressed. Lift up the upper handle (U); push the shears forward with the lower handle so that the plaster fills the throat of the shears. Maintaining a slight pushing force, all the cutting action may be performed with the upper handle, moving it up and down like a beer pump.

65. **Using a plaster saw (1):** Plaster saws may be used for removing or cutting windows in plasters, but they should be used with caution and treated with respect. Do not use a plaster saw unless there is a layer of wool between the plaster and the skin. Do not use it over bony prominences and do not use if the blade is bent, broken or blunt. *Note:* the blade does not rotate but oscillates.

66. **Using a plaster saw (2):** Electric saws are noisy, and the apprehensive patient should be reassured. Cut down through the plaster at one level (1); the note will change as soon as it is through; remove the saw (2) and shift it laterally about an inch (2.5 cm) (3) and repeat (4). *Do not* slide the saw laterally in shallow cuts; the cutting movement should be up and down.

**67. Polymer resin casts:** Plaster of Paris is the most frequently used casting material, although there are alternatives. Most use bandages of cotton (e.g. Bayer's Baycast®) or fibreglass (Smith & Nephew's Dynacast XR®), impregnated with a resin which hardens on contact with water. Advantages include: (1) strength combined with lightness, (2) rapid setting (5–10 min) and curing, reaching maximum strength in 30 min (cf. plasters whose slow 'drying out' period of about 48 hours may lead if unprotected to cracking), (3) water resistance combined with porosity, (4) radiolucence. Disadvantages include: (1) high item cost—but their durability reduces demands on staff and transport, (2) they mould less well than plaster, and are unyielding.

After acute injuries, where further swelling is likely, plaster is generally the more suitable casting material; it can be carefully moulded to the part giving particularly good support, and where necessary it can be applied in the form of a slab. When swelling subsides, and the stability of the fracture is not in doubt, a resin cast may be substituted. Where little swelling is anticipated in a stable fresh fracture, a resin cast may be used from the outset. Where a cast is likely to be abused (e.g. in wet weather where an extroverted teenager requires support for an ankle injury) there is much to be said for using a resin cast, and of course it is possible to reinforce an ordinary plaster cast with an outer resin bandage.

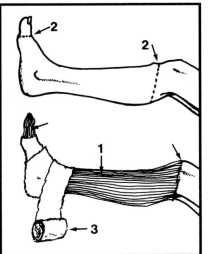

**68. Application (1):** Apply conforming stockingette (1) to the limb: ensure that it extends 3–5 cm (1–2″) beyond the proposed limits of the cast itself (2). Next, apply a layer of padding (3), paying particular care to protect the bony prominences. Where it is necessary to resist exposure to water or to moisture, a synthetic water-resistant orthopaedic padding may be used (e.g. Smith & Nephew's Soffban®).

**69. Application (2):** Open each bandage pack only as required to avoid premature curing. Wear gloves to prevent the resin adhering to your skin or causing sensitisation. Immerse the bandage in warm water for 2–5 seconds, squeezing it two to four times to accelerate setting. Fewer bandages will be required than with plaster—e.g. a below-knee cast in an adult may be applied with two 7.5 cm (3″) and one to two 10 cm (4″) bandages. Use the smaller sizes for the areas requiring a high degree of conformity (e.g. the ankle).

**70. Application (3):** Ensure the limb is correctly positioned, and apply each turn so that it overlaps the one beneath by half a width (1). It is permissible to use a figure-of-eight (2) round the ankle, elbow and knee to assist the bandage to lie neatly in conformity with the contours of the limb beneath. Turn back the stockingette (3) before applying the top layers of the bandage, and make quite certain that there will be no sharp or hard cast edges which can cause ulceration of the skin.

**71. Application (4):** In some cases close moulding of the cast may be encouraged by the temporary application of a firm external bandage. For this a thick cotton or crepe bandage may be used. This is first wetted, and then wrapped tightly round the limb. This will also be found helpful in retaining the last turn or two of the resin bandages, which often have a disturbing tendency to peel away before they set.

Remove the wet overbandage once the cast has set.

**72. Removal of resin casts:** Because of their inherent springiness, resin casts cannot be cracked open after they have been cut down one side as can plasters. In most cases it is necessary to bivalve by cutting down both sides. In the case of leg casts, it is best to turn down the sole piece first (see 58, 63). Either shears or an oscillating saw may be used; in the latter case, a dust extractor should be employed to avoid the inhalation of resin dust. Resin casts are less likely to break after windowing than plasters.

**73. Assessment of union (1):** Union in a fracture cannot be expected until a certain amount of time has elapsed, and it is pointless to start looking too soon. (See individual fractures for guidelines.) When it is reasonable to assess union, the limb should be examined out of plaster. Persistent oedema at the fracture site suggests union is incomplete.

**74. Assessment of union (2):** Examine the limb carefully for tenderness. Persistent tenderness localised to the fracture site is again suggestive of incomplete union.

**75. Assessment of union (3):** Persistent mobility at the fracture site is certain evidence of incomplete union. Support the limb close to the fracture with one hand, and with the other attempt to move the distal part in both the anterior and lateral planes. In a uniting fracture this is not a painful procedure.

**76. Assessment of union (4):** Although clinical assessment is often adequate in many fractures of cancellous bone, it is advisable in the case of the shafts of the femur, tibia, humerus, radius and ulna to have up-to-date radiographs of the region. The illustration is of a double fracture of the femur at 14 weeks. In the proximal fracture, the fracture line is blurred and there is external bridging callus of good quality; union here is fairly far advanced. In the distal fracture, the fracture line is still clearly visible, and bridging callus is patchy. Union is incomplete, and certainly not sufficient to allow unprotected weight bearing.

In assessing radiographs for union, be suspicious of unevenly distributed bridging callus, of a persistent gap, and of sclerosis or broadening of the bone ends. Note that where a particularly rigid system of internal fixation has been employed, bridging callus may be minimal or absent, and endosteal callus may be very slow to appear.

If in doubt regarding the adequacy of union, continue with fixation and re-examine in 4 weeks.

Note that in all cases you must assess whether the forces the limb is exposed to will result in displacement or angulation of the fracture, or cause such mobility that union will be prevented: you must balance the following equation:

$$\text{external forces} < (\text{degree of union} + \text{support supplied by any internal fixation device} \\ \text{and/or external splintage}).$$

# 4. Open fractures: internal fixation

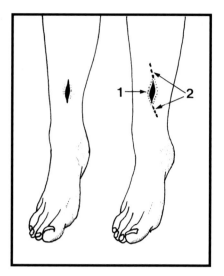

1. **Open fractures: immediate care:** When the case first presents, ensure that the following procedures are carried out in every case: (1) Take a bacteriology swab from the wound. (2) Commence a short course of appropriate antibiotics (see p. 42). (3) Cover the wound with care using sterile dressings (to reduce the risks of secondary (hospital) infection). (4) Apply temporary splintage (e.g. a plaster back shell, or if appropriate, an inflatable splint.

2. **Type I, technically open fractures:** (1) The risks of infection are slight and are unlikely to be lessened by wide exposure (although this is advocated by some). The wound should be thoroughly cleaned (2) and a sterile dressing applied locally (3). Thereafter the method of supporting the fracture must be decided (see p. 42 and also Regional Injuries). If a plaster cast is being applied there *must* be allowance for swelling, e.g. by using a backshell or by splitting a cast applied over copious wool.

3. **Type I, open from within out:** (1) The wound is small with clean or minimally bruised, viable edges (1). The skin edges may be minimally excised, and the wound extended (2) to allow a thorough inspection. It is unlikely that much will be required in the form of excision of contaminated or avascular tissue to achieve a thorough debridement. *Advantage may be taken of the exposure to allow an accurate open reduction of the fracture.*

4. **Type I ctd:** A thorough lavage of the wound should then be carried out. For this up to 10 litres of normal saline may be used, followed by 2 litres of bacitracin–polymixin solution (1). If the wound is being left open (the generally recommended safest procedure), it may be helpful to use anchoring sutures at strategic points (2) to prevent undue retraction that might interfere with any secondary suture. Apply a dressing which ensures the tissues remain moist (e.g. saline-soaked swabs over vaseline gauze). Primary closure of the skin is not advocated. Now fix the fracture.

5. **Type I ctd:** Inspect the wound on the second or third day; if necessary, carry out any revision (secondary debridement). If the wound remains clean, the aim should be to carry out a (delayed primary) wound closure under repeat antibiotic cover at 5–7 days (1). If the wound cannot be closed without tension, any remaining defect should be covered with a split-skin meshed graft (2). If the wound is dirty, then it should be treated by radical excision of all necrotic and infected tissue every 2–3 days until clean and ready to receive meshed grafts.

6. **Type II open fractures** should be managed along similar lines. *In Type III* injuries a vigorous debridement should be carried out with copious wound lavage. All foreign material must be removed along with any completely devitalised tissue (including small bone fragments). The wound should be left open but dressed so as to prevent the underlying tissues from drying out. To facilitate further wound management (conducted along the lines suggested in Frame 5) an external fixator may be the best way to hold the fracture.

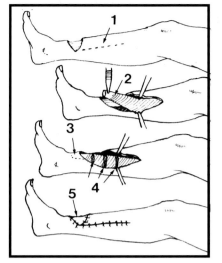

7. **Type III ctd:** If bone is exposed, the aim should be to get it covered as early as possible (certainly under 2 weeks) to avoid the risks of resistant secondary infection. In the case of the tibia it may be possible to carry out a soleus flap immediately or after a short delay. The skin wound may have to be extended (1); the muscle is detached 1 cm distal to its musculo-tendinous junction, transposed (2) and anchored distally (3); added length may be obtained by making several transverse incisions in its sheath (4). At a suitable time, its outer surface may be covered with split skin grafts (Frame 5).

8. **Type III ctd:** Again in the case of the tibia, for wounds situated beyond the reach of the extended soleus, extensor digitorum communis can be used if reversed.

Where much tissue has been lost and greater cover than that afforded by split skin is required in the region of the fracture, the following procedures are available:

(i)   The gastrocnemius myocutaneous flap: this can provide local cover for most skin defects between the lower leg and the lower thigh: either the medial or lateral heads may be used, and the procedure for each is similar. (The muscle belly is isolated from soleus, its attachment to the Achilles tendon divided, and it is freed from its other head before the flap is swung.)

(ii)  The fasciocutaneous flap: this type of local flap includes the skin, the subcutaneous fat and fascia, but not muscle. (Note that whole thickness skin flaps in the lower limb which do not include the fascial layer have a poor record of success. Careful planning of the flap outlines is required, and the secondary defect is covered at the same time with split skin grafts.

(iii) Free microvascular flaps: the commonest and most useful sources are from the latissimus dorsi or rectus abdominis; skin may be tranferred with the graft. The techniques are highly specialised. Failure when it occurs is generally due to vascular problems including infection at the recipient site.

Where bone grafting is required this should be carried out as soon as it is safe to do so. In the case of Type I and Type II open fractures, this can be considered 2–3 weeks after wound healing has been achieved. In the case of Type III open fractures, grafting should be delayed for 6 weeks after healing has been obtained.

*Type IIIc open fractures* have the highest failure and amputation rate, due to difficulties encountered in restoring the circulation or from infection. In handling these cases the fracture must be soundly fixed and any arterial repair (e.g. by an interpositional graft) achieved within 4–6 hours; the vascular problem should be dealt with by an experienced vascular surgeon, and not delegated. Prophylactic fasciotomies should be carried out.

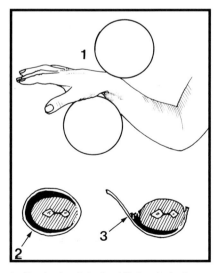

9. **Degloving injuries (1):** In a degloving injury, an extensive area of skin is torn from its underlying attachments and thereby deprived of its blood supply. In the hand or arm it is commonly caused by the limb being crushed between rollers (1); in the leg it may result from the shearing effect of a vehicle wheel passing over the limb in a run-over accident.

10. **Degloving injuries (2):** The skin may remain unbroken (2 in Frame 9), in which case the limb feels like a fluid-containing bag, owing to the presence of an extensive haematoma between the skin and fascia. If the skin is torn (3 in Frame 9), the effect is the creation of a large flap of full-thickness skin. In either case, massive sloughing is likely unless the injury is properly managed. A number of plastic surgical procedures are available. Probably the best method, if facilities are to hand, is the following: (a) The flap should be excised, first marking it (and the defect) so that it may be re-orientated later. (b) The flap is stored in a sterile container in a refrigerator (storage temperature is important). (c) The wound should be debrided, and the conditions optimised for the formation of a local bed of granulation tissue. (d) After 1–2 weeks the stored skin is replaced as a single sheet graft, after the deeper layers have been removed using special equipment.

It any open injury it is vital to keep in mind the risks of serious, life-threatening infections, particularly tetanus and gas gangrene, and the appropriate protective measures must be taken.

## 11.  Principles of internal fixation and common fixation methods

When it is intended to implant materials for the treatment of fractures, the following criteria must be satisfied:

**1.  Freedom from tissue reaction:** It is self-evident that if foreign material is being implanted in the tissues it should be biologically inert, and not give rise to toxic reactions, local inflammatory changes, fibrosis, foreign body giant cell reactions, etc., which in turn are likely to produce local pain, swelling and impairment of function. There is evidence of an extremely low but apparently clear incidence of local, and possibly distal, metal induced neoplasia. In consequence, in the younger patient (under age 40), internal fixation devices are removed routinely once they have served their purpose.

**2.  Freedom from corrosion:** Implanted materials should not corrode. Where stainless steel is used it should be of an accepted grade and free from inpurities; steps should be taken to avoid the initiation of corrosion problems by fretting occurring at the point of contact between the separate components of an implant. It is essential to avoid electrolytic degradation, and in practice this means that if more than one implant is used at the same side (e.g. a plate and screws) that identical materials are employed.

**3.  Freedom from mechanical failure:** Implants must satisfy the purposes for which they are intended. To withstand the forces to which they will be subjected demands a satisfactory compromise between the materials used and the design of the implant. In the treatment of fractures, implants generally must have great mechanical strength in association with small physical bulk; consequently most are made of metal. Of the suitable metals, the most frequently employed are: (1) certain stainless steels, (2) alloys of chromium, cobalt and molybdenum (e.g. Vitallium®, Vinertia®, (3) titanium. The chrome–cobalt alloys are biologically very inert, but are difficult to machine so that most implants, including screws, are microcast using the lost wax technique; this adds to their cost. The stainless steels are less inert, but are easier to machine and are cheaper. In certain situations other materials are sometimes used; e.g. in fractures of the femur in the region of the stems of hip replacements it is possible to employ nylon plates held in position with nylon cerclage straps. At the ankle, biodegradable plastic dowels may be used to treat certain malleolar fractures, and have the advantage that their slow absorbtion obviates any need for their later removal. Sensitivity to these implants (in the form of a low grade inflammatory response) is, however, a not uncommon occurrence. Where it is desirable to have a certain amount of flexibility in a plate to encourage the formation of some external bridging callus, carbon fibre plates are sometimes used.

**Fixation devices and systems:** Fractures vary enormously in pattern; bones vary in their size, texture and strength. To cope with even the most common situations and be a match for every subtle variation of circumstance requires an impressive range of devices and instruments for their insertion. The design of fixation devices has in the past been somewhat haphazard, and aimed at the treatment either of one fracture or the solution of a single fixation problem. There have been attempts to produce integrated systems of fracture fixation: sets of devices which can contend with any fracture situation. The most outstanding system, now firmly established, is that developed by the

Association for the Study of Internal Fixation [ASIF or AO (Arbeitgemeinschaft für Osteosynthesefragen)]. (This group of general and orthopaedic surgeons was founded in 1956 by Maurice E. Müller to research certain concepts propounded by Robert Danis). As a result of their work, apart from the development of a series of screws, plates and other devices, and the corresponding instrumentation, the Association is responsible for some change in emphasis in the philosophy of fracture treatment. They feel that the common aim, a return to full function in the shortest time, can often best be achieved by the use of internal fixation devices, of such strength and design that external splintage can frequently be discarded permitting immediate joint freedom, early weight bearing, short-term hospitalisation, and early return to work and other activities. These ideals are often achieved, but it must be stressed that optimum results cannot be obtained without the necessary technical knowledge of the system and a degree of mechanical aptitude, both of which can be acquired by appropriate training and experience.

With any form of internal fixation great importance must always be placed on recognising which cases are best treated in this way. It is equally important to recognise which cases are not suited to treatment by internal fixation, and those which may be dealt with either surgically or conservatively.

It is in the last group that there is often some difficulty, and it is important to remember the hazards of infection; even though it may be uncommon, it must always be a feared complication which on occasion can turn a comparatively minor fracture into a disaster. As in many branches of surgery, the core problem is in deciding how many excellent results are required to balance the occasional serious failure, and the compromise to be made between the particulars of a case and the outlook and judgement of the surgeon.

**12. Principles of internal fixation and common devices: Cortical bone screws (1):** The AO cortical bone screw enjoys widespread use and is probably the commonest of all internal fixation devices. The standard screw has an outside diameter of 4.5 mm (1) and a core diameter of 3.0 mm (2). The thread form is a modified buttress (3), of 1.75 mm pitch (circa 15 TPI). The large head has a hemispherical undersurface (4) and contains a hexagon socket (5) which is used for its insertion.

**13. Cortical bone screws (2):** To insert an AO screw, the bone is drilled with a 3.2 mm drill (1), preferably using a guide to maintain its perpendicularity. The hole is then tapped (2) and sized, so that the correct length of screw (from a wide range) can be chosen. This is then inserted using a hex screwdriver (3). In certain circumstances it is necessary to use smaller screws (e.g. in dealing with phalangeal fractures) and screws of 3.5, 2.7, 2 and 1.5 mm are available in the AO range.

**14. Cortical bone screws (3):** When two bone fragments are being approximated with a screw, it is usually desirable to do so in such a manner that the adjacent surfaces are compressed one against the other — this improves the quality of the fixation, reduces the risks of non-union, and may be essential if the fracture will otherwise be unsupported (e.g. if a cast is not being applied). To do this, a clearance (or gliding) hole is drilled in the nearest fragment; tightening the screw draws the two fragments together: the so-called lag screw principle.

**15. Cortical bone screws (4):** *Placing the screws.* Two mutually exclusive screw positionings may be used: (a) to obtain the most effective compression, and to avoid side thrusts which might displace the alignment of bone fragments, screws should be inserted at right angles to the plane of the fracture (1); (b) to offer the maximum resistance to torsional forces, screws should be inserted at right angles to the cortex (2). In practice, a combination of these two placements may be employed with effect (3).

**16. Cortical bone screws (5):** In long bones, one or more screws may be used to hold a fracture in perfect alignment (Illus.). Such an arrangement can seldom suffice without additional support: this may be in the form of plaster cast, but commonly a plate is used to neutralise any torsional or bending stresses that the fracture might be subjected to. (Neutralising plate). Note that if the stresses are great (e.g. unsupported weight bearing) that some of the load *must* be carried by the bone, otherwise eventual fatigue fracture of the plate is likely.

**17. Common devices: Plates (1):** There are many different types of plate. Some are quite lightweight and occupy little space (1), being used only to hold major bone fragments in alignment, while others are heavy (2) and sufficiently rigid to allow all external splintage to be discarded. For these to be successful and to encourage endosteal callus formation the bone surfaces should be brought together under a degree of compression. One way of doing this is to use a tensioning device (3) before inserting the screws on the second side of the fracture.

**18. Plates (2):** Another and more commonly used method of achieving compression is to use a dynamic compression plate (1). This has specially contoured slots (2), rather than plain round holes, for the cortical screws which are inserted eccentrically after using an offset drill guide (3). When the screws are tightened (4) their heads pinch the plate (5), causing the plate to slide slightly so that fracture surfaces are brought together in compression (6).

**19. Plates (3):** Plates should be placed on the tension side of a fracture so that compression loads are taken by bone (1), and tension effects are neutralised by the plate (2). In practice this means that plates should be applied to the lateral side of the femur. In the tibia, either side can be in tension: most commonly plates are fixed to the anteromedial surface (unless damage to the overlying skin dictates otherwise). An absolute minimum of two screws should be inserted in each main fragment; preferably three or more should be used, when the end screws may be allowed to engage the near cortex only so that stresses may be spread (3).

**20. Plates (4):** When a flat plate is applied to a bone using any system to obtain compression, this tends to occur in an uneven manner; the far side may open up as compression occurs on the nearside (1). To avoid this, it is common practice to pre-bend the plate at the level of the fracture (2). Then the far side compresses first (3), before the rest of the fracture line becomes involved, with the plate tending to straighten out (4). Note too that with the use of appropriate clamps plates may be individually bent to fit snugly against the contours of a bone (5).

**21. Plates (5):** Plates come in a great variety of shapes and sizes; some have been designed to cope with a specific fracture, while others have been developed to overcome certain inherent problems associated with the use of plates of a standard pattern.

*The low-contact dynamic compression plate (LC-DCP)* is relieved on its undersurface (1) so that the bone with which it is in direct contact is reduced in area: this minimises the amount of periosteum and bone which may be deprived of its blood supply by pressure from the plate. The screw slots are shaped in such a manner that interfragmentary bone compression screws may be inserted at angles up to 40° (2).

*Reconstruction plates* have V-cuts (3) between the screw holes which allow the plates to be bent in zig-zag fashion (4) (as well as in other planes) so that they can be used in special situations (e.g. in certain pelvic fractures).

*T- and L- buttress plates* (5) are of particular value in dealing with fractures of the proximal tibia. Lateral tibial head (*hockey stick*) plates (7) are also used in the proximal tibial area. *Cloverleaf* (8) plates are used mainly for the distal tibia. *Hook plates* [e.g. Zuelzer (9), AO] may be used when one fragment is not particularly suited to receiving a screw [e.g. fractures of the medial malleolus (10) or certain spinal fractures].

*Carbon fibre plates* (which can only be contoured at the time of manufacture) are slightly flexible and allow the formation of bridging callus. For the same reason, *wave plates* (plates with spring necks) may be used.

**22. Plates (6):** *The Eggar plate*, now only occasionally used, is a lightweight plate which is readily contoured to fit the bone to which it is being applied. Additional support (e.g. with an external plaster cast) is generally required. The plate is fixed to the bone with self-tapping screws which are not fully tightened. This permits slight axial movement, so that as bone absorption at the fracture site occurs the bone ends are not kept apart and union is thereby encouraged.

**23. Cancellous bone screws (1):** Screws designed for insertion in cancellous bone have a coarse pitch and a narrow thread angle, a combination which at its extremes produces auger forms. *AO cancellous bone screws* (with diameters of 6.5 or 4 mm) may be *partially threaded* (for use as lag screws) (1), or *fully threaded* (2) (when used to fix plates in the metaphyseal regions of long bones). When they are being inserted, the near cortex only is usually threaded, the end of the screw being used to cut its own path in the cancellous bone (3).

**24. Cancellous bone screws (2):** In the illustration a cancellous screw has been used in the treatment of a tibio-fibular diastasis. (In this condition the inferior tibio-fibular ligaments are torn, and the two bones become separated.) A clearance hole for the screw shank would have been drilled in the fibula and the threaded end of the screw, with its good grip in the metaphysis, would enable the tibia and fibula to be drawn together in the fashion of a lag screw. Note the washer used to spread the loads under the head of the screw and prevent it sinking into the fibula.

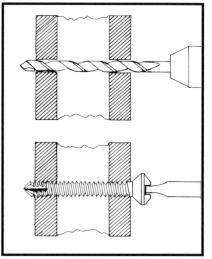

**25. Cancellous bone screws (3):** In the metaphyseal regions cancellous screws get the best grip if they engage the thin bone of the opposite cortex (which may have to be tapped) (1). If a reduction has been held with a Kirschner wire (2), *cannulated* 3.5 and 6.5 mm screws may be used when premature removal of the wire might threaten the reduction. The near cortex is drilled with a cannulated drill (3) and the screw inserted (4) over the wire which is then removed.

**26. Cancellous bone screws (4):** Partially threaded *malleolar screws* have been designed to secure small malleolar bone fragments by getting a purchase on the firm cancellous bone of the distal tibial metaphysis. They have an outside diameter of 4.5 mm and have fluted self-tapping tips. Because of this they are generally inserted without preliminary tapping.

**27. Self-tapping screws:** Where the bone cortex is very thin, self-tapping screws get a better grip than tapped screws. (Note also that prior to the development of the AO range of bone screws, self-tapping screws were in universal use for all forms of internal fixation; their main disadvantage was that they could be difficult to insert in dense cortical bone.) With the Sherman screw [9/64″ (3.6 mm) OD] a pilot hole marginally larger than the core diameter [in practice 7/64″ (2.8 mm)] is drilled before insertion of the screw.

**28. Blade plates:** These are most commonly used at either end of the femur when there is insufficient bone on the epiphyseal side of a fracture to allow an ordinary plate to be used. Blade plates come in a variety of angles and forms: the plate portion (1) is screwed to the shaft of the bone after the blade or spline (2) has been inserted into the bone. Cancellous bone screws (3) may be used for interfragmentary compression.

**29. Dynamic hip screw/dynamic condylar screw:** The principle feature of this device is a large diameter cancellous bone screw (1) which can be drawn [with a small screw (2)] into the sleeve (3) of a plate which is screwed to the shaft of the femur (4). In the case of the neck of the femur the soft bone of the head is gripped and the fracture can be compressed; at the distal end of the femur (5) it is of particular value in treating T- or Y-fractures, allowing the articular fragments to be drawn together (a blade plate in such circumstances is harder to insert and less effective).

**30. Intramedullary nails (1):** These are used to treat diaphyseal fractures, particularly of the femur and tibia. In many (but not all) cases the operation can be performed without exposing the fracture. A reduction is obtained using skeletal traction (1) under image intensifier control (2). Through a proximal incision (3) the medullary canal is located (4). Usually a reaming rod (5) is then passed across the fracture and the canal reamed (6) to allow the passage of a close-fitting nail (7) of suitable length and diameter over a guide rod (8).

**31. Intramedullary nails (2):** Interlocking of the fragments, a well-reamed canal and a close-fitting nail may suffice to resist torsional forces which might jeopardise the quality of the fixation. Bone absorption at the fracture site is usually taken up by telescoping (1). If torsional control is poor, an interlocking nail may be used; with this device twisting forces are neutralised by transversely running locking bolts (2) which pass through holes (3) or slots (4) in the intramedullary nail. Where reaming is undesirable (e.g. in certain open fractures) solid IM nails may be used.

**32. Tension band wiring:** This is used most frequently in olecranon and patellar fractures. The surfaces away from the articular side of the fracture (1) are drawn together and pre-loaded with a high tensile wire (2), while muscle pull (3) acting against the fulcrum of the coronoid (or femoral condyle) brings the rest together (4). The wire is twisted to tighten it (5), and Kirschner wires (6) may be used if required to preserve longitudinal alignment.

**33. External fixators:** There are many types to deal with a wide range of bone sizes. *The pins* must be rigid (flat-threaded Schanz pins are popular) and inserted through 'safe' areas to avoid damage to underlying nerves or blood vessels. Single-side (unilateral or cantilever) systems give the best access for dressing open wounds, with bilateral systems being now reserved mainly for arthrodeses. *The skin* must be meticulously cleaned, and sealed round the pins with suitable dressings to reduce the risks of pin-track infection.

## 34. Internal fixation in open fractures:

The use of internal fixation devices in open fractures is a controversial subject, but cases which pose real difficulty for the uncommitted are in practice rather uncommon. The following points should be noted:

1. In children, internal fixation seldom needs to be considered; in most fractures, if angulation and axial rotation are controlled, the remarkable powers of remodelling can usually be relied upon, and an anatomical reduction is only occasionally required.
It is useful to remember, as in the adult, that if the wound is more than technical, advantage should be taken of it to reduce the fracture under vision; a stable reduction is often attainable.

2. In the adult, where a fracture is undisplaced, conservative methods of treatment can generally be followed without difficulty; once skin healing has occurred, any secondary procedure can be carried out with comparative security.

3. Where a fracture is unstable, and is open from within out with minimal tissue contamination (Type I open fractures), internal fixation may be carried out in reasonable safety once the wound has been adequately dealt with. *In the case of the tibia* intramedullary nailing with reaming may be undertaken without especial risk of infection in Type II open fractures of the tibia. In Type III open fractures the use of intramedullary nails is said to carry no greater risks than other methods of treatment, although many would advocate the use of a solid intramedullary nail without reaming, or seek an alternative method of holding the fracture (such as with an external fixator). *In the case of the femur* intramedullary nailing with reaming may be attempted in both Type I and II fractures; but this procedure carries a very high risk of serious infection in Type III injuries, and is contraindicated.

4. Where there has been extensive skin and soft-tissue damage or loss, and the wound has been badly contaminated, as a general rule internal fixation should be avoided; the fracture should be supported by a plaster cast or by an external fixator; in the case of the femur, skeletal traction in a Thomas splint may be used. (Note that if an external fixator has been applied, and there has been a pin-track infection, reamed intramedullary nailing at a later date is contraindicated: the risks of infection are unacceptably high. When an external fixator is employed, it should be retained until the fracture is united, or until a supporting plaster cast can be substituted.)

Difficulty tends to occur in the handling of the unstable fracture where skin cover is perhaps poor and/or the risks of infection are appreciable but not certain. *Against* the use of internal fixation in these circumstances is:

   (i)  the risk of wider dissemination of infection into uncontaminated tissue by the greater exposure required for the insertion of some internal fixation devices

  (ii)  the greater risks of wound breakdown

 (iii)  the greater difficulty in obtaining healing if infection becomes established, because of the presence of the fixation device acting as a foreign body.

*In favour* of internal fixation are the following:

  (i)  the chance of obtaining a good reduction
 (ii)  the possibility of holding that reduction for as long as required
(iii)  the better prospects of securing bone union.

It is also important to note that *in the case of multiple injuries* the prognosis is best when the circumstances allow early rigid fixation of all lower limb long bone fractures. (This is mainly due to the avoidance of respiratory complications by early mobilisation.) The eventual decision rests on the particular circumstances of the case, and the surgeon's individual assessment of the factors discussed.

## 35. Gunshot wounds

The pattern of injury and the treatment required is dependent on the type of missile; the general principle is that of delayed suture and early split skin grafting.

**Low velocity gunshot wounds (e.g. handgun wounds):** Principles of treatment of uncomplicated wounds:

(a) The margins of the entry and exit wounds should be excised.
(b) The track should be thoroughly irrigated with saline or hydrogen peroxide.
(c) A saline-soaked gauze swab should if possible be passed through and through and then removed.
(d) The track should be lightly packed open with vaseline gauze.
(e) The wound should then be covered with saline soaked dressings, dry gauze and wool, secured with crepe bandages.
(f) The wound should then be inspected at about 5 days, and if clean, sutured.

If there is a bullet in the tissues, the need for its removal should be carefully balanced against the risks of exploration. It should be noted that if a bullet remains in a joint, the toxicity of its metallic elements will have a disastrous effect on the articular cartilage. It is strongly advised that the affected joint should be thoroughly irrigated and every attempt made to remove the foreign body.

**Plastic bullets:** These tend to produce localised blunt injuries, and seldom cause fractures; if by any chance there is an accompanying fracture, this can usually be dealt with by normal closed methods of treatment.

**High velocity gunshot wounds:** These are characterised by small entry and large exit wounds. Shock waves may cause extensive tissue destruction and even fracture at a distance from the direct tract of the missile. A temporary wave of negative pressure within the wound may suck in clothing and other debris. If bone is struck, a multifragmentary fracture results.

These injuries must be treated with great respect along the lines of other Type IIIB open fractures. A full exploration with removal of all devitalised tissues is essential, and primary closure is contraindicated. In many cases prophylactic compartmental fasciotomies are advisable. The fracture is often best fixed with an external fixator applied in such a way as to give good access to the wound. (If it is likely that a myocutaneous or other flap will be required, the pins must be positioned so that this is possible, and a preliminary consultation with a plastic surgeon is often helpful.)

**Explosions:** The severity of the injuries is inversely proportional to the distance between the victim and the source; the initial shock wave is followed by a short-lived fireball, but the accompanying blast wave causes most of the damage. Death or traumatic amputation may result; there may also be accompanying respiratory and auditory damage, and falling masonry or flying debris may cause crush or other injuries. The variety of tissue damage knows no limits, and the treatment is dependent on the exact nature of the injuries sustained.

Where there are multiple casualties, Major Incident or Disaster Routines are generally followed where the most important principles include the establishment of good communications so that the size of the emergency and the call-out can be determined, and in the hospital, differentiating between minor cases (which do not require immediate treatment), severely injured cases (where resources should be concentrated), and the dead and dying: this initial triage would normally be carried out by the most experienced surgeon present. In the Belfast explosion experience (unlike certain other disaster situations) site medical teams have been thought to hinder rather than help the smooth running of the Police, Fire and Ambulance services.

Resuscitative procedures as always precede formal investigation of injuries and arrangements for definitive treatment.

# 5. Factors affecting healing; complications; pathological fractures

## 1. Factors affecting the rate of healing of a fracture

**(1) Type of bone:** *(a) Cancellous bone (spongy bone):* Healing in cancellous bone is generally well advanced 6 weeks from the time of the injury, and protection of the fracture can almost invariably be abandoned by that time. This applies to fractures of bones which are composed principally of cancellous tissue, and also to fractures involving the cancellous bone to be found at the ends of long bones. This rule is illustrated in the following examples:

(i) Weight bearing after a fracture of the calcaneus may be permitted after about 6 weeks.

(ii) A patient with a traumatic wedge fracture of a vertebral body may be allowed up after 6 weeks.

(iii) Plaster fixation may be discarded after 5–6 weeks following a Colles fracture.

(iv) Weight may be allowed through the leg 6 weeks after a fracture of the tibial table.

(v) Bed rest for 6 weeks is usually advised for any substantial fracture of the pelvis, etc.

*(b) Cortical bone (Compact bone):* Endosteal callus may take many months to become reasonably well established, and many uncomplicated long bone fractures may take 9–18 weeks to unite. In some cases, however, abundant external bridging callus may allow an earlier return of function. For example (i) the average time to union of a fracture of the tibial shaft treated conservatively is 16 weeks; (ii) fractures of the humeral shaft can often be left unsupported after 10 weeks; (iii) on the other hand, fractures of the metatarsals, metacarpals and phalanges, where external bridging callus is usually substantial, are usually quite firm in 4–5 weeks.

**(2) The patient's age:** In children, union of fractures is rapid. The speed of union decreases as age increases until skeletal maturity is reached. There is then not a great deal of difference in the rate between young adults and the elderly. For example, in a child, union may be expected in a fractured femur a little after the number of weeks equivalent to its numerical age have passed: viz. a fractured femur in a child of 3 years is usually united after 4 weeks: a fractured femur in a child of 8 is usually sound after 9 weeks. In contrast, a fracture of the femoral shaft in an adult may take 3–6 months to unite.

Apart from great rapidity of union it should be noted that children have remarkable powers of remodelling fractures. These powers are excellent as far

1. Supracondylar fracture of humerus with soft tissue between bone ends.

2. Chronic bone infection and failure of union of tibia following plating (plate removed).

as displacement is concerned, and are often good for slight to moderate angulation. Remodelling is poor in the case of axial rotation. The power to remodel decreases rapidly once adolescence is reached and epiphyseal fusion is imminent.

**(3) Mobility at the fracture site:** Excessive mobility persisting at the fracture site (due, for example, to poor fixation) may interfere with vascularisation of the fracture haematoma; it may lead to disruption of early bridging callus and may prevent endosteal new bone growth. One of the main aims of all forms of internal and external splintage is to reduce mobility at the fracture site, and hence encourage union. If splintage is inadequate, union may be delayed or prevented.

**(4) Separation of the bone ends:** Union will be delayed or prevented if the bone ends are separated, for this interferes with the normal mechanisms of healing. Separation may occur under several circumstances:

*(a) Interposition of soft tissue between the bone ends:* For example, in fractures of the femoral shaft, one of the bone ends may become isolated from the other by herniating through some of the surrounding muscle mass, thereby delaying or preventing union. Fractures of the medial malleolus may fail to unite due to infolding of a layer of periosteum between the fragments.

*(b) Excessive traction:* Excessive traction employed in the maintenance of a reduction may lead to separation of the bone ends and non-union. This may occur, for example, in femoral shaft fractures, particularly those treated by skeletal traction.

*(c) Following internal fixation:* In some situations where internal fixation is used to hold a fracture, resorption of bone may occur at the fracture site; the fixation device may continue to hold the bone fragments in such a way that they are prevented from coming together.

**(5) Infection:** Infection in the region of a fracture may delay or prevent union. This is especially the case if, in addition, movement is allowed to occur at the fracture. Infection of the fracture site is extremely rare in conservatively treated closed fractures; infection, if it occurs, follows either an open injury or one treated by internal fixation. Where infection becomes well established in the presence of an internal fixation device, it is often difficult to achieve healing without removal of the device which acts as a foreign body and a nidus for persisting infection. This is especially the case if there is breakdown of the overlying skin and the establishment of a sinus. Not infrequently the situation arises where cast fixation alone is unable to provide the degree of fixation necessary for union if the device is removed, and where infection is likely to remain if it is not. In such circumstances it is usually wiser to retain the fixation device until union is reasonably well advanced, or to consider using an external fixator.

**(6) Disturbance of blood supply:** It is obvious that for the normal multiplication of bone cells and their precursors an adequate blood supply is required. Where the blood supply to an area is reduced, or where there is interference with the blood supply to both major fragments—e.g. in radio necrosis of bone—healing may be interfered with. On the other hand, reduction of the blood supply to one fragment, especially if cancellous bone is involved, may not interfere with union; indeed, in some situations it may apparently stimulate it. The most striking examples of this are fractures of the femoral neck and scaphoid, where the phenomenon of avascular necrosis is most frequently discovered in soundly united fractures. Interference with the blood supply to one fragment at the time of injury leads to immediate bone death; this is frequently followed by sound union of the fracture. Collapse of necrotic bone beyond the level of union is observed at a later date.

**(7) Properties of the bone involved:** Fracture healing is also affected by a number of imperfectly understood factors which lead to variations in the speed of union. The clavicle is a spectacular example; non-union is extremely rare, the time to clinical union is unexcelled by any other part of the skeleton, yet movement at the fracture site cannot be controlled with any efficiency. Union of the tibia is often slow to a degree that is difficult to explain even when the influence of its nutrient artery and fracture mobility are taken into account.

**(8) Joint involvement:** When a fracture involves a joint, union is occasionally delayed. This may be due to dilution of the fracture haematoma by synovial fluid.

**(9) Bone pathology:** Many of the commonest causes of pathological fracture do not seem to delay union in a material way. (Union may progress quite normally in, for example, osteoporosis, osteomalacia, Paget's disease and most simple bone tumours.) Some primary and secondary malignant bone tumours may delay or prevent union (see pp. 91–94).

### 2. The complications of fractures

Complications which may occur in a patient who has suffered a fracture or dislocation may be grouped in the following way:

**(1) The complications of any tissue damage:** These include (a) internal and external haemorrhage, oligaemic shock, etc., (b) infection (in compound injuries), (c) electrolyte shifts, protein breakdown and other metabolic responses of trauma.

**(2) The complications of prolonged recumbency:** These include (a) hypostatic pneumonia, (b) pressure sores, (c) deep venous thrombosis, (d) muscle wasting, (e) skeletal decalcification and formation of urinary tract calculi, (f) urinary tract infections, etc.

**(3) The complications of anaesthesia and surgery:** These include (a) atelectasis and pneumonia, (b) blood loss leading to anaemia or shock with their secondary effects, (c) wound infection, mechanical failure of internal fixation devices, etc.

**(4) The complications peculiar to fractures:** These include (a) disorders involving the rate and quality of union, (b) joint stiffness, (c) Sudeck's atrophy, (d) avascular necrosis, (e) myositis ossificans, (f) infections, (g) neurological, vascular and visceral complications, (h) implant complications

The last group will be considered in more detail.

**(1) Slow union:** In slow union, the fracture takes longer than usual to unite, but passes through the stages of healing without any departure from normal clinically or radiologically.

3.  Hypertrophic non-union of the ulna.

4.  Atrophic non-union of the humerus.

**(2)  Delayed union:** In delayed union, union fails to occur within the expected time. As distinct from slow union, radiographs of the part may show abnormal bone changes. Typically there is absorption of bone at the level of the fracture, with the production of a gap between the bone ends. External bridging callus may be restricted to a localised area and be of poor quality. There is, however, no sclerosis of the bone ends.

**(3)  Non-union:** In non-union, the fracture has failed to unite, and there are radiological changes which indicate that this situation will be permanent— i.e. the fracture will never unite—unless there is some fundamental alteration in the line of treatment. Two types of non-union are recognised:

*(a)  In hypertrophic non-union* the bone ends appear sclerotic, and are flared out so that the diameter of the bone fragments at the level of the fracture is increased ('elephant's foot' appearance). The fracture line is clearly visible, the gap being filled with cartilage and fibrous tissue cells. The increase in bone density is somewhat misleading, and conceals the fact that the blood supply is good.

*(b)  In atrophic non-union* there is no evidence of cellular activity at the level of the fracture. The bone ends are narrow, rounded and osteoporotic; they are frequently avascular.

**Treatment:** *(a)  Slow union:* Assuming that the fracture is adequately supported, patience should ultimately be rewarded with sound bony union.

*(b)  Delayed union:* The difficult problem in this field is to differentiate between delayed union, which is going to proceed with proper encouragement to union, and delayed union, which is going to go on to non-union. The only sure arbiter is time, but the disadvantage of delay is that it tends to encourage irreversible stiffness in those joints which are immobilised with the fracture (besides frequently creating problems from prolonged hospitalisation and absence from work).

If union has not occurred within the time normally required (or certainly if the fracture is ununited by 4 months) or if gross mobility is still present at 2 months there should be a careful appraisal of the radiographs and the methods of fixation. As the commonest cause of delayed union is inadequate fixation, particular attention should be paid to this aspect of the case. If the radiographs show the changes of slow or delayed union, but none of the changes of non-union, and the fracture is well supported, immobilisation should be continued and the situation re-assessed, with further radiographs, in 4–6 weeks. Improvement in the radiological appearance will then be an encouraging sign, suggesting that persistence in the established line of treatment will lead to union. If there is no change, or if there is deterioration, this is an indication for more active treatment (e.g. rigid internal fixation).

*(c)  Hypertrophic non-union:* If the fracture can be fixed with absolute rigidity by mechanical means (which substitute for the primary bridging callus which is wanting) the cartilaginous and fibrous tissue between the bone ends will mineralise and be converted to bone (by induction). In the femur, this may be accomplished by careful reaming of the medullary canal and the introduction of a stout, large-diameter intramedullary nail. The bone ends are not disturbed. In the tibia and the other long bones, rigid fixation may usually be obtained by compression plating.

There is some evidence that the process of induction which results in the

5. Mal-union of tibia with potential stressing of ankle joint.

6. Mal-union of femur leading to shortening.

conversion of the tissue at the fracture into bone may also be stimulated by the creation of small electric currents in the gap between the bone ends. This may be achieved by embedding percutaneous electrodes in the fracture gap, or by placing field coils round the limb. Treatment by this method is lengthy (extending over several months) but can often be administered on an out-patient basis and is particularly indicated where it is desirable to avoid surgery (e.g. in the presence of continued infection).

*(d) Atrophic non-union:* Treatment for atrophic non-union is less easy or reliable, and involves four important aspects:

(i)     The fracture must be held rigidly; this usually implies internal fixation (e.g. the use of a large-diameter intramedullary nail or a rigid compression plate).

(ii)    Fibrous tissue should be removed from between the bone ends which should be 'freshened' by a limited local trimming with an osteotome.

(iii)   The bone ends should be decorticated from the level of the fracture back to healthy bone; fine interrupted cuts are made in the outer surface of the bone cortex until it has a feathered or shingled appearance.

(iv)   The area round the fracture is packed circumferentially with cancellous bone grafts.

**(4) Mal-union:** In theory the term mal-union could be applied to any fracture which has united in less than anatomical position. In practice, it is used in the following circumstances:

(a) Where a fracture has united in a position of persistent angulation or rotation which is of a degree that gives the limb a displeasing appearance or affects its function. For example, mal-union in a Colles fracture may lead to undue prominence of the distal ulna. The cosmetic effect may cause the patient some distress, although functionally the result may be good. Again, persistent angulation in a fracture of the femur may not be particularly conspicuous, but will lead to impairment of function in the limb as a result of shortening and the effects of abnormal stresses on the knee and hip (leading possibly ultimately to secondary osteoarthritis in these joints).

(b) Where a fracture has united with a little persistent deformity in a situation where even the slightest displacement or angulation is a potential source of trouble. This applied particularly to fractures involving joints. For example, slight persistent deformity in a fracture of the ankle may predispose to early secondary osteoarthritis.

*Treatment:* In treating fractures, one of the main objectives is adequate reduction and avoidance of mal-union. Regrettably, mal-union is sometimes a sign of poor management.

If detected before union has become complete, angulation may sometimes be corrected by wedging of a plaster (see p. 309) or forcible manipulation under anaesthesia—i.e. manipulation which refractures the limb through the early callus. If union is already complete, an osteotomy may be considered if the deformity is particularly severe.

**(5) Shortening:** This is generally a sequel of mal-union. It occurs in transverse fractures which are off-ended, and often in spiral or oblique fractures which are displaced. It also results from marked angulation of a fracture.

In children, bone growth is always accelerated in the injured limb, presumably as a result of the epiphyses being stimulated by the increased blood supply. Any discrepancy in limb length is usually quickly made up. For example, a fracture of the femoral shaft in a child may heal with the fragments overlapping and with perhaps 3–4 cm of shortening. After a year, the leg lengths may be equal—or the injured leg may even be a little longer than the other.

In adults, shortening in the lower limb is seen most frequently after fractures of the tibial shaft. It is also seen after fractures of the shaft of the femur, and of the femoral neck where there is persistent coxa vara.

Shortening of 1.5 cm is easily tolerated, being compensated for by tilting of the pelvis. Shortening in excess of this should be dealt with by alteration of the footwear: for example, 3.5 cm of shortening may be corrected by a 2 cm raise to the affected heel, some of which can be given by a cork lift within the shoe. Where shortening is due to severe, persistent angulation of a fracture, a corrective osteotomy may be indicated not only to correct the shortening but also to reduce abnormal stresses on the related joints.

In the upper limb, shortening seldom causes any problem other than to the patient's tailor. (Note, however, that shortening of either the radius or the ulna, while leading to little overall shortening, may cause severe disability at the wrist or elbow.)

**(6)  Traumatic epiphyseal arrest:** The epiphyseal plate may be damaged as a result of trauma. If the whole width of the plate is affected, then growth may be arrested at that level, leading to progressive shortening of the limb. The final discrepancy in limb lengths is dependent on the epiphysis affected and the child's age at the time of injury; obviously the younger the child, the greater are the potential growth and potential shortening.

More commonly the epiphyseal plate is incompletely affected so that growth continues more or less normally at one side while at the other it may be severely retarded or arrested. This irregularity of growth leads to some shortening of the limb and to distortion of the associated joint which can only be partly corrected by remodelling. In practice there may be progressive tilting of the axis of movement of the joint. For example, a supracondylar fracture may be followed by a cubitus varus deformity as a result of a degree of mal-union. This deformity may become more severe as (uneven) growth continues. Traumatic epiphyseal arrest also occurs after compound injuries, where the delicate epiphyseal plate is damaged, especially by friction. This is seen in road traffic accidents when a child is dragged along by a vehicle, sustaining skin loss and progressive abrasion of the deeper tissues by friction against the road surface.

In all cases of suspected epiphyseal damage a careful follow-up is necessary. The child should be seen every 6–12 months, and any residual deformity carefully assessed by clinical and radiological measurement. In the upper limb, if the deformity is progressive it may produce an unsightly appearance and may be responsible for delayed neurological involvement. In the lower limb, abnormal stresses may be produced in the weight bearing joints, ultimately giving rise to pain, stiffness, instability and often a rapidly progressive secondary osteoarthritis.

*Treatment:* It is sometimes possible to treat this problem with an epiphyseolysis. In this procedure the abnormal block of bone bridging the

7. Traumatic epiphseal arrest of radius leading to its shortening.

8. Mal-union of acetabular fracture causing joint stiffness and secondary osteo-arthritis.

9. Mal-union of fracture–dislocation of elbow (Monteggia) leading to loss of pronation and supination.

epiphyseal plate is excised, and the defect plugged with fat or bone wax to prevent recurrence. In late cases, a corrective osteotomy may be indicated.

**(7) Joint stiffness:** This is a common complication. It must be borne in mind at every stage of fracture treatment in order that its effects may be minimised. Stiffness may result from a combination of factors which include pathology (a) within the joint, (b) close to the joint, (c) remote from the joint.

*Intra-articular causes of stiffness:* (a) Intra-articular adhesions: fibrous adhesions may form within a joint as a result of (i) organisation of a haemarthrosis or fracture haematoma produced, for example, when a fracture runs into a joint, (ii) damage to the articulating (cartilaginous) surfaces with subsequent organisation within the joint, (iii) prolonged immobilisation leading to degenerative changes in articular cartilage.

(b) Mechanical restrictions: (i) the fracture may disrupt the joint to such an extent that there is mechanical restriction of movement—e.g. bony fragments may block part of the range of movements in a joint. (ii) Movements may be restricted by the formation of loose bodies.

(c) Osteo-arthritis (osteo-arthrosis): joint movements may be restricted as a result of (secondary) osteo-arthritis. This may be caused by (i) irregularity of the joint surfaces (caused, for example, by displacement of a fracture which runs into a joint; it may also follow damage to sub-chondral bone, which may not show on routine radiographs but be detectable by MRI scans), (ii) avascular necrosis (produced as result of damage to the blood supply of an intra-articular fragment of bone), (iii) mal-union of a fracture (leading to abnormal stresses on the joint from persistent angulation).

*Peri-articular causes of stiffness:* (a) Joint capsules and musculo-tendinous cuffs may become functionally impaired, leading to joint stiffness. There are many causes which include (i) fibrosis resulting from direct injury, passive stretching or disuse, (ii) oedema, often encouraged by dependency, disuse, or Sudeck's atrophy.

(b) Persistent displacement of a fracture lying close to a joint may lead to a mechanical block to movement.

(c) Persistent angulation of a fracture lying close to a joint may lead to loss of part of a range of movements (sometimes with a corresponding gain elsewhere). For example, persisting anterior angulation in a Colles fracture will result in loss of some palmar flexion. There is sometimes a corresponding gain in dorsiflexion.

(d) In a fracture lying close to a joint, movement may be restricted by adhesions forming between the fracture and overlying muscle or tendon. This leads to tethering of these structures with inevitable restriction of movements. As a general rule, the closer a fracture is to a joint, the greater the danger or movements being restricted in this way. Restriction of movements by tendon tethering is a particular problem in phalangeal fractures.

(e) Myositis ossificans, if present, will act as a mechanical block to movement.

*Stiffness from causes remote from a joint:* (a) Stiffness may result from tethering or entrapment of muscle by adhesions forming between a fracture and overlying muscle. This is commonly seen in fractures of the femoral shaft where the quadriceps muscle may become tethered to the bone, and may sometimes be aggravated by surgery, where exposure of the fracture requires further muscle division. This effect may be minimised by early mobilisation.

(b) Muscle ischaemia, followed by replacement fibrosis and contractures, may occur when there is a vascular injury accompanying the fracture. Deformity of the distal parts is common, and there may be restriction of passive as well as active movements (e.g. Volkmann's ischaemic contracture of the forearm or calf leading to restriction of movements in the hand and foot, respectively).

*Avoidance of stiffness:* Some of the basic principles in the avoidance of joint stiffness are as follows:

a. Accurate reduction of the fracture wherever possible.
b. Splintage of the minimal number of joints compatible with security.
c. Splintage of the fracture for the shortest time compatible with the relief of pain and fracture healing.
d. Urgent mobilisation of all unsplinted joints in the limb; e.g. a patient with a Colles fracture should practise finger, elbow and shoulder movements from the day of injury.
e. Elevation of the injured part during the initial stages to decrease joint oedema.
f. Where applicable, supporting the joints in such a position that restoration of movement on discarding splintage will be encouraged.
g. Where a fracture involves articular surfaces, early movement becomes particularly important if an adequate range is to be regained.
h. Where stiffness is present or anticipated, physiotherapy and where appropriate, occupational therapy should be started as early as possible.
i. Anticipate complications and avoid procrastination, especially with regard to non-union.
j. When internal fixation is being contemplated, there is some merit in selecting techniques and devices which will support the fracture to such an extent that the limb may be exercised without external support.

**(8) Sudeck's atrophy (post-traumatic osteo-dystrophy):** The condition is essentially one of chronic post-traumatic pain with associated autonomic changes. (Causalgia, whose effects follow a peripheral nerve injury, is considered to be a related condition.) This fracture complication is seen most frequently after Colles fractures of the wrist. In most cases it is not recognised until removal of the plaster at the end of the normal 4–6 weeks' period of immobilisation. There is swelling of the hand and fingers, and the skin is warm, pink and glazed in appearance. There is striking restriction of movements in the fingers, and diffuse tenderness over the wrist and carpus. This tenderness may at first suggest that the fracture is ununited, but check radiographs will show that this is not the case. Typically the radiographs demonstrate union of the fracture, with diffuse, osteoporotic mottling of the carpus. Although seen most frequently after Colles fractures, Sudeck's atrophy may follow scaphoid fractures or indeed any injury about the wrist. The condition is also seen in the lower limb, the foot being similarly affected after, for example, an ankle fracture. About the knee, the effects can be particularly severe.

The causal mechanisms of the condition, where there is an unusual sympathetic response to trauma, are uncertain. It may follow the use of

10. Sudeck's atrophy: note the patchy decalcification.

11. Avascular necrosis of the proximal pole of the scaphoid.

splintage which is too tight or too slack; it may occur in association with prolonged elevation of pressure within the muscle compartments of a limb; it may appear when the affected part has had a prolonged period of dependence. It is usually self-limiting, the abnormalities of circulation and decalcification resolving slowly over a period of 4–12 months. Nevertheless, restriction of movements may be permanent; to minimise this, intensive physiotherapy is usually prescribed and continued to resolution. In the more severe cases additional treatment may be advised.

*Diagnosis:* The diagnosis is not often in doubt, but a number of tests are considered to be of value for confirmation, especially if aggressive forms of treatment are being contemplated; these include (i) 3-phase radionuclide scintigraphy (which may show asymmetrical blood flow and increased periarticular uptake; this seems to be of greatest value in the early stages of the disease), (ii) thermography, (iii) the measurement of vasomotor and sudomotor responses, and (iv) synovial biopsy (which may show non-specific subsynovial fibrosis with synovial proliferation).

It is considered, however, that relief of symptoms and signs by sympathetic blockade is of the greatest diagnostic value. Regional sympathetic blockade should produce relief of pain; in the upper limb the stellate ganglion may be injected, and in the lower limb, the lumbar sympathetic chain. Alternatively, a regional perfusion technique may be employed. To do this, a cannula is inserted in a superficial vein and a tourniquet is applied to the limb. The limb is exsanguinated with an Esmarch bandage before the cuff is inflated to 250 mmHg. 20 mg of guanethidine sulphate in a 40 ml solution is then injected, and the tourniquet released after 20 minutes. Relief of pain and an improvement in the clinical signs for 1–4 days after the perfusion is regarded as being diagnostic, even although it is recognised that peripheral vasodilatation is the main effect of guanethedine.

*Additional treatment.* Regional perfusion with guanethidine may be repeated, with or without the use of oral sympatholytic drugs (such as prazocin or phenoxybenzamine); nifedipine is also sometimes tried, and good results have been claimed following the empirical use of prednisolone. Only rarely are surgical or chemical sympathectomy advised.

In the case of Sudeck's atrophy affecting the knee, a particularly aggressive approach is advocated which it is said may often lead to rapid and complete resolution. After confirmation of the diagnosis as described above, an epidural blockade is maintained for 4 days, during which time the limb is mobilised vigorously by measures which include continuous passive motion, alternating hot and cold soaks, muscle stimulation and manipulation.

**(9) Avascular necrosis:** Avascular necrosis is death of bone due to interference with its blood supply. It is an important and serious complication of certain fractures.

There is no doubt that in many comminuted fractures fragments of bone are often completely detached from their surrounding tissues and deprived of their blood supply. If the fragments are small, healing is usually uneventful. If the fragments are larger, healing may be delayed, but it is often difficult to attribute the relative effects of avascularity and the poorer immobilisation associated with comminution. It is not, however, with the shafts of long bones that this complication is most closely associated. Avascular necrosis is seen in the femoral head after some intracapsular fractures of the femoral neck or after dislocation of the hip. It is found in the scaphoid after certain fractures of the proximal half of that bone. It sometimes occurs in the talus after fractures or dislocations. In the lunate it may follow frank dislocations or apparently occur without any obvious previous trauma.

The importance of avascular necrosis is that the affected bone becomes soft and distorted in shape, leading to pain, stiffness, and secondary osteo-arthritis. The following points are of some importance:

(a) Interference with the blood supply to the bone is a direct result of the fracture: the fracture shears those blood vessels which are travelling within the bone towards its articular surface.

(b) As the fracture is responsible for the disruption of the blood supply, it follows that the disruption is attributable to the injury, and dates from the time of injury.

(c) Restoration of the microcirculation within the bone cannot be effected by treatment.

(d) The greater the displacement of the fracture, the greater is the vessel disturbance and the greater the chance of this complication ensuing.

(e) When an injury has occurred at one of the high-risk sites, the chances are that any patent circulatory channels are highly vulnerable. Reduction should be carried out with minimal force and delay if there is to be any hope of avoiding this complication.

(f) Avascular necrosis is quite distinct from non-union. In the majority of femoral neck and scaphoid fractures with avascular necrosis, *the fracture has united*.

(g) Clear-cut radiological evidence of this complication may be quite slow in appearing, especially in the case of the femoral head. Symptoms of pain and stiffness usually *precede* the radiological changes. In the case of femoral neck fractures it is common practice to look for avascular necrosis for up to 3 years after the injury.

*Treatment:* The natural course of avascular necrosis is for the slow revascularisation of necrotic bone from the periphery. This process takes 6–18 months, but in spite of it secondary osteo-arthritic changes in the affected joints are inevitable. In the lower limb, deformity of the avascular bone may be minimised by the avoidance of weight bearing, and this is of some value at least in the case of the talus; otherwise treatment has little influence on the condition.

If symptoms are commanding and secondary osteo-arthritis is well established, surgery may be required (e.g. hip replacement in the case of femoral neck fractures—see under appropriate sections).

**(10) Myositis ossificans:** Myositis ossificans is a complication of trauma. In its commonest form, a calcified mass appears in the tissues near a joint, leading generally to considerable restriction of movements because of its mechanical effects.

The commonest site is the elbow. It may, for example, develop some weeks after a supracondylar fracture, especially where there has been difficulty in reduction and manipulation has been repeated. Myositis ossificans is also found in the elbow after dislocations or fractures of the radial head. It is thought that these injuries result in haematoma formation in the brachialis

12. Myositis ossificans at the elbow.

muscle at the front of the joint, and that this is dealt with by the tissues in the same way as a fracture haematoma—i.e. by calcification and ossification.

The ensuing mass may be as large as a plum, and will greatly restrict flexion of the elbow. It is known that myositis ossificans can follow passive stretching of joints and in the past it was frequently seen in cases where, in good faith, this treatment had been carried out to encourage movement after injury. The risks of this complication are so great, however, that passive stretching must never be practised round the elbow.

Myositis ossificans is also seen at other sites, especially the shoulder, hip and knee. It is found particularly frequently in patients suffering from head injuries or paraplegia. In some cases, especially where there is limb spasticity, routine passive joint movements may be a causal factor.

*Treatment:* Early excision of the mass gives bad results, being almost always followed by massive recurrence. Late excision (say after 6–12 months) is often successful in removing the mechanical obstruction to movement with less risk of recurrence.

**(11)  Osteitis:** Infection in closed fractures (due to systemic spread of organisms) is rare and seldom diagnosed until infection is well established. It is sometimes seen in patients suffering from rheumatoid arthritis who have been treated with anti-inflammatory preparations. Recurrent pyrexia, a raised sedimentation rate and white count, and unduly prolonged pain, local tenderness and swelling should arouse suspicion. Radiological changes may not be diagnostic and are slow in appearing.

Bone infection is a feared complication of open fractures, and is also seen on occasion after the internal fixation of closed fractures. The symptoms and signs are as detailed above. In addition, there will usually be a purulent wound discharge with staining of the plaster or dressings which become foul smelling.

*Treatment:* (a) The risk of this complication should always be kept in mind in the handling of compound injuries or when internal fixation is planned, so that the techniques practised may be above criticism.

(b)  Once firmly established, bone infections are peculiarly resistant to treatment, and may become virtually incurable. Delay must therefore be avoided at all costs.

(c)  If possible, a sample of pus should be obtained so that the bacteriology and antibiotic sensitivity may be firmly established. The appropriate antibiotic must then be administered in adequate dose for an adequate time (usually 4 weeks as a minimum). If a choice is available, preference should be given to an antibiotic which may achieve high concentration levels in bone. In patients being treated in plaster casts, access to the wound may be obtained by windowing of the plaster.

(d)  Unless discovered early, drainage should be established, and regular dressings performed with aseptic precautions in an attempt to allow healing by granulation tissue.

(e)  Although discharge from the wound may persist until any internal fixation device is removed, this should be delayed until fracture healing is well advanced.

(f)  When infection is well established and unresponsive, more radical measures may be called for. These include:

(i) Saucerisation of the area, with radical excision of all infected bone and open packing of the wound.

(ii) Raising the local concentrate of antibiotics by the implantation of irrigation tubes or acrylic beads impregnated with gentamycin or other antibiotics.

(iii) Rarely, amputation may have to be considered where there is profound toxaemia with deterioration of the patient's general condition, uninfluenced by treatment or where there is widespread bone destruction or avascularity, poor control of the infection, and certain continued infection and non-union.

**(12)  Acute arterial arrest:** The arterial blood flow distal to a fracture is occasionally interrupted, and assessment of the circulation in a fractured limb is an essential part of the examination. Arterial arrest results in loss of the distal pulses, pallor and coldness of the skin, loss of the capillary responses, severe pain in the limb, paraesthesiae and eventually muscle paralysis. The commonest cause is kinking of the main arterial trunks by the displacement of a fracture or dislocation. In these cases, the circulation is immediately restored by correction of the deformity, and this should always be carried out as expeditiously as possible. In closed fractures other arterial disturbances are found, but these are relatively uncommon. A ragged bone edge may cause arterial rupture, leading to the rapid formation of a large haematoma. A fracture may also give rise to profound arterial spasm, aneurysm, or intimal stripping. In open fractures, arterial rupture often declares itself by the nature and the extent of the accompanying haemorrhage.

*Diagnosis:* If the pulses distal to the injury site cannot be palpated, the patient should be resuscitated and reassessed within an hour. The most reliable guide to the situation is the Doppler pressure. To take this, a sphygomanometer cuff should be positioned above the injury site and the Doppler signal located. The cuff is then inflated; the pressure at which the signal disappears is the Doppler pressure. Repeat the examination on the good side.

If the pressures are not equal, the advice of a vascular surgeon should be sought *immediately*. If no Doppler equipment is available, then advice should be sought, again without delay, should the peripheral pulses on the injured side be reduced or absent.

*Treatment:* It is obvious that the survival of a useful limb is dependent on restoration of the circulation. Where this is not achieved by reduction of the fracture, exploration of the affected vessel is mandatory. Treatment is then dependent on the findings. If the artery is cleanly divided, an end-to-end anastomosis may be performed. In the presence of a deficit, an in-line reversed vein graft is often used. In either case, to prevent damage to the suture line, internal fixation of the fracture is an essential part of the procedure and is often performed first.

Most of those cases which appear to be due to arterial spasm are in fact associated with intimal damage. Opening of the vessel is necessary to elucidate this, although preliminary irrigation with papaverine is sometimes tried. If intimal damage is confirmed, resection of the affected segment with grafting may be required.

Arterial obstruction leading to muscle death and nerve palsy may also result from swelling within the muscle compartments of a limb. For example in the anterior compartment of the leg haemorrhage, or oedema of muscles following trauma or overactivity, may lead to an inexorable rise of pressure beyond the systolic blood pressure. This will result in muscle necrosis, loss of conduction in the deep peroneal nerve, sensory disturbance in the foot and foot drop. Prompt splitting of the roof of the affected compartment may avert this complication.

**(13) Immediate neurological disturbance:** Neurological complications occurring immediately after fractures and dislocations are comparatively uncommon. Nevertheless, in certain situations a nerve may be stretched over a bone edge in a displaced fracture, or over a bone end in a dislocation. If prolonged this will lead to local ischaemia and interruption of nerve conduction. If stretching is more severe there may be rupture of axons or of neural tubes: actual nerve division is rare, being seen mainly in association with compound injuries (especially gunshot wounds). The commoner fractures and dislocations associated with nerve palsies include the following:

| | |
|---|---|
| Dislocation of the shoulder | Axillary nerve palsy: rarely other brachial plexus lesions |
| Fracture of the shaft of the humerus | Radial nerve palsy |
| Dislocation of the elbow | Ulnar nerve palsy; sometimes median nerve affected |
| Fractures round the elbow | Median nerve palsy; less commonly, ulnar nerve, or posterior interosseous nerve |
| Dislocation of the hip | Sciatic nerve palsy |
| Dislocation of the knee or rupture of lateral ligament of the knee and fracture of medial tibial table | Common peroneal nerve palsy |

*Treatment:* The majority of nerve lesions are in continuity. Assuming that the fracture or dislocation has been reduced, recovery often begins after 6 weeks, progressing quite rapidly thereafter. *The skin* must be protected during the recovery period against friction, burns and other trauma so long as sensation remains materially impaired. *The joints* should be exercised passively to avoid stiffness. *Deformity* due to overactivity of unaffected muscles should be prevented: this applies particularly to the drop wrist of radial palsy, and the drop foot where the sciatic or common peroneal nerves are involved. Lively splintage may be particularly helpful in these circumstances.

Where there is a nerve palsy accompanying a fracture which is going to be treated surgically, opportunity may be taken to inspect the affected nerve. This will often help in establishing a prognosis, and may also permit definitive treatment of the injury (e.g. by removing any local pressure on the nerve).

When an expected recovery does not occur, electromyography and nerve conduction studies may be of occasional diagnostic value, but exploration is often required.

In the case of nerve injury complicating a fresh injury, primary suture should be undertaken if the risks of infection are judged to be slight and facilities are good. Otherwise the nerve ends should be approximated with radio-opaque sutures or markers, and elective repair delayed until sound wound healing has been obtained. If nerve repair is not possible, reconstructive surgery or orthotic support of the paralysed part may be required.

**(14) Delayed neurological disturbance:** Sometimes a nerve palsy gradually develops long after a fracture has healed.

*(a) Tardy ulnar nerve palsy* is the most striking example of this process. In a typical case the patient gradually develops over a period of a few months an ulnar nerve palsy which may become complete. The injury responsible is usually a supracondylar fracture or a Monteggia fracture–dislocation. The striking feature is the interval between the fracture and the nerve palsy. It is usually in the order of several years, and indeed may be as much as 60.

In a number of these cases there is a cubitus valgus deformity, and the resultant stretching of the nerve is usually regarded as being responsible for the onset of the palsy. Nevertheless, tardy ulnar nerve palsy also occurs in the presence of cubitus varus, so that progressive ischaemia of the nerve has come to be considered as another possible factor.

**Treatment:** Tardy ulnar nerve palsy is usually treated by early transposition of the ulnar nerve. (The nerve is mobilised from its exposed position behind the medial epicondyle, brought round to the front of the elbow and buried in the flexor muscles of the forearm just beyond their point of origin.)

*(b) Median nerve palsy:* Signs of median nerve compression may gradually develop a few months after a Colles fracture of the wrist. This is generally akin to the partial nerve lesions seen in the carpal tunnel syndrome. Some residual displacement of the fracture may reduce the space available in the carpal tunnel leading to pressure on the nerve and an incomplete palsy.

*Treatment:* Symptoms are usually relieved by carpal tunnel decompression (by dividing the flexor retinaculum).

**(15) Delayed tendon rupture:** This uncommon fracture complication is seen most frequently at the wrist where, after a Colles fracture, a patient loses the ability to extend the terminal joint of the thumb. This is due to rupture of the extensor pollicis longus tendon some weeks or months after the fracture. The rupture may result from the gradual fraying of the tendon as it rubs against the healing fracture, or it may be caused by traumatic or fibrotic interference with its arterial blood supply, resulting in local sloughing of the tendon.

*Treatment:* In the case of the thumb, the best results are obtained by transposition and suture of the tendon of extensor indicis to the distal segment of extensor pollicis longus (but see 177, 45).

**(16) Visceral complications:** (i) Rupture of the urethra or bladder and perforation of the rectal wall may complicate fractures of the pelvis.

(ii) Rupture of the spleen, kidney or liver may follow severe local trauma, abdominal compression or crushing (such as, for example, run-over injuries).

(iii) Rupture of the intestines or tearing of the mesenteric attachments may also follow abdominal compression.

(iv) *Paralytic ileus*: Paralytic ileus is occasionally seen following fractures of the pelvis and lumbar spine, the most likely cause being disturbance of the autonomic control of the bowel from retroperitoneal haematoma. Distension of the abdomen, absent or faintly tympanitic bowel sounds and vomiting are the usual features. It is, of course, imperative to exclude the possibility of perforation, especially when there is a history of a run-over injury. The diagnosis may be made on the basis of the history and clinical findings, but plain radiographs of the abdomen, abdominal paracentesis, laparoscopy or laparotomy may be necessary where there is a history of direct injury.

13. Paralytic ileus secondary to pelvic fracture: note the air distension of bowel loops in plain abdominal film.

*Treatment:* (a) Nasogastric suction. (b) Intravenous fluids—the quantity and proportions being determined by the amount of aspirate and other losses, and serum electrolyte estimations. In the majority of cases, bowel sounds return within 36 hours, and intravenous fluids and suction may be discontinued shortly afterwards.

*(v) The cast syndrome:* Abdominal distension and vomiting sometimes occur in patients being treated in plaster jackets, hip spicas, or plaster beds, especially if the spine is hyperextended. When the onset is extremely rapid leading to shock and prostration, the superior mesenteric artery or cast syndrome may be suspected (i.e. there is a high intestinal obstruction due to duodenal compression by the superior mesenteric artery).

*Treatment:* (a) If a plaster jacket has been applied, it should be removed. A patient being nursed in a plaster bed should be transferred to an ordinary bed or a Stryker frame. (b) A large-bore gastric tube should be passed. (c) Fluid replacement therapy may be required.

**(17) Fat embolism:** This complication is usually thought to be due to microparticles of marrow fat escaping into the circulation from the region of the fracture. The pathology is by no means clear cut, and disturbance of lipid metabolism may account for certain features of the condition.

It occurs most frequently after fractures of the femoral shaft and pelvis. Excessive mobility at the fracture site may be a contributory factor. There is commonly an unexplained deterioration in the condition of a patient a few days after sustaining such an injury. There may be a slight pyrexia, petechial haemorrhages appear in the skin, the patient may become confused, aggressive or comatose and there may be evidence of renal insufficiency. Radiographs of the chest often show mottling of the lung fields; these changes are generally considered to be due to fat embolisation of the lungs. The systemic effects on the brain, kidneys and skin are less easy to explain unless cardiac septal defects are more common than supposed.

*Prevention:* The risks of this complication are reduced when (i) fluid replacement during and after surgery is impeccable; (ii) when in cases of multiple injury any femoral fracture is rigidly fixed: in practice this generally implies intramedullary nailing.

*Treatment:* (i) Carry out all routine measures such as the administration of oxygen and intravenous fluids. If indicated by the blood gas levels, proceed to endotracheal intubation; (ii) if there is progressive deterioration in blood gas levels, surgical stabilisation of any femoral fracture is advocated. After such a procedure the patient should be left on a ventilator for not less than 24 hours; this may be discontinued when the blood gases improve, and there is an improvement in the tidal volume and the patient's level of consciousness.

**(18) Osteo-arthritis:** See under causes of joint stiffness (p. 81).

**(19) Implant complications:** *Mechanical effects:* Plates and intramedullary nails reduce the natural elasticity of the bone in the area that they lie. As a result, the loads to which a bone is subjected are not absorbed evenly throughout its length; stress concentrations tend to occur at the ends of internal fixation devices. In some cases this may lead to susceptibility to fracture which may occur with less violence than is needed in a normal bone. It is well known that after a plated fracture of the tibia has united, comparatively minor violence may result in a further fracture of the limb at either end of the plate. Similarly, after a minor fall on the side, the forces which would be absorbed by a normal femur may result in a fracture of the femoral neck in someone who has had an intramedullary nailing.

*Corrosion:* No metal implant is completely inert, and the long-term risks of retention of implants within the body have not been fully evaluated. It is not uncommon for the tissues surrounding a stainless steel implant to become discoloured, with the formation of substantial masses of fibrous tissue. This is especially likely to occur if there has been fretting between components (e.g. between a plate and screw). This may be associated with local aching pain, and is an indication for removal of the device, assuming the fracture is soundly healed.

The individual elements in the alloy that has been used for the fabrication of the implant may separate, giving rise to local toxic effects, and having the potential, once they enter the transport systems, of causing problems elsewhere. Stainless steel contains in the order of 13% chromium, and this element is well known for its local irritant effect and its potential for inducing sensitisation. Neoplasia has been reported in bone as the site of plates, and the implants have been considered as being responsible. It is possible that freed metal elements after transportation may be capable of causing neoplasia in the liver and elsewhere. Aluminium is used in certain other alloys used for implants; this is neurotoxic, competing with magnesium in the formation of tubulin, a primary structural protein in the nervous system: this mechanism has been linked with Alzheimer's disease.

*Treatment:* While it must be stressed that problems of the above nature are rare, the risks of any long-term effects should be avoided where possible by routine removal of implants once they have served their purpose; this is the general advice in patients under the age of 40. Over that age the indications are less powerful, but as a general rule intramedullary nails should be removed, as should any other device where there is evidence of local tissue reaction.

### 3. Pathological fractures

A pathological fracture is one which has occurred in a bone which is abnormal or diseased.

In some cases the pathological process leads to progressive weakness of the bone so that fracture may occur spontaneously or after slight injury only. Fracture may occur as an inevitable event in some disease process—e.g. a fracture in course of a destructive, chronic osteitis: always unwelcome, but causing no surprise. On the other hand, the disease process may be unknown to the patient and his practitioner, the trivial nature of the trauma giving concern to both.

Where bone strength is not materially impaired, the causal violence producing the fracture may not cause comment; in these circumstances the radiographs taken after the incident may give the first indication to anyone that something else is amiss. It follows that virtually any condition capable of being detected by radiographs of the skeleton may fall into this category—a limitless range of congenital, metabolic and neoplastic disease. Diagnosis as a result may be difficult, but fortunately there is one important point to take into consideration: where fracture is the presenting feature, the number of conditions commonly responsible is small. These include the following:

14. **Osteoporosis:** This is the commonest cause of pathological fracture, being especially important in the spine, the wrist and the femoral neck. It is most frequently due to lowering of hormone levels in association with age or the menopause: less frequently it follows disuse, rheumatoid arthritis or vitamin C deficiency which lead to a failure of osteoid tissue formation and the translucent appearance of bone on the radiographs. (Illus.: fracture of D6).

15. **Osteomalacia (1):** This is due to a failure in osteoid mineralisation and the radiographic appearances may be difficult to differentiate from osteoporosis. (Illus.: fracture of tibia and fibula.) It is usually secondary to an inability to utilise vitamin D (adult rickets) but is also seen where calcium is deficient in the diet (or excreted in renal acidosis), where phosphate is excreted in excess (Fanconi syndrome) or where vitamin D is not absorbed (e.g. steatorrhoea).

16. **Osteomalacia (2):** Stress fractures are common. Areas of bone translucency (Looser's zones) in the pelvis and long bones are characteristic. (Illus.: note changes in ischium and pubic ramus fracture.) There are disturbances in the blood chemistry: the serum $PO_4$ is reduced, and the serum calcium normal or reduced. If the product of the serum calcium and phosphate is lower than 2.25 (in SI units) the diagnosis is confirmed.

17. **Osteomalacia (3):** Occasionally a triradiate pelvis may be present and also be diagnostic. Osteomalacia may be treated with calciferol 1.25 mg per day, and calcium gluconate 1–2 g per day. The serum calcium, phosphate and urea should be monitored at regular intervals. Hormone replacement (with female sex hormones or anabolic steroids) and calcium dietary supplements may halt the advance of osteoporosis, but cure is less certain. Fracture healing is not materially impaired in either osteomalacia or osteoporosis.

18. **Paget's disease (1):** This common condition is frequently seen in association with fracture, particularly in the tibia and the femur. (Illus.: two healing fractures of the femur.) The radiological picture is complex, with frequently cyst formation, bone thickening, increased bone density and disturbances of bone texture. Stress fractures are common, and complete fractures are usually transverse.

19. **Paget's disease (2):** Increased bone density and deformity may in many situations make the use of internal fixation devices difficult. (Illus.: femoral neck fracture pinned in coxa vara: healing fracture of shaft.) The rate of healing and the soundness of bone union are not, however, usually greatly affected. In many situations conservative methods may be employed with success.

**20. Paget's disease (3):** Note that sarcomatous change (Illus.) in this condition may be followed by fracture as the cortical bone is eroded. Note, too, that the bone changes found in hyperparathyroidism and sometimes in metastatic disease may mimic Paget's disease.

**21. Osteitis:** Sudden collapse of bone secondary to infection is comparatively uncommon as a presenting feature, but is seen where the destructive processes are comparatively low grade. Thorough investigation and appropriate treatment is mandatory. (Illus.: Tuberculosis at the thoracolumbar level.)

**22. Malignant bone tumours (1):** The commonest malignant bone tumour is the metastatic deposit. Secondaries in bone occur most frequently from primary growths in lung or bronchus (Illus.), breast, prostate or kidney. Any bone may be affected, but the spine, subtrochanteric region of the femur and the humeral shaft are amongst the commonest sites.

**25. Malignant bone tumours (4):**
*Treatment:* Note the following points:
(a) Without treatment, union of a fracture occurring at the site of a malignant bone tumour seldom occurs.

(b) If the tumour is responsive to local radiotherapy or to chemotherapy, healing may occur with appropriate splintage, but will be slow.

(c) In the case of metastatic disease, internal fixation has much to recommend it unless the patient is moribund. Acrylic cement is sometimes used to reinforce a bone defect.

(d) In the case of primary malignant bone tumours, the occurrence of fracture may be a factor in some circumstances in the advocation of amputation.

**23. Malignant bone tumours (2):**
Multiple myeloma in the pelvis (Illus.: with fracture of the femoral neck and a destructive lesion of the ilium) may sometimes be confused with secondary deposits from carcinoma of the prostate or other organs; full investigation is essential.

**24. Malignant bone tumours (3):** Primary malignant tumours of bone generally present with pain and swelling rather than fracture, but this is not always the case, especially perhaps in Ewing's tumour (Illus.: radiograph prior to fracture) and osteosarcoma. The aggressive, locally malignant osteoclastoma again usually presents with pain and swelling rather than fracture.

**26. Simple bone tumours and cysts (1):**
In the metacarpals, metatarsals (Illus.) and phalanges (Illus.), enchondromata are frequently encountered as a cause of pathological fracture. These are generally best treated by exploration, curettage and the packing of the resultant cavity in the bone with cancellous bone grafts.

**27. Simple bone tumours and cysts (2):**
In children between 5 and 15 years, unicameral bone cyst is one of the most frequent causes of pathological fracture, especially in the proximal humeral shaft. The bone cortex may be thinned, but expansion is rare. The fracture should be treated conservatively. (If the fracture fails to heal and the cyst disappear, curette and pack with bone grafts.)

**28. Osteogenesis imperfecta:** This hereditary disorder (dominant transmission) is characterised by bone fragility leading to bowing of the long bones, deformities of modelling, pathological fractures and stunting of growth. (Illus.: fracture of humerus: note deformities of ribs.) Deafness and blue sclerotics are commonly associated. The condition generally declares itself in infancy or childhood, but occasionally may not be diagnosed until skeletal demineralisation is noted later in life. Fracture healing is usually quite rapid, and most fractures may be treated successfully by conservative methods. Occasionally in the severer forms of this condition which present in childhood, internal fixation of the long bones by intramedullary nailing may be advocated as a prophylaxis against further fracture and to lessen bowing and other deformities of the legs.

*Investigation of pathological fractures:*
Investigation of a pathological fracture may require some or all of the following:
a. A full personal and family history.
b. Full clinical examination, including pelvic examination.
c. Radiographs of the chest.
d. Radiographs of the pelvis.
e. Radiographs of the skull and skeletal survey.
f. Estimation of the sedimentation rate.
g. A full blood count, including a differential cell count.
h. Estimation of the serum calcium, phosphate, alkaline phosphatase and where appropriate, the acid phosphatase.
i. Estimation of the serum proteins.
j. Serum electrophoresis.
k. Examination of the urine for Bence-Jones proteose.
l. A bone scan.
m. Marrow biopsy.
n. Bone biopsy.
o. Occasionally, radiographs of parents or sibs.

### 4. **Recording and communicating:** Some suggested guidelines:

**Records:** Careful note-taking in good patient management should already be recognised and practised, but in a field of medicine where evidence for insurance claims and litigation is commonly required, it is of particular importance. There are a number of areas where inadequacy is commonly found: these include the following:

(a) Not infrequently when the handling of a case is being studied some time after the event, problems arise because entries or letters have been *undated*; and if, as is often the case that they are on separate sheets, the time that they have been made cannot be determined by their context. It is vital that any entry is clearly dated, and in the seriously ill patient whose condition is rapidly changing during the first few hours after admission, the *time* should be clearly stated as well.

(b) Illegible handwriting is always a problem, but there should be no excuse for numerals and capital letters which are so badly formed that they cannot be read by others or even by the orginator. When contractions are used (and these can be helpful in providing oases of upper-case meaningful clarity) only those in common use should be employed.

(c) Paucity of notes (often very unfairly) suggests a similarly brief, and by implication, incomplete examination. In the heat of dealing with a seriously ill patient there is no time for detailed note-taking, but as soon as pressure eases, a full record should be made, and certainly this should be done *on the day of the admission.*

(d) The interpretation of radiographs should be included in the notes, giving negative as well as positive findings. With the growing tendency to practice a degree of defensive medicine, radiographs should certainly be taken if there is any doubt about the nature or severity of an injury, and if radiographs are not taken, it is perhaps wise to say at the time why this has not been thought to be necessary.

If there is something that you are not sure of, indicate what this is (so that it cannot be claimed later that you had not considered it), and state the course you tend to take (with if appropriate the reasons for doing so).

**Telephoning:** Be clear whether the purpose of your call is to inform, to ask for advice, or to seek assistance: and have all the appropriate information at your finger tips. It is necessary to be able to describe a fracture patient in an unequivocal fashion, so that an unconfused picture of the problem is conveyed. There are undeniably different styles of doing this, but the following method is suggested: (i) preamble; (ii) precise fracture details; (iii) particular qualifiers; (iv) reason for call.

*Preamble:* After any niceties, including if necessary stating exactly who you are, give the age and sex of the patient along with any special attributes which bear directly on the reason for the call: e.g."I have just admitted a 35-year-old man who is a professional ice skater. He has been in a road traffic accident and his main problem is . . . " (Note that it is probably best to avoid contractions such as "RTA" as they have to be translated, and may grate when used over the telephone.

*Precise fracture details:* The description of the fracture should always start with whether it is open or closed, and be followed by the bone involved and at what level; then the pattern of the fracture, and any displacement or angulation should be given: e.g. ". . . an open fracture of his right tibia in midshaft. It's a transverse fracture, but it's displaced medially and there's some lateral angulation. There's some shortening, and there's no bony contact."

*Particular qualifiers:* Where relevant these would include the following:

(a)  Complications of the local injury: this would include a description of the size, nature, location and potential contamination of a wound. It would also include details of any vascular or neurological problem.

(b)  Details of any other injuries sustained: e.g. other fractures, head injury, chest or abdominal injuries.

(c)  General condition of the patient, with, if appropriate, the time when he would be considered fit enough for anaesthesia and surgery.

(d)  Details of any treatment already carried out—e.g. fluid replacement, splintage etc: e.g. ". . . The fracture is from within out, and the wound is 1 cm in length. It looks pretty clean, and there's no neurological or circulatory problem, and he has had no other injury. His general condition's fine; he seems to have had very little blood loss and his pulse and BP are OK. I've set up an IV line and put him in a back splint. He's not had anything by mouth for the last 6 hours. He's been seen by the anaesthetist who is happy to do him any time."

*Reason for call:* (a) When this is to inform only, the details of the treatment carried out and what is further proposed could with profit be expanded: e.g. "I am planning to take him to theatre to debride the wound. I think I'll be able to get a good stable reduction under vision and I'll put the limb in plaster afterwards."

(b)  When advice is sought, the nature of the problem should be clearly stated: e.g. "I think this fracture might do best if internally fixed, but I'm wondering whether this should be done right away, or whether I should just reduce it and splint it, and add it to the beginning of tomorrow's list." (Not generally the best solution!)

(c)  When help is required, this should be clearly stated: e.g. "I think this is one you would want to treat by closed intramedullary nailing, and I've laid on theatre for seven thirty."

For suggestions on the making of follow-up notes, see Chapter 16, 'Fracture Clinics'.

# Section B:
# Regional injuries

# 6.  The shoulder girdle and humerus

1. **Clavicular injuries: Mechanism of injury:** Most (94%) clavicular injuries result from a direct blow on the point of the shoulder, generally from a fall on the side (A). Less commonly force may be transmitted up the arm from a fall on the outstretched hand (B).

*Fracture* is commonest at the junction of the middle and outer thirds (1) but is also common throughout the middle third (2) and to a lesser extent the outer third (3). *Subluxations* and *dislocations* may involve the acromioclavicular joint (4) and the sternoclavicular joint (5).

2. **Common patterns of fracture (1):** Greenstick fractures are common, particularly at the junction between the middle and outer thirds. Fractures may not be particularly obvious on the radiographs and it is often helpful in children to have both shoulders included for comparison. The only abnormality visible in many cases is local kinking of the clavicular contours. (Illus. Fracture of right clavicle.) Healing of this type of fracture is *rapid*, and *reduction* is *not required*.

3. **Common patterns of fracture (2):** In the adult, undisplaced fractures are also common, and are comparatively stable injuries. Late slipping is rare. Symptoms settle rapidly and minimal treatment is required.

4. **Common patterns of fracture (3):** With greater violence, there is separation of the bone ends. The proximal end under the pull of sternomastoid often becomes elevated (1). The shoulder loses the prop-like effect of the clavicle, so that it tends to sag downwards and forwards (2). Note (3) the glenoid, (4) the coracoid, (5) the acromion.

5. **Common patterns of fracture (4):** With greater displacement of the distal fragment, there is overlapping and shortening. In spite of the off-ending, union is rapid, and remodelling, even in the adults, is so effective that strenuous attempts at reduction are unnecessary. Pathological fracture may result from radionecrosis (following radiotherapy for breast carcinoma) and may be mistaken for local recurrence.

6. **Diagnosis:** Clinically there is tenderness at the fracture site; sometimes there is obvious deformity with local swelling, and the patient may support the injured limb with the other hand. In cases seen some days after injury, local bruising is often a striking feature. Diagnosis is confirmed by appropriate radiographs; a single AP projection of the shoulder is usually adequate in the adult.

7. **Treatment (1):** The most important aspect of treatment is to provide support for the weight of the arm which has lost its clavicular tie. As a rule this is best achieved with a broad arm sling (1). Additional fixation may be obtained by wearing the sling under the clothes (2). No other treatment is needed in greenstick or undisplaced fractures.

8. **Treatment (2):** Where there is marked displacement of a clavicular fracture it is usual practice to attempt to correct the anterior drift of the scapula round the chest wall (1). There is no simple way of achieving this. All methods attempt to apply pressure on the front of the shoulder (2) and although they are comparatively ineffective in terms of reduction, are helpful in reducing pain.

9. **Treatment (3): Ring or Quoit method:** Narrow gauge stockingette is cut into two lengths of about a metre each (1). The central portions are stuffed with cotton wool (2). One of the strips is taken and the padded area positioned over the front of the shoulder and tied firmly behind (3).

10. **Treatment (4):** The second strip is applied in a similar manner to the other shoulder (4). The patient is then advised to brace the shoulders back and the free ends of the ring pads are tied together (5). A pad of gamgee (sandwich gauze/cotton wool) may be placed as a cushion beneath the knots (6).

11. **Treatment (5): Figure-of-eight bandage:** Pads of gamgee or cotton wool alone are carefully positioned round both shoulders (1). The patient, who should be sitting on a stool, is asked to brace back the shoulders; a wool roll bandage is then applied in a figure-of-eight fashion (2). For added security the layers may be lightly stitched together at the crossover (3).

12. **Treatment (6):** Commercially available clavicle rings, covered with chamois leather, may be applied and secured with a web strap and buckle. With all these methods care must be taken to avoid pressure on the axillary structures and the additional support of a sling is desirable for the first 2 weeks or so. Note that elderly patients tolerate clavicular bracing methods poorly, and sling support only may be advisable.

13. **After care:** 1. Clavicular braces of all types require careful supervision and, at least initially, may require inspection and possible tightening every 2–4 days. 2. Where braces are used in conjunction with a sling, the sling may usually be discarded after 2 weeks. 3. All supports may be removed as soon as tenderness disappears from the fracture site. 4. Physiotherapy is seldom required except in the elderly patient who has developed shoulder stiffness. 5. A child's mother should always be advised that the prominent callous round the fracture is a normal occurrence, and that it will disappear in a few months with remodelling.

Note: If there is evidence of *torticollis* accompanying a clavicular fracture, further investigation of the cervical spine is indicated, as this finding may indicate a coincidental injury at the C1–2 level (locked facet joints). If plain radiographs are insufficient to clarify the situation, a CAT scan should if possible be carried out.

14. **Acromioclavicular joint injuries:** Injury to the acromioclavicular joint usually results from a fall in which the patient rolls on the shoulder. Note that the clavicle is normally attached to the scapula by (1) acromioclavicular, (2) conoid and (3) trapezoid ligaments. The scapular component of shoulder abduction requires free acromio-clavicular movement.

15. **Pathology:** Note that: (1) in subluxations and sprains, damage is confined to the acromioclavicular ligaments, and the clavicle preserves some contact with the acromion. In dislocations (2) the clavicle loses all connection with the scapula, the conoid and trapezoid ligaments tearing away from the inferior border of the clavicle. The displacement may be severe, and the ensuing haematoma may ossify (3).

16. **Diagnosis (1):** The patient should be standing and the shoulders compared. The outer end of the clavicle will be prominent, and in cases of damage to the conoid and trapezoid ligaments the prominence may be quite striking. Local tenderness is always present.

17. **Diagnosis (2):** Confirm any subluxation by supporting the elbow with one hand gently pushing the clavicle down with the other. Improvement in the contour of the outer end of the clavicle will confirm the diagnosis of subluxation or dislocation.

18. **Diagnosis (3):** Now stand behind the patient and abduct the arm to 90°. Flex and extend the shoulder while gently palpating the acromioclavicular joint. *Failure of the outer end of the clavicle to accompany the acromion indicates rupture of the conoid and trapezoid ligaments.*

19. **Radiographs (1):** Displacement of the clavicle by a diameter or more relative to the acromion (Illus.) suggests rupture of the conoid and trapezoid ligaments. The radiographs however are often fallacious in indicating the severity of the injury (and indeed may not show it). The reason is that spontaneous reduction tends to occur in recumbency—the position in which AP radiographs are normally taken.

20. **Radiographs (2):** It must be clearly indicated on the radiograph request form that the acromioclavicular joint is suspect. The radiographs should then be taken with the patient standing. The weight of the limb is often sufficient to show up the dislocation, but it is common practice to have the patient hold weights in both hands, and to include both shoulders for comparison.

21. **Treatment (1):** If there is no gross instability, treat by the use of broad arm sling under the clothes for 4—6 weeks. Physiotherapy is seldom required and an excellent result is the rule.
*NB:* Subluxations are easily reduced and held by adhesive strapping, but this treatment should *not* be employed as early skin reactions will always force abandonment.

22. **Treatment (2):** In cases of gross instability, good results usually follow conservative management; although complications are common after surgery, this should be considered in patients who are engaged in work which is heavy or involves prolonged elevation of the arms. The preferred method is to bring the clavicle down into alignment with the acromion, using a lag screw (1) run into the coracoid. Note the washer (2) used to spread local stresses. The clavicle should be drilled with an ample clearance hole, and some advise reinforcement of the fixation with absorbable transarticular sutures (3) in the acromioclavicular joint. Any tears in the deltoid or trapezius should also be repaired.

**Treatment (3):** Other methods of internal fixation include figure-of-eight acromioclavicular wiring. Kirshner wires passed across the joint tend to migrate, and their use is not recommended. In all cases there is a strong tendency for the devices to cut out, and it is imperative that there is the additional support of a broad arm sling (under the clothes or with a body bandage). *Internal fixation devices must be removed 6–8 weeks before mobilisation.*

**23. Treatment (4):** If a dislocation reduces with the arm in abduction, a shoulder spica for 6–8 weeks may be used as an alternative to surgery. Complications: Symptoms from acromioclavicular osteo-arthritis may be relieved by acromionectomy or excision of the outer 2 cm of the clavicle. (2) Fascial reconstruction of the coracoclavicular ligaments can be used for persistent instability.

**24. Fractures of the outer third of the clavicle:** Displacement is generally minimal as the coracoclavicular ligaments are not usually torn. When these ligaments are damaged, however, displacement may be marked and give rise (rarely) to non-union. These injuries should be treated along similar lines to acromioclavicular joint injuries: clavicular bracing is valueless and a sling under the clothes for 4–5 weeks is usually quite adequate.

**Complications of clavicular fractures:** 1. Glenohumeral joint stiffness in the elderly may require physiotherapy. 2. Even after normal remodelling (which continues for many months) a persistent sharp clavicular spike may cause discomfort against the clothes and require excision. 3. Non-union is rare, but if causing symptoms is treated by bone grafting and internal fixation by (a) a reconstruction plate applied superiorly, (b) a dynamic compression plate applied anteriorly, or (c) a T-plate in outer-third fractures. A lag screw between the medial fragment and coracoid may also be used.

**25. Sternoclavicular dislocation.** This is sometimes seen without any history of trauma, but generally the commonest lesion, a minor subluxation, follows a fall or blow on the front of the shoulder (1) or fall on the outstretched hand. *There is asymmetry of the inner ends of the clavicles* (2) due to the clavicle on the affected side subluxing downwards and forwards. There is local tenderness. *The diagnosis is essentially a clinical one.*

**26. Radiographs:** AP and oblique radiographs are difficult to interpret but are nevertheless usually performed; they may confirm the diagnosis when there is a major dislocation and the inner end of the clavicle is displaced onto the sternum. Note that in rare cases (illustrated) the clavicle passes *behind* the sternum where it may endanger the great vessels. As a rule tomographs or CAT scans may be more useful in elucidating these injuries.

**27. Treatment (1):** Minor subluxations should be accepted. The clavicle stabilises in the subluxed position; some prominence of the inner end of the clavicle may persist, with some asymmetry of the suprasternal notch, but a pain-free result is usual. The arm should be rested in a sling for 2–3 weeks until acute pain has settled.

**28. Treatment (2):** Gross displacements should be reduced under general anaesthesia. A sandbag (1) is placed between the shoulders which are firmly pressed backwards (2). Clavicular braces are then applied (see 101, 102, 8–12) along with a broad arm sling for 4–5 weeks. Should the reduction be extremely unstable, surgical repair with fascia lata slings should be considered. The rare irreducible dislocation may require open reduction, which may be hazardous.

**29. Scapular fractures (1):** Fractures of the blade of the scapula are usually caused by direct violence. Even when comminuted and angled (Illus.) healing is usually extremely rapid and an excellent outcome is the rule. Treatment is by use of a broad arm sling and analgesics. Mobilisation is commenced as soon as acute symptoms have settled, and is usually possible after 2 weeks.

**30. Scapular fractures (2):** Fractures of the scapular neck are associated with much bruising and swelling. Comminution is common, sometimes with involvement of the glenohumeral joint. If so, the position of the humeral head should be checked. In spite of frequently daunting radiographs, a good outcome is the rule, provided mobilisation is commenced as early as possible. (Treat as 105, 29) Fractures of the spine or coracoid are dealt with similarly.

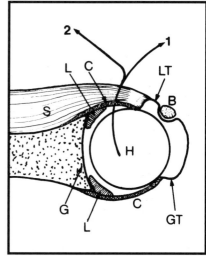

**31. Dislocation of the shoulder:** When the shoulder dislocates, the head of the humerus may come to lie *mainly* (1) in front of the glenoid (anterior dislocation of the shoulder), (2) behind the glenoid (posterior dislocation of the shoulder) or (3) beneath the glenoid (luxatio erecta). Anterior dislocation is *by far* the commonest of these.

**32. Anterior dislocation (1):** This most commonly results from a fall leading to external rotation of the shoulder (e.g. the trunk internally rotating over a fixed hand). It is rare in children, common in the 18–25 years age group (from motorcycle and athletic injuries) and comparatively common in the elderly, where the stability of the shoulder may be impaired by muscle degeneration and where falls are common.

**33. Anterior dislocation (2):** The head of the humerus externally rotates out of the glenoid (1) and, having become free, comes to lie medially in front of the scapula (2). B = biceps tendons; C = capsule; G = glenoid; GT = greater tuberosity; H = head of humerus; L = glenoid labrum; LT = lesser tuberosity; S = subscapularis.

**34. Anterior dislocation (3):** Anterior dislocation is inevitably associated with damage to the anterior structures. Commonly the capsule is torn away from its attachment to the glenoid (1). This is the so-called Bankart lesion, although the frequent simultaneous displacement of the glenoid labrum (2) usually attracts this term.

**35. Anterior dislocation (4):** In the older patient especially, there may be tearing or stretching of the anterior capsule (3), sometimes with associated damage to the shoulder cuff, especially subscapularis (4). The greater tuberosity may fracture (5) and occasionally there is damage to the axillary artery or brachial plexus (6).

**36. Diagnosis (1):** The shoulder is very painful: the patient resents movement, and to prevent this often holds the injured limb at the elbow with the other hand. The arm does not always lie into the side, appearing to be in slight abduction. The outer contour of the shoulder may appear to be slightly kinked due to the displacement of the humeral head.

**37. Diagnosis (2):** Palpate under the edge of the acromion. The usual resistance offered by the humeral head will be absent. If in doubt, compare the two sides. The displaced humeral head may be palpable lying anteriorly.

**38. Diagnosis (3):** Nevertheless the acromion and clavicle make examination difficult. In the doubtful case, it may be helpful to try to assess the relative positions of the humeral head and glenoid by palpation in the axilla.

**39. Diagnosis (4):** Axillary (circumflex) nerve palsy is the commonest neurological complication. Test for integrity of the nerve by assessing sensation to pin prick (1) in its distribution over the 'regimental badge' area. (The shoulder is usually too painful to assess deltoid activity with certainty.) Look for other (rare) involvement of the radial portion of the posterior cord (2) and involvement of the axillary artery (3).

40. **Radiographs (1):** The majority of anterior dislocations of the shoulder show quite clearly on the standard AP radiographs of the shoulder. The humeral head is displaced anteriorly and medially; in its final position it may be described as lying (a) preglenoid (b) subcoracoid, (c) subclavicular. This classification is of little practical importance; the important diagnostic feature is the loss of congruity between the humeral head and the glenoid as illustrated.

41. **Radiographs (2):** This radiograph of a normal shoulder is include for comparison. In both films you should be able to identify the following features: (1) the glenoid, (2) the humeral head, (3) the coracoid, (4) the acromion, (5) the clavicle, (6) the vertebral border of the scapula and, less clearly, (7) the axillary border of the scapula and (8) the spine of the scapula.

42. **Radiographs (3):** *A second radiographic projection is essential if the diagnosis is in doubt.* Note that if the humeral head has minimal medial displacement the AP view may appear *normal*. (This is especially the case in posterior shoulder dislocations.) The most useful additional projection is the axial lateral (sometimes called the tangenital lateral). (Illus.: the *normal* appearances in such films.)

43. **Radiographs (4):** The axial lateral is usually taken with the patient lying on his back with the arm abducted to 90°. The X-ray tube is adjusted so that it lies roughly parallel to the trunk; the central ray passes through the axilla to the plate which is placed above the shoulder. The bony features are easy to identify (the numerical key is the same as 107, 41).

44. **Radiographs (5):** Unfortunately the shoulder may be too painful to allow the taking of an axial lateral. *If so, obtain an apical oblique projection;* the landmarks are similar to those seen in the AP projection, but the glenohumeral relationship is easier to interpret. Alternatively, if the patient is not overweight, a *translateral* projection, truly at right angles to the plane of the AP, may be helpful. This view is often difficult to interpret, but note that in the *normal* shoulder (Illus.) the posterior border of the humerus and the axillary border of the scapula form a *shallow parabolic curve* (c f. Frame 60).

**45. Radiographs (6):** An associated fracture of the greater tuberosity is not uncommon (see 106, 35 for mechanism). This does not influence the initial treatment of the dislocation by reduction, but may require subsequent attention (see 109, 56). The radiographs of an acute dislocation may show evidence of previous episodes (for description see 112, 70).

**46. Radiographs (7): Subluxation of the glenohumeral joint:** Note that if any painful lesion of the arm is treated in a sling for several weeks wasting in the shoulder girdle will commonly result in a minor subluxation; this is most obvious if the AP radiograph is taken with the patient erect; no active treatment is required, but frank dislocation should be excluded by a lateral projection.

**47. Treatment: Reduction by Kocher's method (1):** This, the most popular of reduction methods, may often be successfully carried out in the older patient after the administration of intravenous diazepam, or in the younger patient after a substantial does of intramuscular pethidine. Severe pain or a muscular patient are indications for general anaesthesia. Apply traction (1) and begin to rotate the arm externally (2).

**48. Kocher's method (2):** Take plenty of time over external rotation. In the conscious patient, if muscle resistance is felt, stop for a moment and then continue, distracting the patient's attention with conversation. It should be possible to reach 90° of external rotation. (If severe pain and muscle spasm prevent rotation, general anaesthesia will be required.)

**49. Kocher's method (3):** The shoulder frequently reduces with a clear 'clunking sensation during the external rotation procedure, but if this does not happen adduct the shoulders so that the elbow starts to come across the chest. (This and the following movements may be carried out rapidly.)

**50. Kocher's method (4):** Now internally rotate the shoulder, bringing the patient's hand towards the opposite shoulder. If reduction has not occurred, repeat all stages, attempting to get more external rotation in stage 2. If doubt remains, repeat radiographs should be taken. Complete failure is rare under general anaesthesia. In the sedated patient, failure is an indication for general anaesthesia.

**51. Alternative methods of reduction: Hippocratic method:** The principle is that traction is applied to the arm and the head of the humerus is levered back into position. The stockinged heel is placed against the chest (without being pressed hard into the axilla) to act as a fulcrum, while the arm is adducted.

**52. Gravitational traction:** The patient is given a generous dose of a powerful analgesic (e.g. 200 mg of pethidine in a fit athletic male). A sandbag is placed under the clavicle and the arm allowed to hang over the side of the couch. With muscle relaxation secondary to the analgesia, and the gravitational traction, the shoulder may reduce spontaneously within an hour. Failure is an indication for general anaesthesia.

**53. After care (1):** Check radiographs should be taken. This should be done before any anaesthetic is discontinued if there is doubt about the reduction. The arm should be supported after reduction to lessen the risks of immediate redislocation. Begin by placing a gamgee or wool pad in the axilla (for perspiration) (1) and apply a broad arm sling (2).

**54. After care ctd:** External rotation should be prevented by a body bandage (1), stretchable net (Netelast®) (2) or less securely by the outside clothes (3). The supports may require changing for the sake of hygiene from time to time until they are discarded. If there is some residual pain, an outside sling may be worn for a further week. Mobilisation is usually rapid without physiotherapy being required.

**55. After care (2):** In the younger patient, there is a comparatively high incidence (about 50%) of recurrence within 2 years. The common practice is to continue supporting the limb as described for a *4-week period*, the rationale being that this gives the torn tissues time to heal.

The efficacy of prolonged fixation in this respect is in doubt, and where there are other factors present which make early mobilisation particularly desirable it would seem wise to curtail the period of post-reduction support. Certainly if the shoulder has been dislocated four times or more the patient should be considered to be suffering from recurrent dislocation, and be assessed for reconstructive surgery.

**After care (3):** In the elderly patient the risks of recurrent dislocation are minimal, but the risks of stiffness are great. A sling support under the clothes should be applied initially and discarded as soon as pain will permit. Mobilisation of both the shoulder and the elbow may usually be started after 1–2 weeks. Referral for physiotherapy is advisable in nearly all cases of dislocation in the older patient. In some elderly patients there may be joint instability problems due to damage to the shoulder cuff. If this is suspected it may be confirmed by arthroscopy, and good results have been claimed for subsequent secondary repairs.

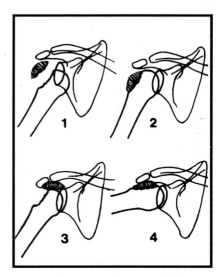

**56. After care (4):** If there has been an associated fracture of the greater tuberosity (1) this generally reduces adequately with the dislocation (2). Again, mobilisation should be commenced as soon as pain will permit (usually after 3–4 weeks). If the tuberosity remains seriously displaced—e.g. under the arcomion (3)—and cannot be reduced by placing the arm in abduction (4) it should be openly replaced and fixed with a screw (see also 115, 90 and 118, 106).

**57. After care (5):** Where there has been an axillary nerve palsy with loss of deltoid function, physiotherapy will be required. Although the lesion is usually in continuity and full recovery may occur, this may take several months and is not invariable. Assisted movements will be required—either normally, with the aid of slings and perhaps weights or by hydrotherapy.

**58. Posterior dislocation of the shoulder (1):** This may result from a fall on the outstretched, internally rotated hand or from a direct blow on the front of the shoulder. The head of the humerus is displaced directly backwards and, because of this, a single AP projection may show little or no abnormality as illustrated here. Nevertheless, clinically there is pain, deformity and local tenderness. *Note:* Posterior dislocation may accompany (and be missed) in obstetrical and Erb's palsies.

**59. Posterior dislocation (2):** The frequently apparently normal AP projection makes it essential for an additional lateral view to be obtained when there is any suspicion of posterior dislocation. Where pain is not severe (as for example if the dislocation occurs as a complication of a neurological disorder) a tangential lateral may show the humeral head lying clearly behind the glenoid.

**60. Posterior dislocation (3):** Generally, however, pain will permit a translateral projection only. The parabolic curve, shaped like the path of a comet, formed by the shaft of the humerus and the edge of the scapula will be broken and further study will show the humeral head to lie behind the glenoid shadow (compare with 107, 44).

**61. Treatment (1):** Reduction is usually easily accomplished by applying traction to the arm in a position of 90° abduction (1) and then externally rotating the limb (2). If the reduction appears quite stable the arm should be rested in a sling as described for anterior dislocation of the shoulder.

**62. Treatment (2):** If the reduction is unstable, it is essential that the arm be kept in 60° lateral rotation for 4 weeks to give the torn capsule and labrum a reasonable chance of healing. This can only be reasonably achieved by the application of a shoulder spica, with the shoulder abducted to about 40°, externally rotated 60° and fully extended.

63. **Luxatio erecta (1):** In this comparatively rare type of shoulder dislocation, there is obvious deformity, with the arm being held in abduction. The radiographs pose no difficulty in interpretation. The patient should be carefully examined for evidence of neurological or vascular involvement, and reduction carried out without undue delay.

64. **Luxatio erecta (2):** Reduction is usually easily obtained by applying traction in abduction (the position in which the limb is lying) (1) and swinging the arm into adduction (2). The shoulder should be supported after reduction as for anterior dislocation.

65. **Late diagnosed anterior dislocation (1):** The diagnosis may have been overlooked, the dislocation not being discovered until some weeks after the injury. Up until about 6 weeks or so, closed reduction (which is often successful) should be attempted. The forearm should be suspended by a canvas sling or bandage from a ceiling hook or improvised fixture above the table. A general anaesthetic is required, and at the time of the actual manipulation a muscle relaxant may be helpful.

66. **Late diagnosed anterior dislocation (2):** The patient should be on his side and the sling adjusted so that, by using the arm as a lever, an assistant can exert considerable traction through the patient's body weight. The humeral head is then manipulated over the glenoid lip. An image intensifier may give considerable assistance. Mobilisation should be commenced at an early stage (say 1 week).

67. **Late diagnosed anterior dislocation (3):** If closed reduction fails, open reduction may have to be considered. This is seldom an easy procedure, and a substantial blood replacement may well be required. An anterior approach is usually employed (see 112, 71); if the reduction is unstable, temporary pin fixation may be required. If reduction cannot be achieved, resection of the humeral head with or without replacement (excisional arthroplasty, hemi- or total replacement arthroplasty) may have to be considered.

If the dislocation is not discovered until some months after the injury, the dislocation in the older patient should generally be left until the outcome of a prolonged period of physiotherapy has been assessed. (Many become pain-free, albeit with a marked restriction in shoulder movements.) In the younger patient, exploration and open reduction or arthroplasty should be considered.

**Late diagnosed posterior dislocation:** Manipulative reduction should be attempted as late as a year from the time of the dislocation. The same technique as that described for late diagnosed anterior dislocation may be employed, with in the case of posterior dislocation, pressure being applied from behind the shoulder on the posteriorly displaced head. Failure of reduction should be managed in the same way as anterior dislocation, but using a posterior approach for any operative procedure.

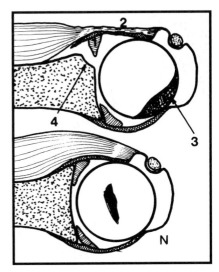

68. **Recurrent dislocation of the shoulder (1):** Even after early adequate treatment, redislocation of the shoulder may occur. Progressively less trauma is required on each occasion: eventually the patient may be able to reduce the dislocation voluntarily. Pathological features may include (1) a Bankart lesion, (2) attrition of the anterior shoulder cuff, (3) a defect with flattening of the posterolateral aspect of the head and (4) rounding of the glenoid margin.

69. **Diagnosis (1)**: The history is usually clear, and clinically external rotation of the shoulder may cause apprehension. Distinguish between *recurrent dislocation* and *habitual* dislocation; in the latter the patients are often psychotic, or suffer from joint laxity. They can often voluntarily dislocate and reduce the joint without pain. Arthroscopy will reveal a lax capsule and capacious joint, but no other features of recurrent dislocation. Treat by bio-feedback re-education of the shoulder muscles and avoid surgery.

70. **Diagnosis (2)**: An axial view may clinch the diagnosis. Posterolateral defects in the humeral head (Illus.) are often striking in recurrent dislocation, but do not occur in habitual dislocation. *Other investigations*:(i) arthroscopy or (ii) an air contrast CAT scan may show bony defects or Bankart lesions (iii); look for abnormal excursion of the humeral head by intensifier examination (or taking stress films) with the shoulder in 90° abduction.

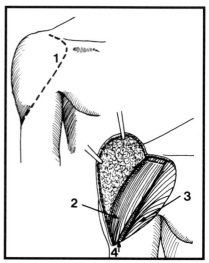

71. **Treatment (1)**: Two surgical repairs are common: the Bankart and the Putti-Platt. In both, the anterior approach to the shoulder is usually employed. An incision is made along the line of the medial border of the deltoid, turning laterally along the clavicle (1). The groove between the deltoid (2) and pectoralis major (3) is identified and opened up; the cephalic vein (4) may need to be ligated.

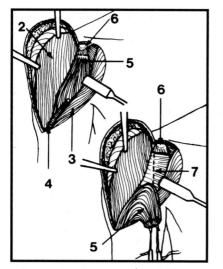

72. **Treatment (2)**: The deltoid is turned back (2) by incising some of its fibres close to the clavicle. The common tendon of the coracobrachialis and the short head of biceps (5) is divided close to the coracoid (6) and turned down, taking care to avoid the musculocutaneous nerve. This reveals the subscapularis (7). (1, 3 and 4 in 112, 71).

73. **Treatment (3): Bankart repair (1)**: The shoulder joint is opened by dividing the subscapularis (1) and the capsule (2). If the glenoid labrum is loose and displaced into the joint (3) it is excised; if not, it is ignored. Access is improved by lateral retraction of the humereal head (4). The glenoid edge is rawed (5) and drilled obliquely to take the anchoring sutures (6).

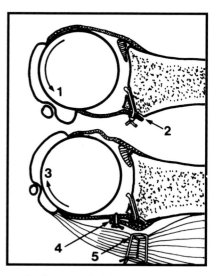

74. **Bankart repair (2)**: Now the shoulder is internally rotated (1) and the sutures which have been passed through bone are used to anchor the lateral part of the capsule to the raw edge of the glenoid (2). With the shoulder in neutral rotation (3) the medial part of the capsule is sewn over the lateral (4). The subscapularis is repaired (5) followed by layer closure. The arm is bandaged to the side for 4 weeks before mobilisation is commenced.

**75. Putti-Platt repair:** Strong mattress sutures are inserted into periosteum, capsule or other intact tissue on the scapular neck (1) and used to anchor the lateral part of the capsule and subscapularis. The medial parts are sewn in front (2), deliberately restricting external rotation and forming a four-layer barrier of tissue in front of the joint. The arm is kept in internal rotation for 4–6 weeks before mobilisation. The failure rate with either procedure is low (< 10%).

**76. Bone-block repair:** A bone graft, fixed to the glenoid, may be used to buttress the joint mechanically in both anterior or posterior dislocations (Illus.) where there is a substantial bony defect. It may also be used in the rare (and generally unrewarding) case where in spite of a joint laxity syndrome or paralytic element to the dislocation there is some strong indication for an attempted repair. In recurrent anterior dislocation the joint may be buttressed anteriorly by a coracoid transfer procedure.

**77. Recurrent posterior dislocation of the shoulder:** Surgical repair of the shoulder (using Bankart or Putti–Platt-like procedures through a posterior approach) may be considered, using criteria similar to those for recurrent anterior dislocation. Recurrent dislocation of the shoulder may also be treated by arthroscopic surgery using several techniques including stapling. There is an appreciable failure rate, and the long term results are not known.

*Fracture–dislocations of the shoulder:*
1. With fracture of the greater tuberosity—see 115, 90 and 118, 106.
2. With fracture of the neck of the humerus—see 119, 110–112.

*Neurological complications of shoulder dislocations:* Any type of brachial plexus lesion may be seen, and most make a good *functional* recovery without surgery. Isolated axillary nerve lesions are the commonest, and have the poorest prognosis in terms of motor recovery. Suprascapular nerve palsies have an excellent recovery rate.

Where there is a diffuse plexus lesion, if joint stiffness is not overcome before neurological resolution occurs, function may be permanently impaired: the lesson is that every effort must be made to mobilise the shoulder as quickly as possible where there is *any* neurological complication.

If no recovery has occurred after 3–5 months in major plexus lesions, exploration is indicated; a wide exposure is generally required to allow, if indicated, nerve resection and free nerve grafting.

**78. Shoulder cuff tears:** With advancing years degenerative changes occur in the shoulder cuff. Minor trauma may then produce small tears which through impingement on the acromion give rise to a painful arc of movement centred at 90° abduction. Physiotherapy in the form of local heat and exercises and local infiltrations of hydrocortisone are usually helpful in relieving symptoms.

More extensive tears may follow the sudden application of traction to the arm, and may give rise to difficulty in abducting the shoulder. There is initial tenderness under the acromion and the shoulder is hunched when the patient tries to abduct the arm; at a later stage he may be able to get over the problem of initiating abduction by means of trick movements. The diagnosis and the extent of the lesion may be confirmed by arthroscopy or air contrast CAT scan. These injuries are usually treated by prolonged physiotherapy once the acute symptoms have settled. If pain remains a problem, surgery may be advised; good results have been obtained as long as 2 years from the onset of symptoms. (Surgery involves an attempt at repairing the rent in the cuff, using plastic surgical techniques if necessary; partial acromionectomy may be performed if the soft tissues are seen to impinge against the acromion. Certain arthroscopic repair techniques are also used.) Surgery may be advised at an earlier stage should the problem arise (as it does only rarely) in the younger patient.

**Fractures of the proximal humerus:** There are many different patterns of fracture which occur in this area; although some are of considerable rarity, they can be important because of the complications which may follow them.

A number of attempts have been made to classify fractures in this region, but in order to accommodate the bewildering array of injuries which occur, simplicity has not been one of the results. (The same outcome is to be seen in the classification of ankle fractures.)

Two general classifications are of importance: one by Neer, and the other by the AO Group. (The latter is placed at the end of this Chapter.) It is suggested that these are used for reference, and that only the bare facts in Frame 79 be committed to memory.

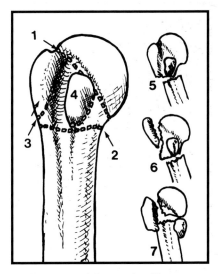

**79. Fractures of the proximal humerus:** Fractures in this region may involve the anatomical neck (rare) (1), the surgical neck (2), the greater tuberosity (3) or the lesser tuberosity (4). Combinations of these injuries are common, and it is customary to describe fractures in this region by the number of fragments involved—e.g. two-part (5), three-part (6) and four-part fractures (7).

**80. Classification of proximal humeral fractures:** In the commonly accepted Neer's classification, proximal humeral fractures are divided into 6 groups.

**Group I:** This group includes *all* fractures in this region (irrespective of the degree of comminution) where there is minimal displacement or angulation. (Minimal displacement is defined as being less than 1 cm; minimal angulation is (surprisingly) defined as being ≤ 45°

**81. Neer's classification: Group II:** This includes all fractures of the anatomical neck displaced by more than 1 cm. These rare injuries may be complicated by avascular necrosis of the humeral head. **Group III:** This includes all appreciably displaced or severely angled fractures of the surgical neck; there are no problems with avascular necrosis. They may be impacted (1), displaced (2) or comminuted (3). Angulation is often anterior, and may give an erroneous impression of abduction or adduction.

**82. Group IV** includes all fractures of the greater tuberosity (1), displaced by the pull of supraspinatus (2). In three-part fractures, a fracture of the surgical neck (3) allows the subscapularis (4) to rotate the head internally so that its articular surface (5) faces mainly posteriorly. **Group V** injuries involve the lesser tuberosity (6). In three-part injuries the humeral head may be abducted and externally rotated so that its articular surface faces anteriorly (7). Four-part injuries (8), identical with four-part injuries of Group IV, may render the head avascular.

**83. Group VI** comprises the fracture–dislocations. Dislocation of the shoulder with an associated greater tuberosity fracture (1) is included in the two-part injuries in Group VI (see also 109, 56). More serious are the dislocations where the two-part fracture of the proximal humerus is through the surgical neck (2). Most difficult of all are the three- and four-part injuries, especially when the humeral head is completely detached and displaced (3), or worse still, split (4).

**84. Children's injuries:** Note that in children the commonest injury is a greenstick fracture of the surgical neck (1); this may be classified as a Neer Group I, two-part fracture. Also common is a slight or moderately displaced proximal humeral epiphyseal injury with an associated juxta-epiphyseal fracture (2) (Salter & Harris Type 2 injury.) This would fit into Group I or II, depending on the displacement and angulation.

**85. Mechanism of injury:** These fractures may be caused by a fall on the side (often leading to impacted, minimally displaced fractures) (1), by direct violence or by a fall on the outstretched hand. The pattern of injury following the latter may be influenced by the direction of motiom of the trunk over the fixed arm (2, 3).

86. **Diagnosis:** The patient tends to support the arm with the other hand (1). There is tenderness over the proximal humerus (2) and in severely angled or displaced fractures there may be obvious deformity. Later, gross bruising gravitating down the arm is an outstanding feature (3). (This may worry the patient unless its occurrence is predicted by the surgeon.)

87. **Radiographs (1):** The diagnosis is established firmly by the radiographs. In a fair number of cases two features may be clear: namely that the fracture involves the cancellous bone of the head and neck and that there is impaction of the fragments. Both these factors contribute to the rapid healing associated with most fractures of proximal humerus. (Illus.: three-part Group I fracture.)

88. **Radiographs (2)** Note that a second radiographic projection of the shoulder is desirable for a clear assessment of these injuries. An apical oblique or a good translateral will generally be able to clarify the relationships of the major elements. The illustration, a translateral, shows complete loss of bony contact between the main elements of a two part fracture.

89. **Radiographs (3):** Note that in children the epiphyseal line is frequently mistaken for a fracture. In many radiographic projections the epiphyseal plate lies obliquely so that instead of appearing as a line it is seen as an oval; as one part of this will be less distinct than the other (see arrow) it may be misinterpreted. (Illus.: normal shoulder.)

90. **Treatment guidelines: Group I injuries (1):** The following classical examples are arranged in order of severity.

*Undisplaced fracture of the greater tuberosity:* This type of injury may occur in isolation or accompany a spontaneously reduced dislocation of the shoulder. The arm should be supported in a collar and cuff sling until the acute symptoms have resolved (1–2 weeks), when mobilisation may be commenced. Watch carefully in case of late displacement.

91. **Treatment guidelines: Group I injuries (2):** Impacted fracture of the surgical neck. (Illus.: three-part fracture involving the greater tuberosity as well as the neck.) There is minimal displacement and angulation showing in this single projection. Prolonged immobilisation is not necessary. Again, a collar and cuff sling should be worn until pain has settled (2–3 weeks usually); shoulder mobilisation may then be commenced. If initial symptoms are severe, proceed as described in 116, 93.

**92. Treatment guidelines: Group I injuries (3):** Unimpacted fracture of the surgical neck (Illus.: two-part fracture involving the surgical neck.) In spite of not being impacted, an appreciable area of cancellous bone is in contact, generally assuring rapid healing. Secondary displacement is unlikely provided the limb has some initial protection (required anyway to relieve the severe pain, aggravated by movement, which often accompanies these injuries). Treat along the lines indicated in (116, 93–97).

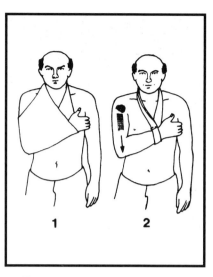

**93. Treatment guidelines: Group I injuries (4):** Slightly displaced and moderately angled humeral neck fractures may be treated satisfactory by external support alone; many other fractures may be managed along similar lines. Firstly, the arm should be supported in a sling. Where disimpaction is undesirable (e.g. 115, 91) a broad arm sling is preferable (1). Where the fracture is disimpacted (e.g. 116, 92), then a collar and cuff sling (2) has some potential for gravitational correction of any angulation.

**94. Treatment guidelines: Group I injuries (5):** In addition, the arm should be protected from rotational stresses by a body bandage (e.g. of crepe bandages) (1) under the clothes (2). Alternatively, an expanding net support may be used (e.g. Netelast® 109, 54) and this is certainly more comfortable in hot weather. Pain is often severe, and analgesics will be required in the first 1–2 weeks.

**95. Treatment guidelines: Group I injuries (6):** After 2 weeks the body bandage may be discarded unless pain is commanding. The sling should be worn under the outer clothes. The patient is advised to commence rocking movements of the shoulder [abduction, flexion (1)] and to remove the arm from the sling three or four times per day to flex and extend the elbow (2).

**96. Treatment guidelines: Group I injuries (7):** At 4 weeks the sling can be placed outside the clothes. Gentle active movements should be practised throughout the day. Over the next 2 weeks the patient should be encouraged to discard the use of the sling in gradual stages.

**97. Treatment guidelines: Group I injuries (8):** At 6 weeks the patient should be referred for physiotherapy if, as is usual, there is considerable restriction of movement. The range of movements (particularly glenohumeral; Illus.) should be recorded at fortnightly intervals, and physiotherapy discontinued when gains cease. Some permanent restriction of glenohumeral movement is common, but seldom incapacitating.

**98. Treatment guidelines: Group II injuries (displaced fractures of the anatomical neck):** These fractures are often complicated by avascular necrosis of the humeral head. Unless the displacement is very severe (e.g. with off-ending), or there is some complication (such as vascular obstruction in the arm) avoid manipulation or open reduction, and treat as in 116, 93–97. If manipulative reduction is required see 117, 100–102. If avascular necrosis ensues, joint replacement may have to be considered.

**99. Treatment guidelines: Group III injuries (severely displaced or angled fractures of the surgical neck):** In the elderly patient a good result can be expected in injuries of this pattern where the deformity is accepted and conservative management is pursued along previously indicated lines (116, 93–97). Nevertheless there will be some restriction of abduction, so where the deformity is particularly severe or the patient very active, manipulative reduction should be attempted.

**100. Treatment guidelines: Group III injuries: Manipulative reduction (1):** The patient is anaesthetised; if an image intensifier is available it should be employed and positioned in such a way that the surgeon has adequate access to the shoulder. Apply traction in the line of the limb (1) and swing the arm into *adduction* (2).

**101. Treatment guidelines: Group III injuries: Manipulative reduction (2):** An assistant maintains traction in adduction (1). Now apply pressure on the humeral shaft, pushing it laterally (3). At the same time, attempt to control the proximal fragment with the other hand, applying firm pressure beneath the acromion.

**102. Treatment guidelines: Group III injuries: Manipulative reduction (3):** If the medial edges of the fracture can be opposed, reduction may be completed by the assistant abducting the arm gently (5) and gradually releasing the traction (6). After reduction of the fracture, the limb should be supported in a broad arm sling and body bandage (see 116, 93–97).

**103. Treatment guidelines: Group III injuries *ctd:*** If closed methods fail, consider open reduction and internal fixation. In the illustration a Rush pin has been used, along with three cortical screws, to hold an additional bone fragment. (Rush pins are solid intramedullary nails with hooked ends; singly they can preserve alignment, but offer poor control of axial rotation; this disadvantage may be overcome if they are used in pairs inserted diametrically opposite one another; unfortunately this is not always possible.)

104. **Treatment guidelines: Group III injuries** *ctd:* The fracture may instead be held with a plate and screws. A good hold in the soft cancellous bone of the proximal humerus may be obtained with cancellous bone screws (1), while the plate may be fixed to shaft with cortical bone screws (2). It is desirable to get at least two screws in the head, and a T-plate may be used to achieve this (3). When this cannot be done without encroaching on the biceps tendon in the groove, an L-plate may be used instead.

105. **Treatment guidelines: Group III injuries** *ctd:* Good results may also be obtained in this class of fracture using an external fixator system. Under image intensifier control a Steinman pin is inserted into the humeral head and the fracture reduced. Two half pins with continuous threads are inserted into the humeral head, and 2–3 pins into the shaft. After connecting the external neutralising bar the Steinman pin is removed.

106. **Treatment guidelines: Group IV injuries (displaced fracture of the greater tuberosity):** Two-part injuries may be reduced by closed methods, but are liable to displace as the result of the unopposed action of the supraspinatus. It is probably best to internally fix these fractures, and this may be done with a single cancellous screw (with a washer under the head). This is also indicated in Group I injuries where there is late displacement.

107. **Treatment guidelines: Group IV injuries** *ctd:* In three-part injuries the articular surface (1) is directed posteriorly by subscapularis. The viability of the head is usually preserved. In the elderly, treat conservatively (see 116, 93–97). In the young and active, consider open reduction and internal fixation. This may be technically difficult, but it may be possible to reduce the three parts of the fracture using a cancellous screw to oppose the head and shaft (2) and a tension band (3) anchored to the screw head, for the tuberosity.

108. **Treatment guidelines: Group V injuries (displaced fractures of the lesser tuberosity):** Two-part injuries (1) are rare and should be treated conservatively. In three part injuries, supraspinatus (2) is unopposed and the humeral head points forwards. Treat as three-part Group IV injuries. Group V four-part injuries (4) are identical with four-part injuries in Group IV; there is a high incidence of avascular necrosis of the detached head. These injuries may also be managed conservatively, and complications dealt with as they arise.

109. **Treatment guidelines: Group VI injuries (fracture–dislocations):** Two-part injuries in which there is a dislocation of the shoulder and a fracture of the greater tuberosity are dealt with as though they were uncomplicated dislocations, i.e. by manipulative reduction. The greater tuberosity usually returns to its normal location, but if it remains severely displaced reduction should be undertaken (see 109, 56; 118, 106).

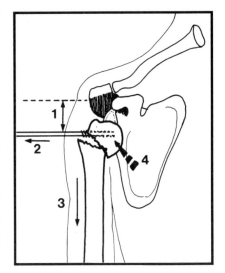

**110. Treatment guidelines: Group VI injuries (fracture-dislocations)** *ctd:* When a two-part injury involves a fracture of the surgical neck of the humerus, the degree of separation of the fragments affects the chances of a satisfactory closed reduction. Where there is little separation (1) an intact periosteal sleeve will generally permit manipulative reduction. Where there is wide separation of the elements (2) closed reduction is difficult.

**111. Treatment guidelines: Group VI injuries** *ctd:* Unless the patient is too frail, reduction should be carried out. Where there is severe separation, the risks of failure are particularly high, and in every case cross-matched blood and full theatre facilities should be available in case an open procedure becomes necessary.

*Closed reduction technique:* Apply strong traction in the neutral position or slight abduction (1) and manual pressure to the head via the axilla and front of the shoulder (2). Avoid hyperabduction.

**112. Treatment guidelines: Group VI injuries** *ctd:* If the previous technique fails, pass a threaded pin into the humeral head (under intensifier control); introduce the pin on the lateral aspect of the arm 3 cm below the acromial arch (1). Apply lateral traction to the pin (2) with slight traction to the arm (3) and manual pressure over the humeral head (4). *After care* is as for Group III injuries.

**113. Treatment guidelines: Group VI injuries** *ctd:* Where closed methods fail, open reduction should be considered unless there are serious contra-indications. In *three-and four-part injuries,* especially where there is splitting of the head fragment, the risks of avascular necrosis with persistent pain and stiffness are high. Under these circumstances, excisional arthroplasty, hemi-arthroplasty or total joint replacement should be considered. (Illus.: four-part fracture–dislocation with an arrow pointing to the humeral head.)

**114. Treatment:** In children, unimpacted fractures may be of adult pattern (Illus.) or Group 2 epiphyseal injures. *Open reduction should be avoided.* Manipulate as described, but if the deformity recurs on bringing the arm to the side apply a shoulder spica in abduction. Bony apposition should be obtained, but persisting angulation in excess of 30° should not induce pessimism as rapid recovery of function through remodelling is the rule.

**115. Complications (1):** Pathological fracture from simple bone cyst is common in the proximal humeral shaft in children. The injury should be treated as an uncomplicated fracture. Healing usually proceeds normally, often with spontaneous disappearance of the cyst. Only rarely (following repeated fracture or cyst expansion) is curettage and packing with bone chips indicated.

116. **Complications (2):** Radionecrosis may follow radiation therapy for breast carcinoma, leading to pathological fracture. Active treatment is difficult due to local fibrosis and vascular change, but joint replacement might be considered in the selected case. (**3**) Arterial obstruction generally responds to reduction of the fracture; if exploration is required, preliminary exposure and taping of the subclavian trunk at the root of the neck must be anticipated.

117. **Fractures of the humeral shaft: Pathology (1):** (a) Fractures of the humeral shaft may result from indirect violence (e.g. a fall on the outstretched hand) or from direct violence (e.g. a fall on the side or blow on the arm). (b) In fractures involving the upper third (Illus.) the proximal fragment tends to be pulled into adduction by the unopposed action of pectoralis major.

118. **Pathology (2):** (c) In fractures involving the mid third, the proximal fragment tends to be abducted due to deltoid pull. (d) Radial nerve palsy, non-union and compounding are commonest in *middle third* fractures.

119. **Diagnosis (1):** The arm is flail and the patient usually supports it with the other hand. Obvious mobility at the fracture site leaves little doubt regarding the diagnosis. Confirmation is obtained by radiographs which seldom give difficulty in interpretation.

120. **Diagnosis (2):** In all cases, look for evidence of radial nerve palsy—drop wrist (1) and sensory impairment dorsum of hand (2). This is in fact an uncommon complication, as a slip of brachialis lies beneath the nerve; this generally prevents it from coming in contact with the musculospiral groove or the fractured bone ends. If, however, radial nerve palsy accompanies an open fracture, exploration is mandatory.

121. **Treatment (1): U-slab method:** Simple, single fractures may be treated by the application of a U-plaster. If angulation is slight, no anaesthetic is required. The patient should be seated (1) and a plaster slab prepared of about eight thicknesses of 15 cm (6") plaster bandage (2). The length should be such as to allow it to stretch from the inside of the arm round the elbow and over the point of the shoulder (3).

122. **Treatment (2):** Wool roll is then applied to the arm (4). Particular attention is paid to the elbow. The padding should extend from the shoulder to a third of the way down the forearm.

123. **Treatment (3):** The slab is now wetted and applied to the arm, starting on the medial side at the axillary fold (5) and then bringing it round the elbow up to the shoulder. The slab should be carefully smoothed down. Overlapping of the edges of the slab anteriorly or posteriorly is of little consequence.

124. **Treatment (4):** The plaster is secured with a wet open weave cotton bandage (6). During the setting of the slab, the fracture may be gently moulded and slight angulation corrected. Thereafter the arm should be supported in a sling (7), which should be worn under the clothes.

125. **Treatment (5):** If the fracture is badly displaced, heavy sedation or general anaesthesia is desirable. An assistant should apply light traction to the arm. A U-slab is applied as before, with careful moulding of the fracture as the plaster sets. A sling is worn under the clothes for additional support.

126. **Treatment (6): Hanging cast method:** The principle of this form of treatment is that the weight of the limb plus the plaster reduce the fracture and maintain reduction (1). A long arm plaster (2) is applied along with a *collar and cuff sling* (3). The patient must be ambulant for this line of treatment to succeed, and it is claimed that there may be a higher rate of non-union from occasional distraction.

127. **Treatment (7):** After the initial pain has settled (say 2–3 weeks) the hanging cast may be replaced by a polythene sleeve or other form of functional bracing, but many prefer to continue using a cast until union. Check for this clinically and radiologically at 9 weeks. If judged sound, a sling may be worn as an additional precaution for 2 weeks, but mobilisation of the shoulder and elbow should be commenced. Depending on progress, the patient should be considered for physiotherapy.

128. **Treatment (8):** Consider internal fixation if (a) there are two or more fractures in the one limb, or if both arms are fractured, or if there are multiple injuries; (b) there is a radial nerve palsy in an open and otherwise suitable fracture, or if the palsy occurs after manipulation. Methods include (i) a pre-bent, broad 4.5 mm AO DCP plate (1) applied posteriorly, with a lag screw across the fracture (2). (ii) Crossed Rush pins (3) inserted through small incisions made on either side of the elbow.

129. **Treatment (9):** (iii) Intramedullary nails (including Rush pins, Enders nails etc.) may be introduced just proximal (1) to the olecranon fossa (2). The patient lies supine; traction is applied (with an olecranon pin) (3) and the hand and forearm supported (4) from an overhead bar. The fracture is visualised and reduced using an image intensifier (5) (for which there is good access). The fixation devices is then inserted through a small triceps splitting incision (6).

130. **Treatment (10):** (iv) Humeral shaft fractures may also be held using intramedullary nails inserted from the region of the greater tuberosity. (Illus.: single Rush pin.) This is used most often in proximal fractures where the exposure may allow simultaneous reduction of the fracture under vision. This method of fixation holds the major fragments in alignment, but offers poor control of rotation. Seidel locked intramedullary humeral nails have a high complication rate, mainly from shoulder impingement.

133. **Complications (2) Radial nerve palsy:** This is generally a lesion in continuity, and recovery often commences 6–8 weeks after the initial injury. If there is no indication for initial exploration (as for example the presence of a radial palsy in an open fracture of the humerus) then the patient should be treated expectantly.

The patient should be provided with a drop-wrist splint, preferably of lively type as soon as possible, and he should attend the physiotherapy department so that he can be encouraged in active and passive movements of the fingers, thumb and wrist. If there is no evidence of recovery in 8 weeks an electromyogram should be taken. If this shows no sign of recovery, exploration of the radial nerve should be undertaken.

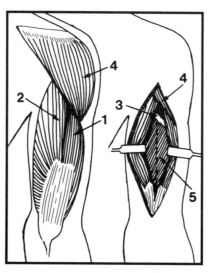

131. **Complications (1): Non-union (1):** This is seen most frequently in middle third fractures, especially in the obese patient where support of the fracture may be difficult or where gravitational distraction of the fracture occurs. Rigid internal fixation (well-fitting Kuntscher nail, compression plating, etc.) and often bone grafting are advised, with postoperative fixation in a plaster shoulder spica.

132. **Non-union (2):** Visualisation of the radial nerve is essential to avoid damage, and a posterior approach is frequently used. A midline posterior incision gives access to the lateral (1) and long heads (2) of triceps, which are separated. The nerve (3) lies close to the deltoid margin (4) and should be identified. The medial head of triceps (5) is split to give access to the humeral shaft.

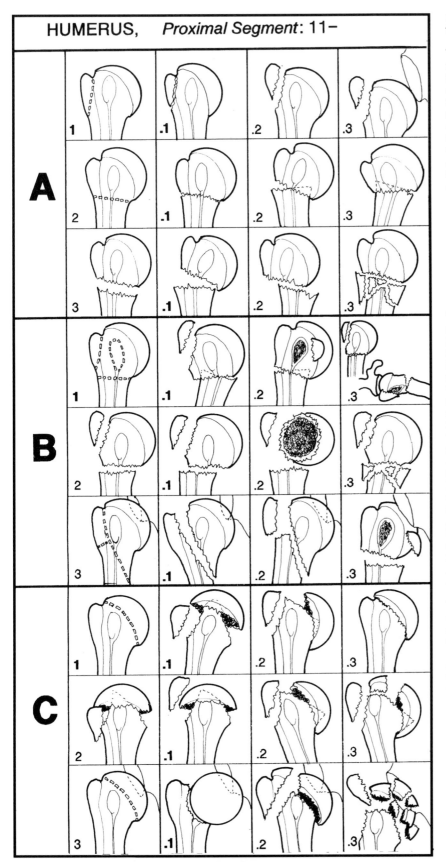

HUMERUS,   *Proximal Segment*: 11–

**134. AO Classification of Fractures of the Humerus, Proximal Segment (11–):**

**Type A** fractures are extra-articular and unifocal, involving either the surgical neck *or* the greater tuberosity *or* the lesser tuberosity. A1 = Fracture of the greater tuberosity: .1 = undisplaced; .2 displaced; .3 with an associated dislocation. A2 = Impacted fracture of the surgical neck: .1 = undisplaced; .2 = with varus deformity; .3 with valgus deformity. A3 = Non-impacted fracture of the surgical neck: .1 with angulation; .2 with displacement; .3 multifragmentary.

**Type B** fractures involve the surgical neck and a tuberosity. B1 = Impacted fracture of the surgical neck of the humerus with a fracture of the greater or lesser tuberosity: .1 with valgus deformity and a fracture of the greater tuberosity; .2 with varus deformity and a fracture of the lesser tuberosity; .3 with anterior angulation and a fracture of the greater tuberosity. B2 = Unimpacted fracture of the surgical neck with a fracture of a tuberosity: .1 without rotation (torsional deformity); .2 with rotation; .3 with a multifragmentary fracture of the metaphysis. B3 = Bifocal fracture with glenohumeral dislocation (fracture dislocation of the shoulder): .1 with the fracture line vertical and greater tuberosity intact (classified atypically here as a bifocal fracture because of the obliquity of the fracture line); .2 vertical fracture line and an associated fracture of the greater tuberosity; .3 posterior dislocation and a fracture of the lesser tuberosity.

**Type C** fractures are articular, with involvement of the anatomical neck and the articular surface. C1 = Slightly displaced articular fracture: .1 with involvement of the anatomical neck and the greater tuberosity, with some valgus deformity; .2 involvement of the anatomical neck and the greater tuberosity, with some varus; .3 solely of the anatomical neck. C2 = Markedly displaced but impacted articular fracture: .1 with involvement of the anatomical neck and the greater tuberosity, and valgus deformity; .2 with involvement of the anatomical neck and the greater tuberosity and varus deformity; .3 with the fracture involving the head and the greater tuberosity, and with varus angulation. C3 = Dislocated articular fracture (anatomical neck fracture–dislocation): .1 unifocal; .2 with tuberosity fractures; .3 multifragmentary of the head.

HUMERUS,    *Diaphyseal Segment:* 12–

**135. AO Classification of Fractures of the Humerus, Diaphyseal Segment (shaft) (12–):**

**Type A** are simple (i.e. there is a circumferential disruption of the bone).
A1 = Spiral fracture; .1 in the proximal zone; .2 in the middle or central zone; .3 in the distal zone.
A2 = Oblique fracture (i.e. fractures where the fracture lies at 30° or more to a line drawn at right angles to the shaft); the Subgroups are the same as in A1.
A3 = Transverse fractures (i.e. the fracture line lies at less than 30° to a line drawn at right angles to the shaft); the Subgroups are the same as in A1.

**Type B** fractures are wedge fractures (i.e. there is a separate (butterfly) segment, but after reduction there is contact between the main fragments (a so-called hitch)).
B1 = Spiral wedge fracture (usually as the result of twisting stresses); .1 in the proximal zone; .2 in the central zone; .3 in the distal zone.
B2 = Bending wedge fracture (usually as the result of bending stresses); the Subgroups are as in B1 above.
B3 = Bending wedge fracture: here the wedge is fragmented. The Subgroups are as in B1 above.

**Type C** fractures are complex (i.e. they have more than two fragments, and even after reduction the pattern is such that there is no contact between the main proximal and distal fragments).
C1 = Complex spiral; .1 with two intermediate fragment; .2 with three intermediate fragments; .3 with more than three intermediate fragments.
C2 = Complex segmental; .1 with one intermediate segment ('double fracture'; .2 with one intermediate segment and an additional wedge fragment; .3 with two intermediate segments.
C3 = Complex, irregular fracture; .1 with two or three intermediate fragments; .2 with shattering of the bone over a length of less than 4 cm; .3 with shattering of the bone over a length of 4 cm or more.

136. What injury and what sequel to injury is shown in this localised radiograph of the shoulder?

137. What is your analysis of this injury?

138. Classify this injury and comment on the position.

139. Describe this injury: what complication might you suspect?

140. What injury is present? Is reduction required?

141. What is this injury? What treatment would normally be advised?

142. What is this injury? What is its commonest neurological complication?

143. What does this radiograph show? What is the prognosis, assuming there is no additional deformity present in the second view? What neurological complication might accompany this injury?

144. Classify this injury. How would it be treated?

136. Acromioclavicular dislocation with massive calcification in the acromioclavicular ligaments (no active treatment is likely to be required apart from physiotherapy).

137. There is a fracture–dislocation of the shoulder (Neer Group VI, three-part injury). The faint shadow of the humeral head is in the medial wall of the axilla, and there is a separate fracture of the greater tuberosity. (AO = 11–C3.2.)

138. This is a greenstick fracture of the proximal humerus. There is no apparent angulation, but a second projection would be necessary to make certain of this. It is probably a Neer Group I, two-part injury. (AO = 11–A2.1.)

139. Fracture of the surgical neck of the humerus; the fracture is of the unstable type, and the shaft is displaced medially so that it has lost contact with the head. The axillary artery and the brachial plexus are at risk. There is a comminuted fracture of the greater tuberosity (Neer Group IV, three-part injury). (AO = 11–B2.1.)

140. This is a greenstick fracture of the clavicle. No reduction is required.

141. Fracture of the glenoid. There is in addition an undisplaced fracture of the acromion. This injury would normally be treated by resting the arm in a sling followed by mobilisation as soon as the acute symptoms had settled.

142. Anterior dislocation of the shoulder (an additional lateral projection would be required to confirm). An axillary nerve palsy might be associated.

143. The radiograph shows a completely off-ended fracture of the humerus in a child. Callus is plentiful, and union is far advanced with considerable shortening. The late result would normally be excellent, with the length discrepancy being made good. Radial nerve palsy is a possible complication in this type of injury. (AO = 12–A1.1; this fracture is slightly spiral in pattern.)

144. Undisplaced fracture of the surgical neck of the humerus in an adult (Neer Group I, two-part fracture). It would be treated conservatively by resting the arm in a sling. (AO = 11–A2.1.)

As an exercise you might care to classify by the AO system the radiographs in these frames: 45, 87, 88, 90, 91, 92, 98, 99, 114, 117, 118.

Answers:
45 = 11–A1.3
87 = 11–B1.1
88 = 11–A3.2
90 = 11–A1.1
91 = 11–B1.1
92 = 11–A3.1
98 = 11–C1.3
99 = 11–A3.1
114 = 11–A3.2
117 = 12–A3.2
118 = 12–A2.2

# 7.  Injuries about the elbow

1. **Definition:** A supracondylar fracture of the humerus is a fracture which occurs in the distal third of the bone. The fracture line lies just proximal to the bone masses of the trochlea (1) and capitulum (capitellum) (2) and often runs through the apices of the coronoid (3) and olecranon fossae. The fracture line is generally transverse.

2. **Occurrence:** The supracondylar fracture is a common fracture of childhood; its incidence reaches a peak about the age of 8 years. It generally results from a fall on the outstretched hand, and should always be suspected when a child complains of pain in the elbow after such an injury.

3. **Diagnosis (1):** The olecranon and medial and lateral epicondyles preserve their normal equilateral triangular relationship (unlike dislocation of the elbow, also common in children). There is tenderness over the distal humerus, there may be marked swelling and deformity, and the child generally resists examination. Radiography is mandatory, but interpretation requires care.

4. **Radiographs (1):** The interpretation of radiographs is made difficult by the changing complexities of the epiphyses. Typical appearances at ages 2, 4, 6 and 9 years are shown.
Note: C = Capitulum—present usually within the first year of life.
R = Radial head—appears 3–5 years.
M = Medial epicondyle—present by 6.
T = Trochlea—appears 7–9.
L = Lateral epicondyle—11–14. (Olecranon—8–11 years.)

5. **Radiographs (2):** Variations in appearances occur, and if there is any difficulty in interpreting the radiographs, there should be no hesitation in having films taken of the other side for direct comparison. These may for example draw attention to (1) the slight cortical irregularity of a minor greenstick fracture.

6. **Radiographs (3):** In fractures associated with more violence, the next detectable sign may be a hairline crack, visible in the AP view only (2). With more violence, the fracture line will be detectable in the lateral projection as well (3). Next, the distal fragment is tilted in a backward direction (4).

7. **Radiographs (4):** With still greater violence there is backward displacement (5), often leading to loss of bony contact. In the AP view there is often medial or lateral shift of the epiphyseal complex (M). The complex may also be rotated relative to the humeral shaft (generally lateral rotation). Rarely, as a result of other mechanisms the distal fragment is displaced and tilted anteriorly (A).

8. **Vascular complications (1):** Where there is appreciable displacement of the fracture, the brachial artery may be affected by the proximal fragment. In the majority of cases this is no more than a kinking of the vessel, but occasionally structural damage to the wall may occur, with the risk of Volkmann's ischaemic contracture. (Rarely the neurovascular bundle is trapped between the fracture and the biceps tendon, with tethering of the overlying skin; this is an indication for exploration.)

9. **Vascular complications (2):** In every case the circulation should be assessed and recorded prior to any manipulation. Note if the radial pulse is absent, and seek other evidence of arterial obstruction (pallor and coldness of the limb, pain and paraesthesiae in the forearm, progressive weakness and paralysis of the forearm muscles). Look for excessive swelling and bruising round the elbow.

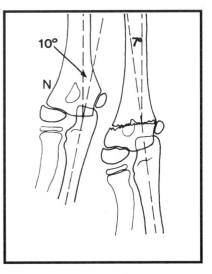

10. **Indications for reduction (1):** Manipulation of the fracture should be undertaken (other things being equal) under the following circumstances:
(1) If there is evidence of arterial obstruction and the fracture is displaced and/or angulated.
(2) If there is off-ending of the fracture.
(3) Ideally if there is less than 50% of bony contact.

11. **Indications for reduction (2):** (4) If there is backward tilting (anterior angulation) of the distal fragment by 15° or more. Note that in the normal elbow the articular surfaces of the distal humerus lie at 45° to the axis of the humerus. (The construction is shown and the actual deformity is 20° (45–25°).) Remodelling of persistent angulation is slow and may be poor, leading to loss of flexion.

12. **Indications for reduction (3):** (5) If there is lateral or medial tilting of 10° or more. Note that the normal 'carrying angle' of the elbow is about 10°. (Illus.: is a cubitus varus deformity of 17° (10 + 7°).) Cubitus varus and cubitus valgus do not remodel well, and may ultimately be associated with tardy ulnar nerve palsy.

**13. Indications for reduction (4):**
Assuming that no vascular complications are present, pure posterior displacement (1), lateral displacement (2) or medial displacement of 50% or less *may be accepted as remodelling is generally rapid and effective*. Severe torsional deformity (axial rotation) (3) should be corrected by manipulation.

**14. Manipulation techniques (1):** The arm should be manipulated under general anaesthesia. Gentle/moderate traction is applied at about 20° of flexion while an assistant applies counter-traction. This leads to disimpaction of the fracture. Some surgeons advise that this and the following stages should be carried out with the arm in supination.

**15. Manipulation (2):** Now maintaining traction and counter-traction (1) flex the elbow to 80° (2). This lifts the distal fragment thereby reducing any posterior displacement and correcting any backward tilting (anterior angulation).

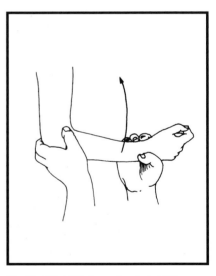

**16. Manipulation (3):** During this manoeuvre, the epiphyseal complex may be further coaxed into position by grasping it in the free hand. The thumb can be used to steady the proximal humeral shaft. Lateral displacement and torsional deformity (axial rotation) may also be corrected in this way.

**17. Fixation (1):** After reduction, the fracture must be maintained in a stable position. Flexion of the elbow stretches the triceps over the fracture, often splinting it most efficiently. *The aim should be to flex the elbow as far as the state of the circulation will permit.*

**18. Fixation (2):** Assuming that at 80° a pulse is present (if present before the manipulation it should still be there, and if absent it will have hopefully been restored) continue flexion of the elbow until the pulse disappears (due to the elbow flexure crease along with the swelling compressing the brachial artery).

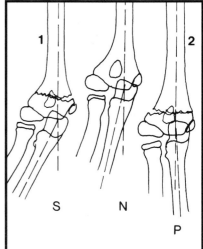

**19. Fixation (3):** Now extend the elbow slowly till the pulse just returns. *This is the position in which the arm should be maintained*. If 110–20° or more of flexion can be preserved, a sling and body bandage, well secured with adhesive strapping, may suffice for fixation.

**20. Fixation (4):** Unfortunately further extension of the elbow may be required to restore the circulation. In such cases, apply a generous layer of wool (1), followed by a long arm plaster slab (2) secured with bandages and a sling (3). *Many surgeons favour this in every case. Warning:* never apply a *complete* plaster because of the risks of swelling.

**21. Fixation (5):** While the slab is being applied, the risks of recurrence of valgus or varus deformity may be reduced by careful positioning of the forearm: viz. if there has been valgus deformity (lateral tilting, medial angulation) (1) place the arm in supination. With varus (2) place the arm in pronation. With insignificant angulation the neutral position may be employed.

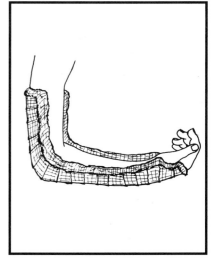

**22. Check radiographs:** Check radiographs must now be taken in two planes. (For interpretation of AP radiographs, see later.) In the lateral projection illustrated there has been a good reduction. Note how all posterior displacement has been corrected (1) and the normal angulation of the epiphyseal complex has been largely restored (2). (F = fracture line; C = capitellum; R = radial head.) If a good reduction has been achieved: (1) the anaesthetic can be discontinued; (2) the child should be admitted for overnight observation; (3) the arm should be elevated in a roller towel or similar device; (4) access should be made in the dressings for observation of the pulse and circulation in the fingers.

**23. Late development of ischaemia:** If while under observation the pulse disappears, and especially if there are other signs of ischaemia, *all* encircling bandages should be cut, and *all* wool in front of the elbow teased out. If this does not lead to improvement, the elbow should be placed in a more extended position (e.g. by cracking the slab and slackening the sling).

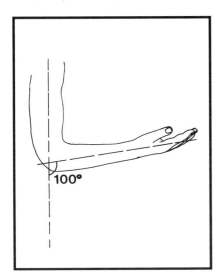

**24. Absent pulse after manipulation:**
Returning to 7.18: If after manipulation the pulse is *not* palpable, the elbow should be flexed to *not more than 100°* and maintained in that position with a sling and a back slab (applied over wool and held with a lightly applied bandage). The anaesthetic should be continued while check radiographs are taken.

**25. Radiographs (1):** If the radiographs show a poor reduction, then two further attempts at manipulation may be permitted under the same anaesthetic. The illustration shows a typical unsatisfactory lateral projection where the distal fragment is completely off-ended and also displaced proximally (compare with 133, 22).

**26. Radiographs (2):** an AP projection should also be taken and checked in every case, although errors in correcting the appearances seen in the lateral are more usual in causing circulatory impairment. As the AP view cannot be taken with the elbow straight, superimposition of the radius, ulna and humerus make interpretation difficult (see 134, 27).

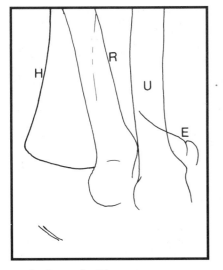

**27. Radiographs (3):** The epiphyseal complex preserves its relationship with the radius and ulna. In turn, with a good reduction, the radius and ulna regain their alignment with the humerus. Note in this unsatisfactory reduction the radius (R), ulna (U) and epiphyseal complex (E) are displaced medially in relationship to the humerus (H).

**28. Radiographs (4):** The preceding case with vascular impairment was remanipulated and the above correction obtained. This is a good reduction, and was accompanied by restoration of the pulse at the wrist, (see 134, 29 for interpretation).

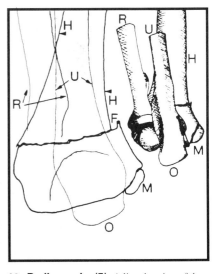

**29. Radiographs (5):** A line drawing of the preceding radiograph is shown along with a sketch of the forearm bones drawn in roughly the same position (compare also with 134, 26). R = radius, U = ulna, H humerus, F = fracture, O = olecranon, M = medial epicondyle.

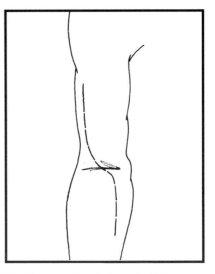

**30. Remanipulation:** If a poor reduction has been obtained and remanipulation is necessary, the preceding technique may be repeated; alternatively, while an assistant applies light traction to the forearm, the distal fragment is pushed forwards with the thumb while the fingers control the proximal fragment. Plaster fixation may be applied as described before.

**31. Absent pulse, adequate circulation:** If a good reduction has been obtained and the pulse remains absent, the circulation should be checked more critically. The use of a pulse oximeter before and after manipulation is often helpful. Clinically, if the hand is warm and pink, with good capillary return in the nails, there is no immediate indication for further intervention. *Admission, elevation and close observation for 24 hours* are essential. (Generally the pulse returns spontaneously over 2–3 days.)

**32. Absent pulse, ischaemia:** If there are incontrovertible signs of gross ischaemia, either in the face of a good reduction or a failed reduction, *exploration of the brachial artery* must now be undertaken. Exposure of the artery is straightforward. (a) A lazy S incision may be used, following the lateral edge of biceps and crossing the elbow near the fold.

**33. Exploration of brachial artery *ctd:*** (b) The skin edges are reflected and the bicipital aponeurosis (1) divided close to the tendon (2). (c) The arm is put in full pronation and the space (5) between brachioradialis laterally (3) and pronator teres medially (4) opened up with the finger tips.

**34. Exploration brachial artery *ctd:*** (d) The brachial artery (A) is found lying close to the biceps tendon. The median nerve (M) lies on its medial side. The fracture lies deep to the brachialis (B) in the floor of the wound. In some cases relief of local pressure on the vessel (e.g. from the fracture) may restore the circulation, but other measures, requiring experience in vascular surgery, may be necessary.

**35. Reduction failure with satisfactory circulation (A):** it is unwise to repeat manipulation beyond the third attempt owing to the risks of increasing swelling. In these circumstances, marked displacement (but not angulation) may be accepted, relying on later remodelling. The fracture illustrated was off-ended in the lateral: after a year, considerable remodelling has occurred, with loss of 15° only of flexion.

**36. Reduction failure (B) (1):** If displacement and angulation are outside acceptable limits, open reduction is not recommended. Instead, continuous traction may be employed (Dunlop traction). This is especially indicated where there is minimal circulatory impairment, and the elbow cannot be flexed, but brachial artery exploration is not indicated. Traction tapes are applied to the limb. W= wool: C = lightly applied crepe bandage.

**37. Reduction failure (B) (2):** The arm is abducted at the shoulder and traction of 1.5 kg applied with the elbow at 60° flexion. Counter-traction of 1 kg is applied directly with a canvas sling. After swelling subsides the situation may be re-appraised, or the traction discontinued and a plaster slab substituted at 2–3 weeks.

**38. Reduction failure (C) (1):** Reduction failure may be avoided in a number of cases if image intensification is available. With this facility the problem may often be seen to be due to excessive instability of the fracture. Under these circumstances reduction may be held by Kirschner wires inserted percutaneously. (Reduction is effected by traction as described.)

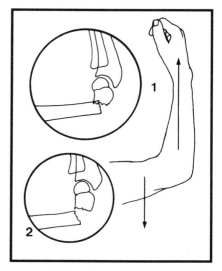

**39. Reduction failure (C) (2):** Two wires must be used, either parallel (1) or crossed (2). The wires are cut short, the ends bent (to avoid migration) and slipped under the skin. A plaster slab is used as additional support for about 4 weeks. The wires are removed at 3 weeks.

**40. The anterior (reversed) supracondylar fracture (1):** Supracondylar fractures in which the distal fragment is displaced anteriorly are comparatively uncommon. The normal angle (45°) between the epiphyseal complex and the shaft is increased. *This deformity is aggravated by flexion of the elbow.*

**41. Anterior supracondylar fracture (2):** An uncommon but related injury is the more distally situated traumatic separation of the epiphyseal complex (Salter & Harris Type 1 or 2) in which the displacement is identical. To reduce either of these injuries, traction is applied to the elbow in the flexed position (1). This disimpacts the fracture (2).

**42. Anterior supracondylar fracture (3):**
Continuing the traction (1) the elbow is slowly extended (2), reducing the angulation (3). The arm is put in a plaster back slab in a position of 10° flexion (4). *This position should not be maintained for more than 3 weeks.* At that stage the elbow should be gently flexed (usually about 70–80° can be achieved) and supported either with a sling or further slab till union.

**43. Anterior supracondylar fracture (4):**
An alternative technique is to apply wool to the limb (1) and disimpact the distal fragment by direct traction on the epiphyseal complex (2). A plaster cuff (3) is then applied by an assistant and allowed to set. Care must be taken to avoid ridging at the distal end (4).

**44. Anterior supracondylar fracture (5):**
The rest of the plaster is quickly applied, and while it is still soft flex to 110° or less and exert pressure on the distal fragment through the forearm; the position is held till the plaster has set. Check radiographs are taken and fixation continued as for a normal supracondylar fracture.

**45. Supracondylar fractures: After care (1):** Assess union at about 3–4 weeks for a child of 4 years, and about 4–5 weeks for a child of 8 by radiographs and fracture site tenderness. A further useful test is to place your thumb over the biceps tendon, and then flex and extend the elbow through a total range of 20°. Spasm of the biceps indicates that the elbow is not yet ready for mobilisation.

**46. Supracondylar fractures: After care (2):** Mobilisation may be commenced from a sling (i.e. the arm is removed from the sling for 10 minutes' active exercises three to four times per day). The sling is discarded as soon as any discomfort has settled. This procedure may also be used where there is a little residual fracture tenderness. Physiotherapy is indicated if after 2 weeks' mobilisation there is still gross restriction.

**47. Supracondylar fractures: After care (3):** The range should be recorded at every clinic attendance; physiotherapy can be safely stopped when a range of 25–120° is reached (normal 0–145°). On no account should passive movements be allowed, and *the parents* should be warned against this. If any cubitus varus or valgus is present it should be recorded and the child assessed yearly regarding deterioration and the need for corrective osteotomy.

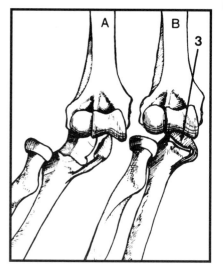

**48. Medial epicondylar injuries: Pathology (1):** The medial epicondyle (1) may be pulled off by the ulnar collateral ligament (2) when the elbow is forcibly abducted (3). It may be injured by direct violence, and possibly avulsed by sudden contraction of the forearm flexors which are attached to it (4). Suspect if there is medial bruising (5) and always test the integrity of the ulnar nerve (6).

**49. Pathology (2):** The most minor degrees of violence result in slight separation of the medial epicondylar epiphysis (1). Comparison films may be helpful in diagnosis. With greater violence the epiphysis is separated and displaced slightly in a distal direction (2). Injuries of these types may be treated by immobilisation in a long arm padded plaster for 2–3 weeks. In some cases tardy ulnar nerve palsy may occur.

**50. Pathology (3):** *The potentially most serious injury is when the medial epicondyle is trapped in the elbow joint.* This may follow dislocation of the elbow (A), which must always be accompanied by rupture of the ulnar collateral ligament or avulsion of the medial epicondyle. In the latter case, when the elbow is reduced (B), the epicondyle may be trapped in the joint (3).

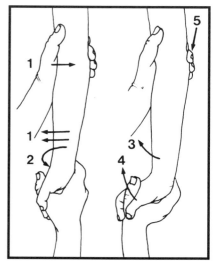

**51. Pathology (4):** A further hazard in diagnosis is when the medial epicondyle is trapped in an elbow which has been momentarily dislocated but has reduced spontaneously. *Note:* (1) If the child is over 6 years and the medial epicondylar epiphysis cannot be seen in the AP view it is probably in the joint. (2) If there is any doubt comparison films should be taken.

**52. Pathology (5):** (3) In the normal lateral projection, the medial epicondyle cannot be seen; if it can, as in the case here, it is lying in the joint. The rules are quite clear: (a) Should the medial epicondyle be visible (i.e. what is the child's age)? (b) Does it show in the AP view? (c) Is it visible in the lateral?

**53. Treatment of trapped medial epicondyle (1):** Removal by manipulation is often successful. Under general anaesthesia, increase valgus (1), supinate (2), extend elbow (3) and jerk wrist into dorsiflexion (4). A finger placed over the medial side of the elbow (5) may detect the medial epicondyle slipping out of the joint. (After care as 138, 49.)

**54. Trapped medial epicondyle (2):** If the previous method fails, the medial epicondyle may be brought out by electrically stimulating the flexor mass. General anaesthesia is required, the elbow *must* be strongly abducted and a good muscle contraction must be obtained. The necessary equipment and expertise in its use may be available through the physiotherapy department.

**55. Trapped medial epicondyle (3):** If both measures fail the medial epicondyle must be extracted through a small anteromedial incision and held in position either by a Kirschner wire (retained for 3 weeks) or soft-tissue suture.

The majority of ulnar nerve palsies found in association with medial epicondylar injuries are lesions of continuity: commencement of recovery can be expected in 3–6 weeks.

**56. Lateral epicondylar injuries in children:** The epiphysis for the lateral epicondyle is inconstant, but usually appears about 11 years, fusing with the main epiphysis 2–3 years later (1). It may, however, ossify by direct extension from the capitellum (2). Detachment may follow adduction stress; rarely it may become trapped in the joint after a dislocation. Treat as for medial epicondyle.

**57. Lateral condylar injuries (1): Pathology (1):** The common pattern of injury involves the *whole of the capitellum and nearly half the trochlea* (1). This large fragment may be displaced by the forearm extensors (2) or the lateral ligament. As the capitellar epiphysis (3) and the shaft (4) may be the only structures visible on the radiographs, *their relationship may be the only clue to injury.*

**58. Lateral condylar injuries (2): Pathology (2):** Fractures of the lateral condyle may be (1) undisplaced, (2) laterally displaced, (3) rotated.
**Treatment** *(1): Undisplaced fractures* should be treated conservatively by a long arm padded back shell and sling for 3–4 weeks. As it is important to make sure no late slip occurs *radiographs should be taken at weekly intervals.*

**59. Lateral condylar injuries (3): Treatment (2):** Where there is slight to moderate lateral shift of the complex, closed reduction may be attempted by applying local pressure (under general anaesthesia). If reduction is successful, a long arm padded back shell should be applied and retained with a sling for 3–4 weeks. Again it is vital to detect any early slipping by weekly radiographs.

**60. Lateral condylar injuries (4): Treatment (3):** Where there is lateral displacement which is unstable or late slipping occurs, Kirschner wire fixation is indicated. Where image intensification is available, it may be possible to do this without open operation, but in many cases this is necessary. Two wires must be used, followed by a plaster shell and sling. The wires may be removed after 2–3 weeks and mobilisation commenced at 4 weeks.

**61. Lateral condylar injuries: Treatment (4):** In injuries where there is rotation of the complex such as illustrated here, closed methods are unlikely to give a satisfactory reduction, so that there is risk of non-union, growth disturbance and progressive cubitus valgus. Open reduction and Kirschner wire fixation are therefore indicated. (After care as above.) (Note that if there is some uncertainty over the position or extent of the epiphyseal fragments, films taken after the injection of a radio-opaque dye into the fracture haematoma may be helpful.)

**62. Adult fractures: Supracondylar fractures (1):** In adults, the fracture line tends to lie a little more proximal than in children; comminution, obliquity or spiralling and medial or lateral tilting are common. Nevertheless, many may be treated successfully as in children by manipulation and plaster fixation; 6–8 weeks' immobilisation is usually required.

**63. Supracondylar fractures (2):** If instability is a problem, it may be possible to control the fracture with percutaneous wires (Illus.). If this fails, or if there are other factors favouring primary internal fixation (e.g. multiple injuries), then this may be carried out using a variety of techniques, e.g. (a) AO plating (cf. 142, 74); (b) twin Rush pins; (c) a single Rush pin and plaster cast. In all cases, early mobilisation is essential to minimise stiffness.

**64. Medial and lateral epicondylar fractures:** Displacement of these fractures is seldom severe and, although potential instability of the joint may be present, symptomatic treatment only is usually required. A crepe bandage applied over wool to limit swelling and a sling for 3–4 weeks is usually adequate. A short period in a long arm plaster is indicated if pain is severe.

**65. Fractures of the capitellum (1):** The cartilaginous and bony surfaces of the capitellum may be damaged by force transmitted up the radius from a fall on the outstretched hand, often in association with radial head injuries. There may be late osteochondritis dissecans and osteo-arthritis.

**Treatment:** Initially symptomatic: later, excise loose bodies and drill the capitellum to encourage revascularisation.

**66. Fractures of the capitellum (2):** A small flake may be detached from the capitellum as a result of force transmitted up the radius; it may come to lie in the front of the joint. It should be treated as a loose body and excised. This may be carried out safely through a small lateral incision (which must not extend as far as three finger breadths below the joint line to avoid damage to the posterior interosseous nerve).

**67. Fracture of the capitellum (3):** A more serious fracture involves the major portion of the anterior half of the articular surface of the capitellum. Generally the corresponding part of the trochlea is involved. Severe disability will result if this is not accurately reduced, and generally exposure through an anterior approach will be necessary. Smillie pins or a Herbert screw may be used for fixation.

**68. Fractures of the capitellum (4):** Occasionally reduction may be achieved by pressure over the fragment while traction is applied to the arm. An imperfect reduction should not be accepted. After reduction, a long arm padded plaster should be retained for approximately 5 weeks before commencement of mobilisation.

**69. Fracture of a single condyle (1):** Fracture of the lateral condyle (1) (AO = 13–B1*) or of the medial condyle (2) (AO = 13–B2) may be caused by the same mechanisms responsible for the more severe Y-fractures. Displacement may be slight or marked (3). Where there is displacement, best results are obtained by open reduction and internal fixation: this can usually be achieved using one or two cancellous lag screws (4).
*See p. 150 for summary of AO Classification of injuries in this region.*

**70. Fracture of a single condyle (2):** If displacement is minimal, as illustrated, or the patient elderly and frail, apply a long arm plaster (over wool) and a sling. The plaster may usually be discarded safely after 4–5 weeks, and mobilisation commenced from the sling. Physiotherapy may be started shortly thereafter.

**71. Intercondylar Y- or T-fractures (1):** This potentially serious injury is caused by the coronoid (1) being driven like a wedge between the two halves of the trochlea (2), often by a fall or blow on the elbow. The vertical split bifurcates (4), and with further violence the two main fragments may separate (3) (AO = 13–C1). Fragmentation (comminution) (5) is often a further problem (AO = 13–C2).

**72. Intercondylar fractures (2):** If there is no separation of the fragments the injury may be treated as for an undisplaced unicondylar fracture (141, 70). If there is separation of the fragments, and open reduction is thought inadvisable (e.g. because of the patient's age, or the impossible technical difficulty of a highly fragmented fracture), apply a long-arm plaster over wool; before this sets, apply traction, and side-to-side pressure. Remove the plaster and mobilise from a sling at an early date (e.g. 4–5 weeks).

**73. Intercondylar fractures (3):** In displaced and moderately fragmented fractures in the younger patient, open reduction should be carried out. *Approaches:* (a) through a lateral incision, (b) through a triceps splitting incision, or (c) through a chevron osteotomy of the olecranon (1) with its proximal reflection (triceps attached) (2). *Reduction:* The articular fragments should be reduced first using Kirschner wires: it may be helpful to manipulate the lateral element using a wire inserted in the retrograde fashion (a, b, c).

**74. Intercondylar fractures (4):** After reduction insert a cannulated screw (1) and compress with a cancellous lag screw (2). The articular complex may then be lined up with the shaft, and temporarily held with Kirschner wires (3). The AO Group then recommend a posterolateral 3.5 mm reconstruction plate (4), and a medial one-third tubular plate (5). Less severe fractures may be held with two cancellous screws and a single plate (6). Defects should be packed with bone grafts (7). (Repair any osteotomy as in 147, 103.) *Mobilise early.*

**75. Dislocation of the elbow (1):** Dislocation of the elbow is common in both children and adults and generally results from a fall on the outstretched hand. It is sometimes confused with a supracondylar fracture. The two may be distinguished clinically by searching for the equilateral triangle formed by the olecranon and epicondyles (1). This is undisturbed in supracondylar fractures (2) but distorted in elbow dislocations (3).

**76. Dislocation of the elbow (2):** Damage to the ulnar nerve, median nerve or brachial artery is uncommon, but nevertheless should always be sought.

A number of motor tests may be used to assess function in both nerves. *In the case of the ulnar nerve* the ability to grip a sheet of paper between the ring and little finger (1) may be used to assess good interosseous muscle function. It is important that the fingers are not allowed to flex at the MP joints. *In the case of the median nerve* contraction and power in abductor pollicis may be assessed by feeling the muscle (2) while the patient attempts to resist the thumb being pressed from a vertical position into the plane of the palm. Sensory function in the areas supplied by the median and ulnar nerves should also be quickly tested (3). *In the case of the brachial artery* the quickest assessment is of course by identification of the radial pulse (4).

**77. Radiographs:** These radiographs show a typical dislocation of the elbow. Note how the radius and ulna are displaced posteriorly and laterally relative to the humerus. This is by far the commonest displacement ('posterolateral dislocation of the elbow'). Fractures accompanying dislocation of the elbow are comparatively uncommon. Nevertheless, in adults in particular, fractures of the coronoid process and of the radial head should be looked for. In children, the epicondyles or the lateral condyle may be involved, and these fractures should be excluded *as a routine*.

**78. Treatment (1):** Reduction should be carried out under general anaesthesia. A fair amount of force is often required, although the use of a muscle relaxant will reduce this. Apply strong traction in the line of the limb, and if necessary slightly flex the elbow while maintaining traction. Success is usually accompanied with a characteristic reduction 'clunk'.

**79. Treatment (2):** If the last manoeuvre is not successful, clasp the humerus from behind and push the olecranon forwards (and medially) (1) while as assistant applies traction in moderate flexion (2). (The fingers apply counter-traction (3).) Always take check radiographs. If a good reduction has been obtained, a padded crepe bandage may be applied and worn with a sling for 2 but not more than 3 weeks (4). Alternatively, apply a plaster back slab and sling with the elbow in 90° flexion (5). Too early or too vigorous mobilisation runs the risk of myositis ossificans, and passive movements must be avoided.

**80. Late diagnosed posterior dislocation in children:** Between 3 weeks and 2 months, open reduction carries an unacceptable risk of myositis; if the dislocation is discovered within that period the injury should be treated conservatively and the elbow just mobilised. A quarter do well and need no further treatment; in the remainder (and in cases discovered later than 2 months) operative reduction should be attempted.

**81. Associated injuries (1):** In children, the medial epicondylar epiphysis may be detached. *On reduction of the elbow*, it will generally be restored to an acceptable position (1 or 2 as in 138, 49) (2 Illus.). A plaster slab and a sling are advised for 4 weeks. (2) *The medial epicondyle may be retained in the joint:* this must always be excluded (see 138, 48 et seq.).

**82. Associated injuries (3): Lateral condylar injury:** Note the following points. (a) The capitellar epiphysis (along with half the cartilaginous trochlea) has been carried medially by the radius, and is slightly rotated. (b) The medial epicondylar epiphysis has just appeared and is not displaced. (c) The *medial* dislocation of the elbow is unusual.

**83. Associated injuries: Lateral condylar injuries** *ctd.* The preceding injury was treated by manipulative reduction; the lateral condylar complex remained displaced. (Reduction could be achieved by firm local pressure, but displacement occurred in this unstable injury as soon as pressure was released.)

**84. Associated injuries: Lateral condylar injuries** *ctd.* Open reduction was therefore carried out and the condylar mass held in position with two Kirschner wires. Note how these pass through the cartilaginous epicondylar region. Note the small bone fragment from the shaft (Salter/Harris Type 2 injury). Fixation was complemented by a long arm plaster back shell for 4 weeks.

**85. Associated injuries (4): Fracture of the coronoid:** Coronoid fractures can be classified into three types: (i) simple avulsions; (ii) fractures involving half or less of the coronoid; (iii) fractures involving more than half. Groups (i) and (ii) may be treated conservatively, commencing mobilisation before 3 weeks. Group (iii) injuries may be internally fixed to reduce the risks of recurrent dislocation. *Established recurrent dislocation* (rare) may be treated by bone block reconstruction of the coronoid and/or repair of the capsule and medial ligament.

**86. Associated injuries (5): Fracture of the radial head:** (a) If there is a highly comminuted fracture of the radial head (Illus.) reduce the elbow dislocation and *delay excision of the radial head for at least 4–8 weeks* to lessen the risks of myositis ossificans. (b) Minor fractures of the radial head should not affect treatment. (c) Fracture of the radial neck: reduce the elbow and proceed as for this injury (149, 115).

**87. Anterior dislocation of the elbow (1):** This is an uncommon injury, but may follow a fall on the elbow which results in the forearm bones being pushed forwards. For dislocation to occur, the olecranon must fracture, and this becomes a potentially very unstable injury (see also 162, 40).

**88. Anterior dislocation (2):** The elbow may be reduced by applying traction and extending the joint. If the reduction is stable, it may then be treated by plaster fixation for a limited period in extension as in an anterior supracondylar fracture. Nevertheless, there is appreciable risk of late subluxation and difficulty in elbow mobilisation so that, on the whole, internal fixation is recommended for this injury (Illus. tension band wiring and a Rush pin).

**89. Anterior dislocation (3):** A more complex form of anterior dislocation is seen in the side swipe injury ('baby car fracture'). This occurs when a driver rests his elbow on his car's window ledge, and he is struck by a passing vehicle. Typically the elements of this injury include (1) anterior dislocation of the elbow with fractures of (2) the olecranon (3), the humerus (4), the ulna and sometimes (5) the radius.

**90. Anterior dislocation (4):** It is vital to reduce the dislocation immediately, and this may be held by immediate internal fixation (Illus.) or plaster fixation in extension for 2–3 weeks prior to delayed internal fixation of the olecranon. The other injuries may be treated with less urgency conservatively or surgically. It is not often possible or wise to attempt immediate fixation of all the elements of this severe injury.

**91. Isolated dislocation of the ulna:** Dislocation of the ulna may occur in association with a fracture of the radial shaft. As such fractures may be quite distal, it is important that adequate radiographs of the forearm are taken. This double injury may be treated by manipulative reduction of the elbow followed by a long arm plaster until union of the radius (assuming a satisfactory reduction). Alternatively, internal fixation of the radius may permit earlier mobilisation.

**92. Isolated dislocation of the radius:** Lateral, anterior or posterior dislocation of the proximal end of the radius is almost invariably part of a Monteggia lesion (but see also forearm injuries) sometimes concealed because the ulnar fracture is of greenstick pattern (Illus.). Great care must be taken in the assessment and treatment of these injuries which is dealt with separately (See Monteggia fracture dislocation p. 162.)

**93. Pulled elbow (1):** This condition is due to the radial head stretching the orbicular (annular) ligament and slipping out from under its cover. It occurs in children in the 2–6 age group, and is normally caused by a parent suddenly pulling on the child's arm (e.g. to prevent it running on to a road). It is also said to occur in wrestlers.

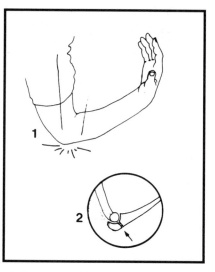

**94. Pulled elbow (2): Diagnosis:** In addition to having the appropriate history of sudden traction on the arm, the child will be found to be fretful. There is tenderness over the lateral aspect of the joint (1) and supination is limited (2). Radiographs are usually normal, there being seldom any detectable increase in the radiohumeral joint space even with comparison films.

**95. Pulled elbow (3): Treatment:** In most cases reduction can be achieved by either (a) placing the wrist in full radial deviation (1) and forcibly supinating the arm (2) or (b) rapidly alternately pronating and supinating the forearm (3).

If these measures fail, the arm should be rested in a sling, when spontaneous reduction usually occurs within 48 hours.

**96. Fractures of the olecranon (1):** The olecranon may be fractured as a result of a fall on the point of the elbow (1). Such fractures may be displaced as a result of triceps contraction (2). The olecranon may also be fractured as a direct result of triceps contraction.

**97. Fracture of the olecranon (2):** Diagnosis is usually straightforward, but beware of the following fallacies: (1) the normal epiphyseal line, (2) duplication of the normal line due to obliquity of the projection, (3) normal bifid olecranon epiphysis (the epiphyses appear between the ages of 8 and 11 and fuse at 14 years), (4) patella cubiti due to ossification in the triceps tendon (note rounded edges).

**98. Treatment (1):** (A) *If the fracture is hair-line and undisplaced,* it may be treated by *immobilisation of the arm in a long arm plaster* (3–4 weeks in a child, 6–8 weeks in an adult). Note in the radiograph the three lines running through the olecranon: the most distal is a fracture, the middle the epiphyseal line, the most proximal either a bifid epiphysis or a fracture of the epiphysis (differentiate by looking for tenderness).

**99. Treatment (2):** (B) If the fracture line is pronounced but still undisplaced, it may be treated in the same way, but radiographs should be taken at weekly intervals during the first 3 weeks in case of (unlikely) late displacement.

(C) Minor epiphyseal separations may also be treated conservatively in a similar manner.

(D) Slight to moderate displacement may be accepted in the frail elderly.

100. **Treatment (3):** (E) In the young adult, where the olecranon fragment is small (a third or less of the articular surface) and significantly displaced (by triceps pull) surgical excision gives excellent results. *Operation:* The operation is performed under a general anaesthetic using a pneumatic tourniquet to obtain a clear bloodless field. The fragment is exposed through a vertical posterior incision and excised. The tear in the triceps insertion is then carefully repaired with horizontal mattress sutures and the wound closed in layers. A pressure bandage (crepe over wool) and a collar and cuff sling are applied (or a plaster back shell and sling may be employed). The elbow may be mobilised after 2 weeks.

101. **Treatment (4):** If there is any doubt regarding the stability of the elbow (i.e. if the olecranon fragment is fairly substantial) this should be tested on the table by attempting to produce an anterior dislocation with the elbow flexed at 90°. If the elbow can in any way be subluxed, the olecranon must be retained.

102. **Treatment (5):** (F) If the olecranon fragment is substantial it must be reduced and held by some form of internal fixation. The methods available include:
(1) a Zuelzer hooked plate and screws.
(2) a Croll olecranon screw, (3) a lag screw (an AO cancellous screw may be used), (4) contoured plating. During the final tightening of a Croll or lag screw it is important to check that elbow movements are not prevented by the fracture components binding like calliper brakes.

103. **Treatment (6):** (5) Tension band wiring: the Kirschner wires control alignment and rotation; the stainless steel wire when twisted compresses the fragments together. The ends of the Kirschner wires are bent over and hammered home. A Rush pin may be used instead. The security of fixation dictates the need for any external fixation and when mobilisation may be safely commenced.

104. **Fractures of the radial head: Mechanics of injury (1):** Although the radial head may be fractured by direct violence, such as a fall or blow on the side of the elbow, injury frequently results from indirect violence (illus.) A fall on the outstretched hand results in force being transmitted up the radius, with the radial head striking the capitellum (capitulum).

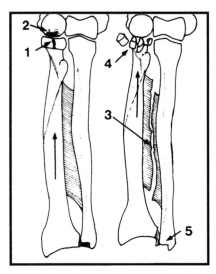

**105. Mechanics of injury (2):** The radial head fractures (1) but may also damage the articular surface of the capitellum (2), prolonging recovery. In some cases, where violence is severe, the interosseous membrane tears (3), severe comminution of the head occurs (4) and there is *subluxation of the distal end of the ulna* (5) due to proximal migration of the radial shaft. (Essex–Lopresti fracture-dislocation.)

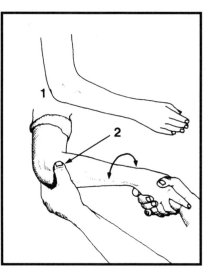

**106. Diagnosis (1):** There is complaint of pain in the elbow and there may be local bruising and swelling (1). In *minor fractures*, tenderness may not be apparent until the damaged portion of the head is rotated under the examining thumb (gently pronate and supinate while palpating the radial head) (2). The range of pronation and supination is often full, but elbow *extension* is usually restricted.

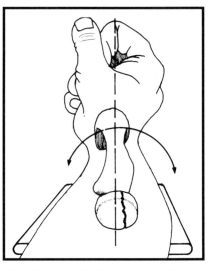

**107. Diagnosis (2): Radiographs:** Most radial head fractures will show in the standard lateral and (supination) AP projections, but if there is clinical evidence of fracture and negative radiographs, *additional* AF projections should be taken in the midprone and full pronation positions, so that all portions of the radial head will be visualised in profile.

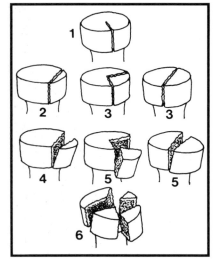

**108. Diagnosis (3):** Assess the type and severity of the fracture from the radiographs: (1) hairline, (2) undisplaced marginal, (3) undisplaced segmental (2 types), (4) displaced marginal, (5) displaced segmental, (6) comminuted.

Always examine the forearm and wrist to exclude an Essex–Lopresti fracture-dislocation.

**109. Treatment (1):** Non-displaced fractures (1–3) should be treated with a light compression bandage and a sling before mobilisation from the sling is commenced after 2–3 weeks. The sling alone may be worn for a further 2 weeks. If pain is very severe initially, a plaster back slab may be used. An excellent outcome is usual, but note that many months may elapse before full *extension* is regained.

**110. Treatment (2):** Severely comminuted fractures (6) should be treated by immediate excision of the radial head. This may be carried out through a lateral incision (see 141, 66) with care to avoid the posterior interosseous nerve. All fragments must be removed. The arm is then rested in a sling for 2–3 weeks before mobilisation. If a primary silastic prosthetic replacement is carried out, mobilisation may be commenced earlier.

**111. Treatment (3):** Sometimes excision of the radial head is followed by proximal drift of the radius (1) so that the distal end of the ulna becomes prominent and painful (2). This in turn may be treated by excision of the distal end of the ulna, albeit with some weakening of the grip. Proximal drift is a feature of the Essex–Lopresti lesion, and may be minimised by delaying radial head excision for 6 weeks. In either case, a silastic prosthetic replacement is sometimes undertaken as a prophylaxis.

**112. Treatment (4):** Displaced marginal and segmental fractures (4 and 5) should be treated conservatively and reassessed after 2–3 months. If pronation, supination and extension are severely restricted, *late excision* of the radial head should be considered. *Note well:* In any case of fracture, excision of the radial head should be performed *either* within the first 48 hours *or* after union (between carries the risk of myositis ossificans). *Late diagnosed injuries should be left till union.*

**113. Fractures of the radial neck (1):** The axis of rotation of the radio-ulnar joints passes through the centre of the radial head (1) and the attachment of the triangular fibrocartilage (2). The axis passes through the centre of the neck (3) and lies at right angles to the plane of the head. Fractures through the neck (4) have the potential to disturb this relationship between the head and the neck.

**114. Fractures of the radial neck (2):** Fractures of the radial neck may result from the same mechanisms as those causing fractures of the radial head, and diagnosis is also similar. Patterns: The fractures may be hair-line and undisplaced (1) or result in slight (2) or gross tilting (3). In children, the epiphysis of the head may be completely separated and widely displaced (4).

**115. Treatment (1):** (a) With slight or no tilting (1 and 2) and up to 30° in children treat conservatively (as 148, 109). (b) With marked tilting (3) (20° or more in adults) manipulate. Do so by applying traction and gently pronate and supinate, feeling for the prominent part of the radial head to present; then apply pressure when the head is at its zenith. (Thereafter treat as 148, 109) Open reduction is indicated if closed methods fail.

**116. Treatment (2):** (c) Where there is gross epiphyseal displacement, operative reduction is indicated. On reduction, the fragments may be found to lock in a stable position. If not, a Kirschner wire may be used for 2–3 weeks to achieve stability. *Note:* In some cases of severe tilting it is possible to obtain a reduction by inserting a temporary percutaneous wire into the radial head and levering it back into position under intensifier control.

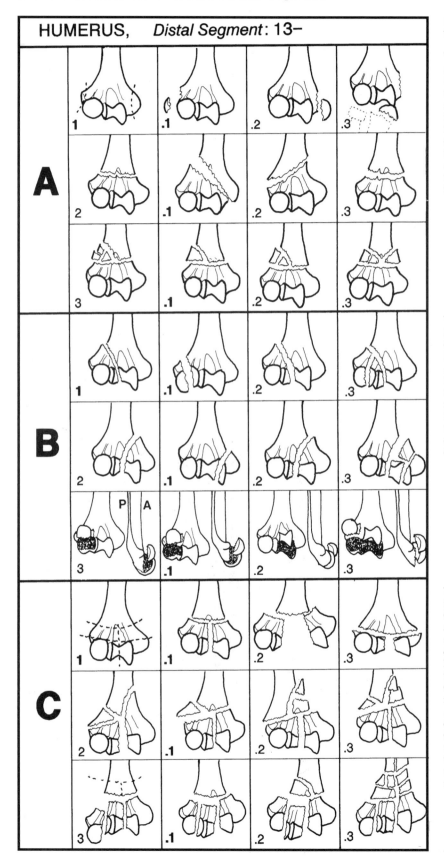

**117. AO Classification of Fractures of the Humerus, Distal Segment (13–):**

**Type A** fractures are totally extra-articular.
A1 = Avulsion fracture (of apophysis): .1 lateral; .2 medial; .3 medial, with the fragment trapped in the joint.
A2 = Simple metaphyseal (supracondylar fracture): .1 with the proximal part of the fracture line lying lateral; .2 with proximal part of the fracture line lying medial; .3 with the fracture line lying transverse.
A3 = Multifragmented metaphyseal; .1 with an unbroken wedge; .2 with the wedge fragment fractured; .3 complex.

**Type B** fractures are partially articular.
B1 = Lateral sagittal (i.e. generally most obvious in the AP radiographic projection): .1 involving the capitellum; .2 simple trochlear; .3 multifragmentary trochlear.
B2 = Medial sagittal: .1 medial side of the trochlea; .2 through the trochlear notch; .3 multifragmentary trochlear.
B3 = Frontal (i.e. generally most obvious in the lateral radiographic projection): .1 of the capitellum; .2 of the trochlea; .3 of both the capitellum and the trochlea.

**Type C** fractures are complete articular fractures, and are multifragmentary.
C1 = Simple fractures of both the epiphysis and the metaphysis (T- and Y-fractures): .1 slight displacement only; .2 with marked displacement; .3 T-fractures with the horizontal limb distally placed so that it is in the epiphysis.
C2 = Simple fracture of the epiphysis, multifragmentary fracture of the metaphysis: .1 wedge intact; .2 wedge fractured; .3 complex.
C3 = Multifragmentary epiphyseal fracture with a simple or multi fragmentary fracture of the metaphysis; .1 metaphysis simple; .2 wedge fracture of the metaphysis; .3 complex metaphyseal fracture.

RADIUS/ULNA, *Proximal Segment*: 21–

118. **AO Classification of Fractures of the Radius/Ulna, Proximal Segment (21–):**

**Type A** fractures are extra-articular.
A1 = Fracture of the ulna only: .1 Avulsion of the triceps insertion (olecranon); .2 simple, of the metaphysis; .3 multifragmentary of the metaphysis.
A2 = Fracture of the radius only: .1 avulsion of the biceps insertion (radial tuberosity); .2 simple fracture of the neck; .3 multifragmentary of the neck.
A3 = Fracture of both the radius and ulna; .1 both simple; .2 one simple and the other multifragmentary; .3 both multifragmentary.

**Type B** fractures are partial articular fractures.
B1 = Articular fracture of the ulna with the radius intact: .1 unifocal, of the olecranon or coronoid; .2 bifocal (olecranon and coronoid) — both simple; .3 bifocal multifragmentary.
B2 = Articular fracture of the radius with the ulna intact: .1 simple fracture of the radial head; .2 multifragmentary fracture of the radial head without depression; .3 depressed multifragmentary fracture of the radial head.
B3 = Articular fracture of one bone, with an extra-articular fracture of the other: .1 simple articular fracture of the ulna; .2 simple articular fracture of the radius; .3 multifragmentary articular fracture of either bone.

**Type C** fractures are complete articular fractures.
C1 = Simple articular fractures of both bones: .1 head of radius and olecranon; .2 head of radius and coronoid. There is no third subgroup here.
C2 = Articular fractures of both bones, one simple and the other multifragmentary: .1 radial head simple, olecranon multifragmentary; .2 olecranon simple, radial head multifragmentary; .3 coronoid simple, radial head multifragmentary.
C3 = 3 both bones multifragmentary; .1 three fragments in each bone; .2 more than three fragments in the ulna; .3 more than three fragments in the radius.

119. Diagnose and suggest treatment. (As an additional exercise you might like to classify this and all the following radiographs using the AO Classification.)

120. What is this injury? Comment on the position.

121. Diagnose and suggest treatment.

122. Comment on this AP radiograph of the elbow. What force has been responsible for the injury?

123. Comment on this supracondylar fracture which has been manipulated and put in plaster.

124. What is this fracture? What complication has occurred?

125. What is this injury? How should it be treated?

126. What does this radiograph show? What treatment will probably be required?

127. What does this radiograph show?

128. What fracture is present? How should this be treated?

129. How would you treat this injury?

119. The radiographs show an undisplaced supracondylar fracture of the humerus in a child. Assuming there were no circulatory problems, a collar and cuff sling under the clothes should suffice for initial treatment. AO = 13–A2.3.

120. Y-fracture of the humerus. There is considerable separation of the two distal components, and open reduction and internal fixation should be considered unless the patient is particularly frail (when repeat manipulation with side-to-side compression may be undertaken). 13–C2.1.

121. Dislocation of the elbow with fracture of the olecranon. The elbow should be reduced and check radiographs taken. Moderate residual displacement of the olecranon should be accepted and it is unlikely that open reduction would be required. Note that the ossification centres for the olecranon have not yet appeared and this really represents a Salter/ Harris Type 2 injury. AO = 21–B1.1.

122. There is a double injury—avulsion of the medial epicondyle and fracture of the radial neck, almost certainly both due to an abduction (valgus) injury. Humerus: AO = 13–A1.2; radius: AO = 21–A2.2.

123. This has been an anterior supracondylar fracture and the reduction is unacceptable. AO = 13–A2.3.

124. Fracture of the lateral condyle with non-union. AO = 13–B1.1.

125. Dislocation of the elbow with highly comminuted fracture of the radial head. Treat by reduction and immediate excision of the radial head, with or without prosthetic replacement. AO = 21–B2.3.

126. Displaced fracture of the capitellum. Open reduction with Kirschner wire or Herbert screw fixation will probably be required. AO = 13–B3.1.

127. A displaced fracture of the head of the radius in a child. Manipulative reduction should be attempted first. AO = 21–A2.2.

128. Undisplaced fracture of the distal humerus involving the elbow; more stress would probably have produced a Y-fracture. Treat by rest in a sling and early mobilisation. AO = 13–B2.2.

129. Undisplaced fracture of the radial head: treat by crepe bandaging and rest in a sling. Mobilise after 2 weeks. AO = 21–B2.1.

# 8. Injuries to the forearm bones

1. **Anatomical features:** The radius and ulna are bound together by (1) the annular (orbicular) ligament, (2) the interosseous membrane, (3) the radio-ulnar ligaments and the triangular fibro-cartilage. This gives the radius and ulna some of the features of (4) a bundle of sticks and (5) a linked parallelogram.

2. **Direct violence:** With direct violence it is possible to fracture either of the forearm bones in isolation. These injuries are comparatively uncommon, but do occur, especially in the ulna when in a fall the shaft strikes a hard edge. They may also occur when the ulna is struck by a weapon as the victim attempts to protect his head with his arms.

3. **Indirect violence:** More commonly the forearm is injured as the result of indirect violence, such as a fall on the back or the front of the outstretched hand. The force of impact on the hand stresses the forearm bones: the most common occurrence is for both to fracture.

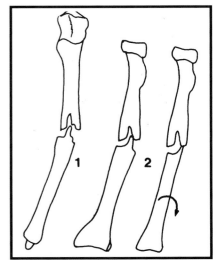

4. **Fracture dislocations (1):** If *one* forearm bone is seen to be fractured and angled, it has inevitably become relatively shorter (1). If its attachments to the wrist and humerus are intact, the other forearm bone *must* be dislocated. The commonest fracture–dislocation of this type is a fracture of the ulna with a dislocation of the radial head. (Monteggia injury) (2).

5. **Fracture dislocation (2):** The same pattern of injury occurs in the Galeazzi fracture–dislocation when a dislocation of the distal ulna accompanies a shaft fracture of the radius. *Never accept a single forearm bone fracture as an entity until a Monteggia or Galeazzi injury has been eliminated.*

6. **Axial rotation (1):** In any forearm injury, when the ulna fractures it may angulate or displace like any other bone (1). When the radius fractures, however, *in addition* to angulation one fragment may rotate relative to the other (axial rotation) (2).

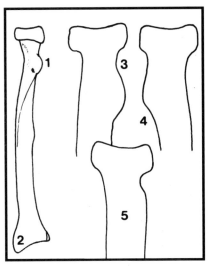

7. **Axial rotation (2):** Axial rotation of the ulna is rare, but always check to see that it is not present. To do so, note that in the lateral projection the olecranon (1), coronoid (2) and styloid process (3) should be clearly visible. This relationship is lost in the presence of axial rotation (4).

8. **Axial rotation (3):** In the case of the radius, note any discrepancy in the widths of the fragments at fracture level. A difference as illustrated indicates the presence of axial rotation.

9. **Axial rotation (4):** Note also the normal relationship between the radial tubercle (1) and the styloid process (2) in this AP view of the radius in full supination. In *full supination* the radial tubercle lies *medially* (3). In *pronation* it lies *laterally* (4). In the mid position it is concealed (5). The position of the radial styloid should always correspond.

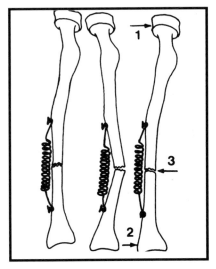

10. **Axial rotation (5): Forces responsible (a):** In all radial shaft fractures, pronator quadratus tends to pronate the distal fragment (1). In all upper (proximal) third fractures, pronator teres helps to pronate the distal fragment (2), assisting pronator quadratus in this movement.

11. **Axial rotation (6): Forces responsible (b):** In upper third fractures, the proximal fragment is fully supinated by biceps (3) while the distal fragment is fully pronated by pronators teres and quadratus (1, 2), (i.e. there is a maximal tendency to axial rotation). In fractures distal to the mid third, biceps is opposed, so the proximal fragment tends to lie in the mid position.

12. **Fracture slipping (1): Greenstick fractures:** In children's greenstick fractures any intact periosteum on the original concave surface of the fracture exerts a constant, springy force which may cause recurrence of angulation if the plaster slackens, impairing three-point fixation. *Frequent check films may be essential in any conservatively treated fracture.*

25. **Treatment (9):** In the unstable injury, check the plaster and the position of the fracture at weekly intervals for 3–4 weeks; if satisfactory, the sling may then be discarded. The plaster is maintained till union (usually after a further 3–4 weeks in a child of 10 years, and a further 1–2 weeks in a child of 4). In stable injuries, fortnightly checks will usually suffice. Mobilisation may be commenced from a sling.

26. **Management of late angulation (1):** (Detected by progress radiographs) (1) Slight angulation of up to 10° may be accepted, especially under the age of 10, but a slack plaster must be changed to prevent *further* angulation. (2) Where angulation is more severe and has been detected before callus has appeared (Illus.) the plaster should be changed under general anaesthesia and the angulation corrected by manipulation.

27. **Management of late angulation (2):** (3) In a young child, if callus has appeared, accept any angulation unless gross (20° or more). (4) In the older child, say 10 years or over, if angulation is marked remanipulation should be considered even in the presence of callus (Illus.), as the powers of remodelling are less good. Union after remanipulation is usually rapid.

28. **Adult fractures:** In the adult displacement is often quite marked, with loss of bony contact between one (Illus.) or both forearm bones. Rotational deformities are a frequent occurrence, and closed reduction is often difficult or impossible to achieve. Even if an acceptable position can be obtained, and a cast successfully applied, late slipping of the fracture is extremely common and difficult to treat.

29. **Adult fractures** *ctd:* The correct treatment for displaced fractures of the forearm bones in the fit adult is open reduction and internal fixation, plating of both bones through separate incisions generally giving very satisfactory results. When rigid fixation has been obtained (e.g. by the use of AO dynamic compression plates) early mobilisation and return of movements can usually be guaranteed, but note that the plates should be retained for not less than 21 months to lessen the risks of re-fracture.

30. **Treatment (1):** The operation is performed under a tourniquet (1). The ulna is subcutaneous along its posterior border; a longitudinal posterior incision, followed by exposure and cleaning of the bone ends, usually permits easy reduction (2). Plating is usually carried out to stabilise the fracture; intramedullary nailing may not always control any (slight) tendency to axial rotation.

**19. Treatment (4): Displaced fractures:** When the fracture is displaced, axial rotation of the fragments should be looked for and the appropriate position in the pronation/ supination range evaluated. The forearm is then placed in that position, and strong traction is applied for a quarter of a minute or so, with the patient well relaxed under a general anaesthetic. The elbow is flexed at a right angle for counter-traction.

**20. Treatment (5): Displaced fractures ctd.:** Assessment of reduction is difficult, but often residual displacement may be detected by feeling the subcutaneous surface of the ulna in the region of the fracture. In the difficult case it is sometimes possible to gain bony apposition by applying traction and *increasing* the deformity before finally correcting it. Only rarely is open reduction and internal fixation indicated.

**21. Treatment (6): Fixation:** To lessen the risks of ischaemia apply a back shell only, maintaining traction while this is done. Wool (1) is followed by the shell (2), held by cotton bandages. Just before the plaster sets give a final moulding (e.g. 3—post-angulation fracture). Review the check radiographs before withdrawing the anaesthetic. (Note that some proximal third fractures in children are only stable with the elbow in extension, and this position can be maintained for 5 weeks with relative safety.)

**22. Radiographs:** (1) Persistent displacement without angulation may be readily accepted. (2) Complete off-ending without angulation: remanipulate but accept if no improvement can be gained. Careful surveillance to detect early angulation is essential. (3) Slight angulation (10° or less) while undesirable *will* correct with remodelling in the younger child, and should be accepted. Marked angulation requires remanipulation.

**23. Treatment (7):** A broad arm sling, keeping the arm well elevated, should be employed, and the fingers exposed. If there is much swelling, or the reduction has been difficult, the patient should be admitted for elevation of the arm and circulatory observation: otherwise the child must be seen within 24 hours of the application of the plaster and the parents given the usual warnings.

**24. Treatment (8):** On review, the fingers should be checked for swelling, colour and active movements. If there is some doubt, slowly and gently extend the fingers—if this produces excessive pain, it is suggestive of ischaemia. If ischaemia is present, the encircling bandages must be split and the situation carefully re-assessed after a short interval. If the circulation is perfect, the plaster may be completed.

**25. Treatment (9):** In the unstable injury, check the plaster and the position of the fracture at weekly intervals for 3–4 weeks; if satisfactory, the sling may then be discarded. The plaster is maintained till union (usually after a further 3–4 weeks in a child of 10 years, and a further 1–2 weeks in a child of 4). In stable injuries, fortnightly checks will usually suffice. Mobilisation may be commenced from a sling.

**26. Management of late angulation (1):** (Detected by progress radiographs) (1) Slight angulation of up to 10° may be accepted, especially under the age of 10, but a slack plaster must be changed to prevent *further* angulation. (2) Where angulation is more severe and has been detected before callus has appeared (Illus.) the plaster should be changed under general anaesthesia and the angulation corrected by manipulation.

**27. Management of late angulation (2):** (3) In a young child, if callus has appeared, accept any angulation unless gross (20° or more). (4) In the older child, say 10 years or over, if angulation is marked remanipulation should be considered even in the presence of callus (Illus.), as the powers of remodelling are less good. Union after remanipulation is usually rapid.

**28. Adult fractures:** In the adult displacement is often quite marked, with loss of bony contact between one (Illus.) or both forearm bones. Rotational deformities are a frequent occurrence, and closed reduction is often difficult or impossible to achieve. Even if an acceptable position can be obtained, and a cast successfully applied, late slipping of the fracture is extremely common and difficult to treat.

**29. Adult fractures *ctd:*** The correct treatment for displaced fractures of the forearm bones in the fit adult is open reduction and internal fixation, plating of both bones through separate incisions generally giving very satisfactory results. When rigid fixation has been obtained (e.g. by the use of AO dynamic compression plates) early mobilisation and return of movements can usually be guaranteed, but note that the plates should be retained for not less than 21 months to lessen the risks of re-fracture.

**30. Treatment (1):** The operation is performed under a tourniquet (1). The ulna is subcutaneous along its posterior border; a longitudinal posterior incision, followed by exposure and cleaning of the bone ends, usually permits easy reduction (2). Plating is usually carried out to stabilise the fracture; intramedullary nailing may not always control any (slight) tendency to axial rotation.

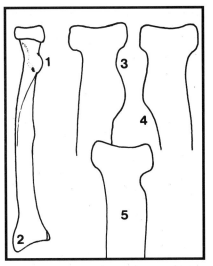

**7. Axial rotation (2):** Axial rotation of the ulna is rare, but always check to see that it is not present. To do so, note that in the lateral projection the olecranon (1), coronoid (2) and styloid process (3) should be clearly visible. This relationship is lost in the presence of axial rotation (4).

**8. Axial rotation (3):** In the case of the radius, note any discrepancy in the widths of the fragments at fracture level. A difference as illustrated indicates the presence of axial rotation.

**9. Axial rotation (4):** Note also the normal relationship between the radial tubercle (1) and the styloid process (2) in this AP view of the radius in full supination. In *full supination* the radial tubercle lies *medially* (3). In *pronation* it lies *laterally* (4). In the mid position it is concealed (5). The position of the radial styloid should always correspond.

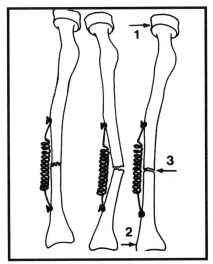

**10. Axial rotation (5): Forces responsible (a):** In all radial shaft fractures, pronator quadratus tends to pronate the distal fragment (1). In all upper (proximal) third fractures, pronator teres helps to pronate the distal fragment (2), assisting pronator quadratus in this movement.

**11. Axial rotation (6): Forces responsible (b):** In upper third fractures, the proximal fragment is fully supinated by biceps (3) while the distal fragment is fully pronated by pronators teres and quadratus (1, 2), (i.e. there is a maximal tendency to axial rotation). In fractures distal to the mid third, biceps is opposed, so the proximal fragment tends to lie in the mid position.

**12. Fracture slipping (1): Greenstick fractures:** In children's greenstick fractures any intact periosteum on the original concave surface of the fracture exerts a constant, springy force which may cause recurrence of angulation if the plaster slackens, impairing three-point fixation. *Frequent check films may be essential in any conservatively treated fracture.*

13. **Fracture slipping (2):** Another contributory cause of fracture slipping is when muscle wasting occurs in a patient in a full arm plaster wearing a collar and cuff sling. Loss of brachialis and brachio-radialis bulk leads to plaster slackening and angulatory deformity. (*Note*: soft tissue shadow 160, 26) *Patients with conservatively treated fractures should be given broad arm slings.*

14. **Fracture of both bones of the forearm in children: Patterns (1):** Most fractures are greenstick in pattern as illustrated. The radiograph shows fractures of the radius and ulna in the middle thirds. The distal fragments are tilted anteriorly (posterior angulation) but there is no displacement. An extensive, intact periosteal hinge can be assumed and reduction of such a fracture involves correction of the angulation only.

15. **Patterns (2):** When there is off-ending of one or both bones there is potential instability. Shortening and angulation are more likely, and axial rotation may occur; reduction may therefore be more difficult.

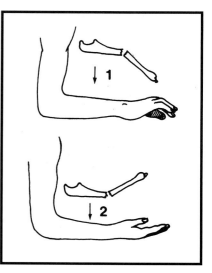

16. **Treatment (1):** In the undisplaced angulated greenstick fracture, the child should be given a general anaesthetic and the angulation corrected. One hand applies a little traction and the corrective force, while the other acts as a fulcrum, under the fracture.

17. **Treatment (2):** If the fracture is overcorrected, the periosteum on the initially concave side of the fracture will be felt to snap. This will immediately give the fracture more mobility: this has the advantage of reducing the risks of late angulation, but has the disadvantage of requiring greater care with respect to the initial positioning in plaster.

18. **Treatment (3):** In the undisplaced greenstick fracture where there is no axial rotation (torsional deformity) of any of the fragments, the position of the forearm is important in preventing re-angulation while in plaster. *Fractures with posterior tilting* (anterior angulation) (1) should be placed in full pronation. *The commonest fractures with anterior tilting* (posterior angulation) (2) should be placed in full supination.

31. **Treatment (2):** Unless the radial fracture is in the distal third, a formal (Henry) exposure is required to avoid damage to the posterior interosseous nerve (1). The biceps tendon (2) is followed down to the tubercle, and the plane between the supinator (3) and the pronator teres (4) located. The supinator is reflected laterally (5) carrying the nerve away from danger. The rest of the shaft may then be exposed safely for reduction and plating.

32. **Treatment (3):** Postoperatively, if the fixation is not rigid (A), a cast may be used until there is reasonable callus formation round both fractures (often about 10 weeks); change the cast and remove the sutures at 3 weeks. With better fixation (B), after few days with a crepe support the arm may be mobilised fully and then a cast provided for a short period after discharge from hospital. *If the internal fixation is rigid, no external support may be necessary and the arm can be fully mobilised from the start.*

33. **Treatment (4):** It is reasonable to treat fractures of the forearm bones in the adult conservatively (Illus.): (a) if the fractures are undisplaced, (b) in the elderly, or in the patient suffering from multiple injuries where the duration of anaesthesia required for open reduction and internal fixation is considered hazardous. If manipulation is required, proceed as 159, 19, with attention to axial rotation.

34. **Treatment (5):** If internal fixation is not employed, the following precautions must be taken. (1) The plaster should be checked weekly for slackness, and changed if necessary. (A complete plaster, applied over wool, should be used in an adult.) (2) Only a broad arm sling should be used. (3) Weekly radiographs are necessary to detect and allow correction of early slipping.

35. **Isolated fracture of the ulna (1):** This injury may result from direct violence (e.g. in warding off a blow from a stick or falling object, or by striking the arm against the sharp edge of, for example, a machine or a step). In all cases, however, the whole of the radial shaft should be visualised to exclude in particular an associated dislocation of the radial head.

36. **Isolated fracture of the ulna (2):** Treatment: Displacement is generally slight, and if this is the case a long arm plaster should be applied with the hand in mid pronation (1). Beware of late slipping. The plaster is retained until union is advancing (usually about 8 weeks). If angulation is marked, then open reduction and internal fixation will have to be considered (2).

**37. The Monteggia fracture–dislocation and related injuries: Mechanisms (1):** Severe angulation of a forearm bone is normally accompanied by fracture or dislocation of the other (see 156, 4). In the Monteggia fracture–dislocation, fracture of the ulna is associated with dislocation of the radial head. The most easily understood mechanism is when a violent fall or blow on the arm fractures the ulna and displaces the radial head anteriorly.

**38. Mechanisms (2):** More commonly the injury results from forced pronation A fall on the outstretched, fully pronated arm (1) is followed by further pronation as the trunk continues to turn over the fixed hand (2). The radius is forced against the ulna, fracturing it (3) and in turn is levered away from the capitellum (4). Rarely the radial head may dislocate without damage to the ulna; *supination* of the arm is needed for reduction.

**39. Patterns (1):** (1) The radial head may dislocate backwards (note that in the normal elbow a line through the axis of the radius cuts the centre of the spherical capitellum), with fracture and posterior angulation of the ulna (posterior Monteggia); or the radial head may dislocate anteriorly, with anterior angulation of the ulna (anterior Monteggia) (2) or (3) the radial head may dislocate laterally, with lateral angulation of the ulna (lateral Monteggia).

**40. Patterns (2):** (4) The radial head may dislocate anteriorly and be as associated with a fracture of the olecranon (Hume fracture). (5) Greenstick fracture of the ulna, often difficult to detect, partly accounts for the fact that Monteggia lesions are frequently overlooked in children. *Always* check the position or the radial head in both views, and *always* look for distortion and kinking of the ulna.

**41. Treatment (1):** The key to successful management of this potentially difficult injury is accurate reduction of the ulnar fracture. In the adult, and in children with displaced fractures, this is best achieved by open reduction and internal fixation. The fracture is easily approached through a posterior incision, and the reduction may be held with a plate applied to the medial aspect of the ulnar shaft with cortical screws.

**42. Treatment (2):** Thereafter the elbow should be placed in right-angled flexion. The position of the radial head should be checked by palpation and by radiographs. Full supination may be required to maintain reduction, but generally the neutral position will be satisfactory in maintaining stability after the ulna has been fixed. If the radial head will not reduce in full supination, it should be exposed, any loose cartilage fragments removed, and any tear in the orbicular ligament sutured.

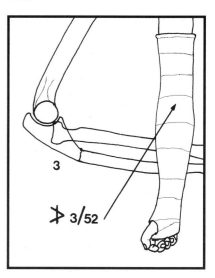

**43. Treatment (4): After care:** (1) The plaster is changed at 3 weeks and the stitches removed. (2) Plaster is finally discarded when on your assessment there is adequate stability. Your opinion will be based on the type of fixation, its technical adequacy, callus formation, etc. In practice, mobilisation from a sling (3) may often be started about 6 weeks. Physiotherapy is often required.

**44. Treatment (6): Monteggia fractures in children (a):** Any green stick angulation of the ulna should be corrected by manipulation (1). Anterior Monteggia fractures should be put up in a position of 90° flexion at the elbow and in supination (2).

**45. Treatment (6): Monteggia fractures in children (b):** Posterior Monteggia fractures (3) are often stable in full extension and may be fixed for not more than 3 weeks in this position; the elbow should be brought into a more flexed position for the remainder of the time in plaster. The position of the radial head must be confirmed by weekly radiographs; if there is any evidence of incongruity, exploration may have to be considered.

**46. Late diagnosed Monteggia lesions:** (1) In the adult, some restriction of elbow movements may be the only complaint. Excision of the radial head may give temporary relief, but is often followed by proximal drift of the radius and troublesome subluxation of the ulna at the wrist. (2) Tardy ulnar nerve palsy may be the patient's first complaint; transposition of the ulnar nerve is often effective in arresting the progress of this condition. (3) In children, excision of the radial head is contra-indicated (it would lead to growth disturbance). In some cases manipulative correction may be possible depending on the delay.

In exceptional circumstances the condition may be very late in being brought to light. In children under the age of 10 good results have been claimed for surgery performed as late as 4 years after the initial injury. (Such late reconstructions involve (1) excision of scar tissue in the region of the radiohumeral joint; (2) proximal ulnar osteotomy; (3) reduction of the radial head; (4) reconstruction of the annular ligament using palmaris longus.

**47. The Galeazzi fracture–dislocation:** This is a fracture of the radius associated with a dislocation of the inferior radio-ulnar joint. Note that in the normal wrist the distal end of the ulna (excluding the styloid process) lies just proximal to the articular surface of the radius, the space between being occupied by the triangular fibrocartilage. If the radius is fractured, always look for subluxation of the ulna.

**48. Isolated fracture of the radius:**
Fracture of the radius can occur without initial involvement of the inferior radio-ulnar joint. This comparatively uncommon situation may follow direct injury to the radius which results in an undisplaced fracture. Nevertheless, late subluxation of the inferior radio-ulnar joint may appear when, as is frequent, late angulation of the fracture occurs.

**49. Galeazzi fracture: Treatment:** (1) In the adult, open reduction and plating of the radius through an anterior incision eliminate the risks of late slipping. Reduction of the radius is followed by spontaneous reduction of the ulnar subluxation, and only in exceptional circumstances does the inferior radio-ulnar joint require opening. With stable internal fixation and an intact ulna, there is less need for additional external fixation.

50.  (2) In the adult, isolated fractures of the radius with no significant angulatory or rotational deformity may be treated in plaster with the arm in supination. Slight axial rotation may be controlled by careful positioning of the forearm; in all cases careful surveillance is vital to detect early slipping, an indication for operative intervention. (3) In children, isolated fractures of the radius should also be treated conservatively. Galeazzi fracture–dislocations should be manipulated and put up in plaster in supination. Open reduction is seldom required. (4) *Late diagnosed Galeazzi lesions:* Prominence of the ulna with pain in the wrist is the commonest complaint and excision of the distal ulna may give relief. (5) Non-union of the radius may be treated by internal fixation and bone grafting.

RADIUS/ULNA, *Diaphyseal Segment : 22–*

A

B

C

51. **AO Classification of Fractures of the Radius/Ulna, Diaphyseal Segment (22–):**

**Type A** are simple (i.e. there is a circumferential disruption of the bone), involving one or both bones.
A1 = Simple fracture of the ulna with an intact radius: .1 oblique; .2 transverse; .3 with dislocation of the radial head (Monteggia fracture dislocation).
A2 = Simple fracture of the radius, with the ulna intact: .1 oblique; .2 transverse; .3 with dislocation of the distal radio-ulnar joint (Galeazzi fracture–dislocation).
A3 = Simple fracture of both bones:
.1 proximal part of radius involved; .2 middle third of radius fractured; .3 fracture of distal radius.

**Type B** fractures are wedge fractures (i.e. there is a separate (butterfly) segment, but after reduction there is contact between the main fragments (a so-called hitch)); one or both bones are involved.
B1 = Wedge fracture of the ulna and an intact radius: .1 wedge intact; .2 multifragmentary wedge; .3 with dislocation of the radial head (Monteggia fracture–dislocation).
B2 = Wedge fracture of the radius and an intact ulna: .1 wedge intact;
.2 multifragmentary wedge; .3 with dislocation of the distal radio-ulnar joint (Galeazzi fracture–dislocation).
B3 = Wedge fracture of one bone, with a simple or wedge fracture of the other:
.1 wedge ulna; .2 wedge radius; .3 wedge fractures of both bones.

**Type C** fractures are complex (i.e. they have more than two fragments, and even after reduction the pattern is such that there is no contact between the main fragments); one or both bones may be involved.
C1 = Complex fracture of the ulna: .1 bifocal with an intact radius; .2 bifocal, with the radius fractured; .3 irregular, with or without fracture of the radius.
C2 = Complex fracture of the radius: .1 bifocal ulna intact; .2 bifocal with a fracture of the ulna; .3 irregular, with or without a fracture of the ulna.
C3 = Complex fracture of both bones;
.1 bifocal of both bones; .2 bifocal of one bone and irregular fracture of the other; .3 irregular fracture of both bones.

52. Describe this fracture. What treatment would you advocate?

53. Interpret this radiograph. How might this appearance be avoided?

54. What is this injury?

55. Describe this injury. How would you treat it?

56. Describe this injury. What treatment would you carry out?

57. Comment on this radiograph.

## Answers to self test

52. Greenstick fractures of the radius and ulna, with anterior angulation. Treat by manipulation under general anaesthesia and the application of long arm plaster slab. AO = 22–A3.3.

53. Cross-union has occurred in this fracture of the radius and ulna. The distal fragments have rotated 90° relative to the proximal fragments (mal-union). No pronation or supination will be possible. This would be avoided by open reduction and internal fixation through separate incisions. AO = 22–A3.3.

54. Hume fracture. (Anterior Monteggia fracture–dislocation where the ulnar fracture is one of the olecranon.) (In the AO Classification this would appear as a special variety of radius/ulnar proximal segment; as there is a small coronoid fracture this would be 21–B1.2.)

55. Adult anterior Monteggia fracture–dislocation, with a fracture of the ulna in the proximal part of its middle third, with anterior angulation; the radial head is dislocated anteriorly. Treatment would be by open reduction and internal fixation of the ulna; reduction of the radial head would then have to be confirmed AO = 22–A1.3.

56. Galeazzi fracture–dislocation in a child; there is a greenstick fracture of the radius with anterior angulation. The distal end of the ulna is dislocated anteriorly. AO = 22–A2.3.

57. The radiograph is of an arm in plaster; there is a fracture of the ulna, apparently in reasonable alignment in this single view but the radial head is dislocated anteriorly: i.e. this is an anterior Monteggia fracture–dislocation which has not been satisfactorily reduced. The arm appears to be in the mid-prone position, and reduction of the radial head might have been achieved if the arm had been placed in supination. Further treatment here is imperative (e.g. remanipulation and placing the arm in supination; should this fail to reduce the dislocation of the radial head, exploration of the radiohumeral joint would have to be considered. AO = 22–A1.3.

# 9.  The wrist and hand

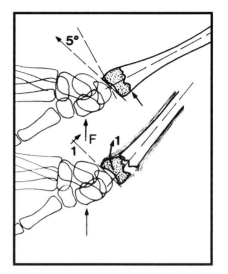

1. **Colles fracture:** A Colles fracture is a fracture of the radius within 2.5 cm of the wrist (1), with a characteristic deformity if displaced. It is the commonest of all fractures. It is seen mainly in middle-aged and elderly women, and osteoporosis is a frequent contributory factor. It generally results from a fall on the outstretched hand (2).

2. **Displacements (1):** The *six* characteristic features of a displaced Colles fracture (see later for details) are shown in this foreshortened view of the pronated right arm, viewed from below. The slight obliquity of impact (F) produces the two most striking features of *dorsal and radial displacement* (D & R) of the distal fragment. (T = triangular fibro-cartilage: U = ulnar styloid)

3. **Displacements (2):** The deformity can be followed by studying the wrist in the two planes in which the radiographs are usually taken. The impact (F) fractures the radius through the cancellous bone of the metaphysis. With greater violence the anterior periosteum tears, and the distal fragment tilts into *anterior angulation* (1) with loss of the 5° forward tilt of the joint surface.

4. **Displacements (3):** With greater violence there is *dorsal displacement of the distal fragment* (2). The shaft of the radius is driven into the distal fragment leading to impaction (3). (The dotted lines indicate the position of the distal fragment prior to any displacement.)

5. **Displacements (4):** The altered contour of the wrist in a badly displaced Colles fracture is striking, and is referred to as a 'dinner fork deformity'. When viewed from the side, the wrist has the same curvature as a fork, with the tines resembling the fingers.

6. **Displacements (5):** This radiograph shows a typical displaced Colles fracture. The anterior angulation, dorsal displacement, and impaction are obvious (Deformities 1, 2, 3).

7. **Displacements (6):** In the AP plane, a small lateral component of the force of impact causes *lateral (radial) displacement of the distal fragment* (4). The distal fragment is attached to the ulnar syloid by the triangular fibro-cartilage, and generally this leads to avulsion of the ulnar styloid. Note that in the AP projection of the normal wrist that the joint surface has a tilt of 22°.

8. **Displacements (7):** Sometimes the triangular fibrocartilage is torn; in either case there is disruption of the inferior radio-ulnar joint. The distal fragment tilts laterally into *ulnar angulation* (5) (reducing the tilt to less than 22°) and impacts. The sixth feature is a rotational or torsional deformity (6) (see 170, 2) not obvious in either AP or lateral projections.

9. **Displacements (8):** In this AP radiograph of a Colles fracture, note the features just mentioned, i.e. radial deviation, ulnar angulation and impaction of the distal fragment.

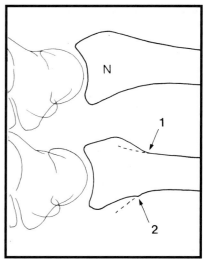

10. **Diagnosis:** (a) If there is pain in the wrist and tenderness over the distal end of the radius after a fall, radiographs must be taken in every case. The site of maximum tenderness will help to differentiate fracture of the scaphoid (but see scaphoid fractures). (b) Where there is marked displacement the characteristic appearance leaves little diagnostic doubt. Note that in the normal wrist the radial styloid lies 1 cm distal to the ulnar.

11. **Radiographs (1):** In the majority of cases the fracture is easily identified.
(2) Sometimes it may be missed because impaction has rendered the fracture line inconspicuous. If in doubt, look at the angle between the distal end of the radius and the shaft in the lateral radiograph. Decrease to less than 0° is suggestive of fracture (but enquire about previous injury).

12. **Radiographs (3):** The minimally displaced fracture will also reveal itself in the lateral projection by an increase in the posterior radial concavity, often with local kinking (1) or by a separate or accompanying break in the smooth curve of the anterior surface of the radius (2).

**13. Radiographs (4):** In the AP view of the wrist, look for any irregularity in the smooth lateral aspect of the radius.

If there is any doubtful radiographic feature suggesting fracture, return to the patient *and confirm whether there is any localised tenderness over the suspect area.*

**14. Diagnosis *ctd:*** A Colles fracture is generally caused by a fall on the outstretched hand—a mechanism common to many upper limb fractures. Although other injuries in the arm occurring in association with Colles fracture are *uncommon,* clinically the scaphoid, elbow and shoulder should be examined, and on the radiographs the scaphoid should be scrutinised. (Special views required if directly suspect.)

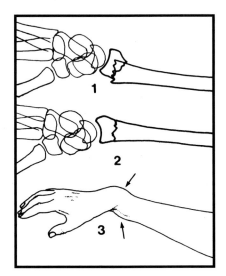

**15. Treatment: Does the fracture require manipulation? (1):** If the fracture is grossly displaced, it obviously should be reduced (1). If undisplaced, no manipulation is needed (2). Between these extremes, the following additional factors may be considered: if there is a readily appreciated naked eye deformity (3) manipulation should be carried out (but distinguish between *swelling* and *deformity.*)

**16. Does the fracture require manipulation? (2):** If there is displacement of the ulnar styloid, this indicates *serious disruption of the inferior radio-ulnar joint.* (Acute ulnar angulation of the distal fragment is also evidence of this.) An attempt at correction should be made *irrespective of other appearances.*

**17. Does the fracture require manipulation? (3):** If the joint line in the lateral projection is tilted 10° or more posteriorly rather than anteriorly, the fracture should be manipulated: but in the very old, frail patient somewhat greater degrees of deformity may be accepted.

**18. Reduction technique (1):** Anaesthesia is necessary for the reduction of this fracture, and either a general anaesthetic or intravenous regional anaesthetic (Bier block) may be used with success. Although the latter has a good safety record, it should not be employed unless facilities for resuscitation are freely available. Where there is a preference for general anaesthesia but the patient attends late at night with a history of recent intake of food or drink, it is permissible and often safer to apply a temporary plaster back shell and an arm sling, and delay reduction of the fracture till morning.

19. **Reduction technique (2):** Before any manipulation, start by preparing a suitable plaster back slab. The *length* should equal the distance from the olecranon to the metacarpal heads (1). The *width* in an adult should be 15 cm (6″), and it should be about eight layers thick. The slab should be trimmed with a tongue (2) for the first web space, a large radial curve to allow elbow flexion (3) and allowance for ulnar deviation (4).

20. **Reduction technique (3):** The essential first stage in the reduction of a Colles fracture is to disimpact the distal radial fragment. The elbow is flexed to a right angle and the arm held by the interlocked fingers of an assistant (1). Traction is applied in the line of the forearm (2).

21. **Reduction technique (4):** Traction need only be applied for a few seconds, and disimpaction may be confirmed by holding the distal fragment between the thumb and index. It should be easy to move anteriorly and posteriorly.

22. **Reduction technique (5):** The elbow is now extended (1). The heel of one hand should be placed over the dorsal surface of the distal radial fragment, and the fingers curled round the patient's wrist and palm (2). This grip allows traction to be re-applied to the disimpacted fracture.

23. **Reduction technique (6):** Now, by using the heel of the other hand as a fulcrum (3) firm pressure directed anteriorly (4) will correct all the remaining deformities normally visible in lateral radiographs of the wrist (posterior displacement, anterior angulation).

24. **Reduction technique (7):** Still maintaining traction, alter the position of the grip so that the heel (here of the right hand) is able to push the distal fragment ulnarwards and correct the radial displacement (5). Ulnar angulation, the other deformity seen in the AP radiograph, is corrected by placing the hand in full ulnar deviation at the wrist.

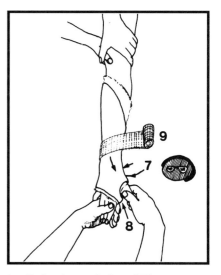

**25. Reduction technique (8):** Change the grip to allow free application of the plaster. Note that one hand holds the thumb fully extended (1). The other holds three fingers (to avoid 'cupping' of the hand) maintaining slight traction (2). The limb should be in full pronation (3), *full* ulnar deviation at the wrist (4) and *slight* palmar flexion.

**26. Reduction technique (9):** Note that the elbow must be *extended* (either by an assistant (5) or by resting the upper arm against the edge of the table) to maintain this position. The skin may be protected with wool roll (6). If stockingette is preferred, it must be applied prior to reduction.

**27. Reduction technique (10):** The wetted slab should now be positioned so that it covers the anterior, lateral and posterior aspects of the radius (7). The tongue should be carefully turned into the palm (8). The slab should be held in position with two wetted 10 cm (4″) open weave bandages (cotton, gauze or Kling® bandages) (9). The end can be secured with a wetted scrap of plaster bandage.

**28. Reduction technique (11):** Before the plaster sets, many surgeons like to apply further pressure over the posterolateral aspect of the distal fragment, and maintain this until setting occurs ('final moulding'). This precaution ensures maintenance of the reduction, but care should be taken not to dent the plaster.

**29. Reduction technique (12):** A collar and cuff sling should be applied (1). Make sure that there is no constriction at the elbow (2) or at the wrist (3), and try to flex the elbow beyond a right angle so that the forearm is not dependent.

**30. Alternative techniques:** It is not unexpected that in this common fracture methods of reduction are legion. As it is generally an easy fracture to reduce, it follows that success can rightly be claimed for many techniques. The method given is logical in so far as it correlates with the pathology as seen on the radiographs.

Note, however: (A) a direct, simple and extremely effective procedure is to disimpact the fracture (173, 20), apply a plaster slab (174, 27) and correct the deformity before the plaster sets by applying pressure on the posterolateral aspect of the distal fragment (as in 174, 28). (B) In the elderly patient, unfit for general anaesthesia (but preferably after intravenous diazepam) a *marked* dorsal displacement may be corrected by quick application of pressure (without previous disimpaction) over a dorsal slab. (C) In the young adult, if a good reduction cannot be secured and held, so that there is recurrence of severe deformity, the use of an external fixator should be considered. A number of techniques may be employed: commonly the proximal segment is held with two pins inserted into the distal third of the radial shaft; and the distal segment by two pins inserted into the lateral aspect of the metacarpal shaft of the index finger. The two half-pin sets are then secured by a suitable linking bar; this is then adjusted to obtain a good correction in all planes.

**24 h**

**2–5 days**

31. **Treatment *ctd:*** Check radiographs should be studied. Severe persisting deformity, *especially in the AP projection* (Illus.) should not be accepted, and remanipulation should be undertaken. If difficulty is anticipated, radiographs may be obtained before discontinuing the anaesthetic. If the position is acceptable, the patient is shown finger exercises and advised regarding normal plaster care.

32. **After care (1):** The patient is seen the next day and the fingers examined for adequacy of the circulation and the degree of swelling (1). The palm, fingers, thumb and elbow are checked for constriction caused by bandaging or elbow flexion, and any adjustments made (2). Thereafter the patient should be seen within the next 2–5 days with a view to completion of the plaster.

33. **After care (2):** At the next review (usually a fracture clinic) finger swelling is checked: if slight, the plaster is completed (if marked, completion is delayed). *Superficial* layers of cotton bandage are removed, the slab retained, and encircling plaster bandages applied. The patient is instructed in elbow and shoulder exercises, and unless there is still a fair amount of swelling the sling may be discarded.

**2/52**

34. **After care (3):** At 2 weeks the plaster is checked for marked slackening (replace), softening (reinforce) and technical faults (175, 35). Movements in the fingers, elbow and shoulder are examined and appropriate advice given or physiotherapy started. In some centres radiographs are taken at this stage; slight slipping is inevitable, but marked slipping may be an indication for remanipulation (not usually a profitable procedure). At this stage too, if desired, the plaster may be replaced by a resin cast.

35. **After care (4): Positional errors:** (1) The commonest fault is lack of ulnar deviation. This should be sadly accepted if discovered at 2 weeks (but replastered in the correct position if discovered earlier). Lack of ulnar deviation increases the risks of late problems arising from disruption of the inferior radio-ulnar joint; non-union of the ulnar styloid is common, with frequently some restriction of pronation and supination and local pain. (2) Excessive wrist flexion is liable to lead to difficulty in recovering dorsiflexion and a useful grip, and if present, the plaster should be re-applied with the wrist in a more extended position. (Full wrist flexion was once advocated in the treatment of Colles fracture—the Cotton–Loder position—but has been abandoned for the reasons given.)

36. **After care (5): Plaster faults:** Errors in plastering technique should not occur, but nevertheless are often discovered at this stage. The following faults are common: (1) The distal edge of the plaster does not follow the normal oblique line of the MP joints, and movements of the little and sometimes the ring finger are restricted. The plaster should be trimmed to the dotted line. (2) All the MP joints are restricted by the plaster which has been continued beyond the palmar crease. Trim to the dotted line. (3) The thumb is restricted by a few turns of plaster bandage. Again the plaster should be trimmed to permit free movement. (4) The plaster is digging into the skin of the first web and should be trimmed back to the dotted line. (5) The plaster is too short. Support of the fracture is greatly impaired; the plaster should be extended to the olecranon behind, and as far in front as will still permit elbow flexion.

37. **After care (6):** The plaster should be removed at 5 weeks (or 6 weeks in badly displaced fractures in the elderly) and the fracture assessed for union. (Radiographs are of limited value.) *If there is marked persisting tenderness,* a fresh plaster should be applied and union re-assessed in a further 2 weeks.

38. **After care (7):** If tenderness is minimal or absent, (1) a circular woven support (e.g. Tubigrip®) or a crepe bandage may be applied (to limit oedema and to some extent increase the patient's confidence). (2) The patient is instructed in wrist and finger exercises and encouraged to practise these frequently and with vigour. (3) Arrangements are made to review the patient in a further 2 weeks.

39. **Need for rehabilitation (1):** At about 7 weeks post injury, you must decide whether to discharge the patient or refer her for rehabilitation. Base your decision on: (a) finger movements, (b) grip strength, (c) wrist movements, (d) the patient's occupation.

For example, (a) if finger 'tuck-in' (i.e. the last few degrees of flexion) cannot be carried out (loss Illus.) physiotherapy should be considered.

**40. Need for rehabilitation (2):** (b) Assess the patient's grip strength by first asking her to squeeze two of your fingers as tightly as possible while you try to withdraw them. Compare one hand with the other. Repeat with a single finger. Marked weakness is an indication for physiotherapy.

**41. Need for rehabilitation (3):** (c) Assess wrist movements. Initially, material restriction of *palmar flexion* is normal and by itself is of little importance. If, however, the total range of *pronation and supination* is less than half normal, physiotherapy is advisable. (d) Where there is only slight restriction of movements and power, rehabilitation may still be indicated through the special requirements of the patient's work.

**42. Complications (1): Persistent deformity or mal-union (a):** Radial drift of the distal fragment results in prominence of the distal radius (1). Radial tilting and bony absorption at the fracture site lead to relative prominence of the distal ulna (2) and tilting of the plane of the wrist as seen in the AP radiographs (3). These deformities may be symptom free, and surgery on purely cosmetic grounds is seldom indicated.

**43. Mal-union (b):** In some cases there is quite marked pain in the region of the distal radio-ulnar joint, owing to its severe disorganisation. There is generally quite *marked local tenderness* and supination in particular is reduced. Physiotherapy in the form of grip strengthening and pronation/supination exercises is indicated. If symptoms remain severe, excision of the distal end of the ulna may be considered.

**44. Mal-union (c):** Uncomplicated persistence of dinner-fork deformity (i.e. persistent deformity in the lateral but not in the AP radiographs) is accompanied by some loss of palmar flexion, but significant functional disturbance is unusual. This type of residual deformity is generally accepted.

**45. Complications (2):** *Delayed rupture of extensor pollicis longus* may follow Colles fracture, and be due to attrition of the tendon by roughness at the fracture site, or by sloughing from interference with its blood supply. Disability is often slight, and spontaneous recovery may occur. There is no urgency regarding treatment, and in the elderly this complaint may be accepted or treated expectantly. In the young, extensor indicis proprius tendon transfer is advocated.

**46. Complications (3): Sudeck's atrophy:** This is often detected about the time the patient comes out of plaster. The fingers are swollen and finger flexion is restricted. The hand and wrist are warm, tender and painful. Radiographs show diffuse osteoporosis (Illus.). *Treatment*. (1) The mainstay of treatment is intensive and prolonged physiotherapy and occupational therapy, but (2) if pain is very severe a further 2–3 weeks rest of the *wrist* in plaster may give sufficient relief to allow commencement of effective finger movements. (3) If the MP joints are stiff in extension and making no headway, manipulation under general anaesthesia followed by fixation in plaster (MP joints flexed, IP joints extended) for 3 weeks only may be effective in initiating recovery. (4) In severe cases, a sympathetic block may be attempted by infiltration of the stellate ganglion, or by regional perfusion with guanethidine sulphate (see p. 82).

**47. Complications (4): Carpal tunnel (median nerve compression) syndrome:** Paraesthesiae in the median distribution is the main presenting symptom, but look for sensory and motor involvement. *If detected before reduction:* (a) Complete lesion: reduce, plaster and re-assess. If no improvement, explore, and divide not only the roof of the carpal tunnel but the antebrachial fascia. (b) Partial lesion: reduce and apply a cast; if motor symptoms remain, or if symptoms persist for a week, decompress.

**48. Median nerve compression syndrome** *ctd: If detected after reduction:* Release the splints, put the wrist in the neutral position, and use Kirschner wires or an external fixator to hold the reduction; if symptoms persist, explore. *If detected after union:* Exploration is generally advised, as symptoms otherwise tend to persist. Note that diagnosis at the late stage may be suggested by the response to tapping over the nerve (Illus.), or by nerve stretching, tourniquet, or nerve conduction tests.

**49. Complications (5): Comminution of the radial fragment:** Sometimes there may be a small vertical crack through the radial fragment, showing in the AP view (1). In other cases the fracture may run horizontally, and the scaphoid or lunate may separate the fragments (2). In the young adult, especially where the main fragments are separated and there is no gross fragmentation, open reduction and internal fixation are indicated.

**50. Complications (5 *ctd*):** For this purpose it may be possible to employ a small T-plate and (small fragment set) screws, but only if the screws can be seen to get a reasonable grip in the articular fragments; otherwise Kirschner wires (Illus.) may be used. Some additional support, either with a cast or an external fixator, will be needed. Some permanent joint stiffness is the rule after injuries of this pattern, and prolonged physiotherapy will generally be required.

**51. Complications (6): Persisting stiffness:** Restriction of movements, even after prolonged physiotherapy, is not uncommon, but is seldom severe enough to impair limb function to a material extent. This is due to compensatory (trick) movements developed by the elbow, shoulder and trunk (e.g. in case of loss of supination.)

**52. Complications (7): Associated scaphoid fracture:** This may be treated by manipulation of the Colles fracture and application of a scaphoid plaster. After the Colles fracture has united, further immobilisation may be required for the scaphoid. Alternatively, the scaphoid fracture may be fixed with an AO lag cancellous screw (Illus.) (or a Herbert screw), the Colles fracture manipulated, and fixation discontinued as soon as the latter has united.

**53. Related fractures (1):** A number of fractures involving the distal end of the radius, produced by falls on the outstretched hand, have certain similarities to the classical Colles fracture. The commonest of these is the *undisplaced greenstick fracture of the radius.* In its most minor form it may be overlooked; the only sign may be slight local buckling.

**54. Undisplaced greenstick fracture of the radius** *ctd:* The level of the fracture is rather variable, and it may be situated fairly proximally. These fractures may be treated like undisplaced Colles fractures by the application of a plaster slab. This may usually be completed after 1–2 days. Fixation for about 3 weeks only is usually all that is necessary.

**55. Related fractures (2): Angulated greenstick fracture of the radius:** In this type of injury there is both clinical and radiological deformity. Manipulation is required as for a Colles fracture, and the after care is similar; the period of plaster fixation may be reduced to 3 or 4 weeks, depending on the age of the child.

**56. Related fractures (3): Overlapping radial fracture (1):** In children the radius often fractures close to the wrist, with off-ending of the fragments. On the ulnar side there may be: (1) detachment of the triangular fibrocartilage; (2) separation of the ulnar epiphysis; (3) fracture and angulation of the distal ulna; (4) fracture and displacement of the distal ulna (Illus.), in effect a fracture of both bones of the forearm; (5) dislocation of the ulna (Galeazzi fracture–dislocation).

**57. Overlapping radial fracture (2):** If the fracture line is transverse (1), reduction is straightforward by traction (2) and local pressure (3). When, however, there is an oblique fracture running daily from front to back (4), reduction by traction is often impossible owing to the integrity of the periosteum on the dorsal surface (5) and the overlapping bony spikes (6).

**58. Overlapping radial fracture (3):** Two closed techniques may be tried. For the first, two assistants are essential to apply *maximal* traction to the limb (1). While this is being strongly maintained, the surgeon should press forcibly with the heel of one hand on the distal fragment (2) and use the other to apply counter-pressure (3). Reduction is achieved by shearing off one of the bone spikes (4).

**59. Overlapping radial fracture (4):** Alternatively, by *increasing* the deformity (1) and applying pressure directly over the distal radial fragment (2), whilst maintaining traction (3), reduction may be achieved. After the fragments have interlocked the angulation is corrected. Thereafter plaster fixation is carried out as in other fractures in this region.

**60. Overlapping radial fracture (5):** If shortening is marked, and closed methods fail, open reduction may be considered. (Performed through a small dorsal incision under a tourniquet; internal fixation is not required, although a Kirschner wire may be used to hold the fracture temporarily—being withdrawn as soon as the plaster has been applied.) Nevertheless, if persisting overlap is reluctantly accepted, a good result from remodelling is the usual outcome (Illus.) *provided* any angulation is corrected.

**61. Related fractures (4): Slipped radial epiphysis:** This injury is common in adolescence, and the displaced distal radial epiphysis is usually associated with a small fracture of the metaphysis (Salter–Harris Type 2 injury). Unless displacement is minimal, manipulation followed by plaster fixation (as for a Colles fracture) is indicated. Growth disturbance is rare, but reduction should be carried out promptly (it is often difficult to reduce after 2 days).

**62. Related fractures (5): Fracture of the radial styloid:** This fracture is sometimes caused by an engine starting-handle kickback as well as by a fall on the outstretched hand. Displacement is usually slight, and manipulation unlikely to be of value. A Colles plaster is usually adequate, although some prefer fixation with a lag screw or Kirschner wires. Physiotherapy is usually required, and Sudeck's atrophy a common complication.

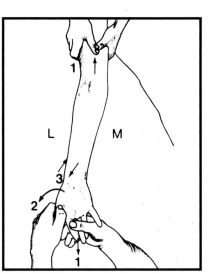

**63. Related fractures (6): Smith's fracture (1):** This injury frequently results from a fall on the back of the hand, although a clear history is not always obtainable. The distal radial fragment is tilted anteriorly (posterior angulation) and may be displaced anteriorly. The fracture is usually impacted.

**64. Smith's fracture (2):** This fracture is frequently referred to as a reversed Colles fracture because the deformities when viewed from the side clinically and radiologically are in the opposite direction to those seen in a Colles fracture. (Note, however, that the two fractures may be identical in AP radiographs.) Comminuted Smith's fractures may involve the articular surface of the radius (Illus.). Greenstick fractures are common (see also 181, 65).

**65. Smith's fracture (3):** To reduce these fractures, traction is applied to the arm (1) in supination (2) until disimpaction is achieved. (This may be confirmed as in a Colles fracture.) Pressure may be applied with the heels of the hands to force the distal fragment dorsally (3).

**66. Smith's fracture (4):** The reduction is difficult to hold, and a long arm plaster is required (1). This may be more conveniently applied in two stages, and best as a complete plaster. The arm is held in full supination and dorsiflexion (2). This is easily maintained with the elbow extended (3). Wool roll is applied to the arm (4) and an anterior slab, trimmed as shown, may be used (5) before completion (6). The fracture may be moulded while setting. It is then extended above the elbow (1). *After care:* (1) Split if necessary. (2) Radiographs should be taken at weekly intervals for the first 3 weeks to detect any significant slipping (treated by remanipulation or moulding). (3) A slack plaster should be changed with care. (4) Six weeks' fixation is usually required, with physiotherapy after removal of the plaster.

**67. Related fractures (7): Barton's fracture:** This is a form of Smith's fracture in which the anterior portion only of the radius is involved. Closed reduction may be attempted along the lines indicated for Smith's fracture, but this may fail with the carpus wedging the fragments apart. If this fails, with the carpus wedging the fragments apart, open reduction and internal fixation are indicated in the younger patient (e.g. by cancellous screw or an Ellis buttress plate).

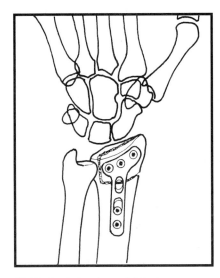

68. **Barton's fracture** *ctd:* In the young patient these potentially unstable and disabling fractures are best treated by open reduction and internal fixation. The most satisfactory procedure is to expose the fracture anteriorly and reduce it under vision; thereafter it is best held with a volar plate (e.g. with an Ellis buttress plate or an AO right angled or oblique T-plate (Illus.)).

69. **Related fractures (8):** Forcible palmar flexion may result in a *minor avulsion fracture of the carpus* at a ligament insertion (Illus.). **(9)** If the wrist is forcibly palmar flexed or dorsiflexed, the carpus impinging on the distal end of the radius may produce a *marginal chip fracture of the radius*.

Symptomatic treatment only is required for any of these injuries (e.g. 2–3 weeks in a plaster back slab).

70. **Fractures of the scaphoid: Mechanisms of injury:** Scaphoid fractures often result from 'kickback' when using starting handles on internal combustion generators, pumps, compressors and inboard marine engines. (The motorist's avoidance of this fracture is his only dividend from the unfortunate abolition of car starting handles.) Otherwise the fracture may be acquired by falls on the outstretched hand.

71. **Fractures of the scaphoid: Diagnosis (1):** Fracture of the scaphoid may be suspected when there is complaint of pain on the lateral aspect of the wrist following any injury (or frequently repeated stress). In those cases which follow starting handle accidents there may be marked and rapid swelling of the hand and wrist.

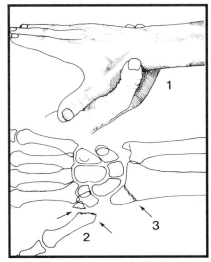

72. **Diagnosis (2):** Tenderness in the anatomical snuff box (1) is suggestive of this injury, but by no means diagnostic. Many wrist sprains without fracture give rise to tenderness in this site. Beware too of tenderness which may be the result of a Bennett's fracture of the thumb metacarpal (2) or of a fracture of the radial styloid (3).

73. **Diagnosis (3):** In a true scaphoid fracture, tenderness will also be elicited on the application of pressure over the *dorsal aspect of the scaphoid,* and also on pressure over the palmar aspect. Tenderness in these additional sites very seldom occurs in other injuries in this area, no matter how severe.

**74. Diagnosis (4): Radiographs:** Radiography is required in all suspect cases. Note the following important points: (1) Request cards should be clearly marked 'scaphoid' and not 'wrist', to ensure that (2) at least three views of the scaphoid are obtained. (Illus.: four views showing fracture of the distal waist.) The fracture is often hairline and hard to see, so that in all suspected but unconfirmed cases radiographs should be repeated at 10–14 days, when local decalcification may reveal a previously hidden fracture. If doubt remains, a bone scan may be helpful. Note that there is a 20% rate of false positive reporting of scaphoid radiographs, and *clinical confirmation of the diagnosis is mandatory.*

**75. Anatomical features (1):** The scaphoid plays a key role in wrist and carpal function, taking part in the radiocarpal joint (1) and in the joint between the proximal and distal rows of the carpus (2). It articulates with the radius (R), trapezium (Tm), trapezoid (Td), capitate (C) and lunate (L). The commonest site for fracture is the waist (50%); 38% of fractures occur in the proximal half and 12% in the distal half. (U = ulna, H = hamate, P = pisiform, TI = triquetral.)

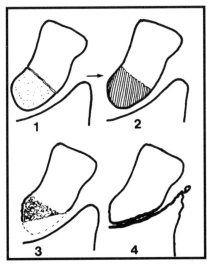

**76. Anatomical features (2):** A number of abnormalities in ossification may be confused with fractures. The *os centrale* may be small (1), large (2) or double (3). The *os radiale externum* (4) lies in the region of the tubercle and in some cases may represent an old, ununited fracture; certainly the so called 'bipartite scaphoid' (5) is now generally regarded as being due to this. (Rounded edges differentiate these from fracture.)

**77. Anatomical features (3):** The blood supply of the scaphoid is through small vessels which enter the ligamentous ridge (1) lying between the two main articular surfaces (2). When these vessels are well scattered (a), ischaemia following fracture is uncommon. If all the vessels enter the distal part of the ridge (b), fractures of the waist (W) and proximal poles (P) may be followed by avascular necrosis.

**78. Anatomical features (4):** Avascular necrosis is of immediate onset, but 1–2 months may elapse before increased density betrays its presence on the radiographs (2). There is usually slow but progressive bony collapse (3) and radiocarpal osteo-arthritis (4). This leads to worsening pain and stiffness in the wrist. This complication occurs in about 30% of fractures of the proximal pole of the scaphoid.

79. **Anatomical features (5):** Because of its role in two major joints (1), movement of the fragments is difficult to control, and non-union may occur in waist fractures. Cystic changes at the fracture site (2) are followed by marginal sclerosis (3). The edges may round off and form a symptomless pseudoarthrosis (4) or osteo-arthritis may supervene (5). Note that non-union can occur without avascular necrosis, and that most fractures with avascular necrosis are united.

80. **Prognostic features:** The prognosis is good in *stable* injuries: these include (Herbert Classification) fractures of the tubercle (A1), and hair-line fractures of the waist (A2). The prognosis is poorer in *unstable* injuries which include oblique fractures of the distal third (B1), displaced fractures of the waist (B2), proximal pole fractures (B3), fractures associated with carpal dislocations (B4) (Illus.: trans-scapho perilunar dislocation of the carpus—see 187, 97) and comminuted fractures (B5).

81. **Treatment of suspected fracture:** When there is local tenderness and normal radiographs, apply a scaphoid plaster and sling. Remove the plaster and re-X-ray at 2 weeks (see also 183,74). Absorption of bone at the site of any hair-line fracture will then reveal it. If a fracture is confirmed, apply a fresh cast and treat as for a frank fracture. If the radiographs are negative, the patient is presumed to have suffered a sprain and is treated accordingly: but if symptoms persist re-examine and X-ray after another 2 weeks.

82. **Fractures of the tuberosity of the scaphoid:** Avascular necrosis never occurs in fractures of this type, and non-union here does not give rise to significant symptoms. Symptomatic treatment only is needed (e.g. crepe bandage or plaster, depending on pain). Some extend this to include all distal pole fractures, but generally plaster fixation is the mainstay of treatment of all fractures through the body of the scaphoid (but see 186, 93).

83. **Treatment of undisplaced fractures of the body of the scaphoid. The classical scaphoid plaster (1):** The position of the hand is of some importance and this should be made quite clear to the patient prior to the application of the plaster. The wrist should be fully pronated (1), radially deviated (2), moderately dorsiflexed (3). In addition, the thumb should be in mid abduction (4).

84. **The scaphoid plaster (2):** An anterior plaster slab, although by no means essential, is frequently used. This may be made from 6–8 layers of 10 cm (4″) plaster bandage, or from a slab dispenser. The proximal corners should be trimmed and a cut-out made to accommodate the swell of the thenar muscles.

85. **The scaphoid plaster (3):** Stockingette is applied from just above the elbow (1) to the proximal phalanges (2), allowing for subsequent turn-down. A smaller gauge may be used for the thumb (or wool roll) (3). A turn of wool is used to protect the bony prominences of the wrist (4). If there is a lot of early swelling suggesting more to come, more generous wool padding is applied round the wrist and hand.

86. **The scaphoid plaster (4):** The plaster slab may then be wetted and applied to the forearm, taking care not to extend it beyond the proximal palmar crease (5). Encircling plaster bandages are then applied, using 15 cm (6″) bandages for the forearm, 10 cm (4″) for the wrist and 7.5 cm (3″) for the thumb (6). The edges of the stockingette are turned down before completion (7).

87. **The scaphoid plaster (5): Common faults:** Plaster including MP joints of fingers, restricting flexion (1). Terminal phalanx of thumb included, preventing interphalangeal joint flexion (2). Plaster too short (3). Plaster restricting flexion of the elbow (4). (Note that to give the best support to a scaphoid fracture there is some questioning of the position of the wrist and the need to include the thumb. Some use a Colles plaster in neutral or slight flexion, without radial deviation.)

88. **Scaphoid fracture: After care (1):** A sling should be worn for the first few days until swelling subsides. Analgesics are usually required initially. The patient is reviewed at 2 weeks (assuming the initial plaster check has been satisfactory). If on this visit the plaster is unduly slack, it should be changed. Any softening in the palm should be reinforced.

89. **After care (2):** At 6 weeks the plaster should be removed and the scaphoid assessed clinically and with radiographs. There are several possibilities: (a) if there is no tenderness over the dorsal surface and in the snuff-box, and the fracture appears united on the radiographs, the wrist should be left free and reviewed in 2 weeks (usually for discharge, or further radiographs if pain recurs).

90. **After care (3):** (b) The fracture line may still show clearly on the radiographs. (c) The radiographs may suggest union, but there is marked local tenderness. (d) There is some uncertainty on either score. These possibilities are all suggestive of delayed union, and a further 6 weeks of plaster fixation is desirable.

91. **After care (4):** At 12 weeks, there may be: (a) evidence of *avascular necrosis* (note density of proximal half in radiograph), (b) clear evidence, clinically and radiologically of *union*.

In these circumstances, there is no need and no advantage in continuing with plaster fixation.

92. **After care (5):** At 12 weeks, there may be: (c) no evidence of union, (d) evidence of established non-union; internal fixation should be considered (e.g. using a Herbert screw which has a different pitch at each end to draw the fragments together). In (d), local bone grafting will also be required. If surgery is refused, or not thought advisable, plaster should be discarded in established non-union. In (c), a further period of plaster immobilisation may be considered if there is marked persistent pain and local tenderness.

93. **Displaced fracture of the scaphoid:** Where there is marked displacement of a fractured scaphoid (Illus.), careful analysis of the radiographs should be made to exclude a carpal dislocation. Where displacement or angulation exceed 1 mm or 15° respectively, open reduction and internal fixation (through an anterior approach to avoid impairing the blood supply of the fragments) is indicated.

94. **Complications (1): Sudeck's atrophy:** Treat as in 178, 48. **(2) Avascular necrosis:** Surgery should be carried out before secondary changes occur in the wrist. (Illus.: the scaphoid is collapsing, and although there is as yet little evidence of osteo-arthritis further delay would be unwise. The scaphoid should be excised, with or without the insertion of a silastic spacer.)

95. **Complications (3): Non-union:** (a) Late diagnosed non-union, seen 3–6 months after injury, may still be effectively treated by plaster fixation and pulsed magnetic fields, *provided* that there is no displacement, carpal collapse, or osteoarthritic change. (b) If there is displacement, or if seen later than 6 months, and symptoms are present, internal fixation and bone grafting may be attempted. (c) If an early impingement osteo-arthritis threatens, satisfactory results may be obtained from excision of the radial styloid even although the midcarpal joint is unaffected by this (Illus.). (d) Symptomless non-union of the scaphoid, sometimes discovered by accident, should have the risks of secondary osteoarthritis assessed; if the appearances indicate that these are insignificant, then no treatment is indicated.

96. **Complications (4): Advanced osteo-arthritis:** This generally occurs as a sequel to avascular necrosis or non-union. The following treatments may be considered: (a) **Wrist joint (radiocarpal) fusion:** Pronation and supination movements are retained, but all other wrist movements are lost. This is the most reliable procedure and is the only one which should be considered in the patient who undertakes heavy manual labour. (b) Where the retention of some wrist movement is essential, excision of the proximal row of the carpus may be considered. The results are a little unpredictable in terms of final range of movements, strength, and freedom from pain. (c) Where surgery is thought inadvisable, good results in terms of relief from pain, with reasonable function may be obtained by the use of a block-leather support, or similar orthotic device.

97. **Dislocations of the carpus:** These may result from a fall on the outstretched hand, and are comparatively uncommon. There are two main groups. In the first, the metacarpals (m), the distal row of the carpus (d) and part of the proximal row (p) dislocate backwards. In classifying injuries within this group, the prefix 'peri' is used to describe undisplaced structures in the proximal row. Occasionally one of the carpal bones fractures, part remaining in alignment and part displacing with the distal row of the carpus. Note in the illustrations that structures drawn in feint lines are *displaced* (N = normal appearance from the side or *volar* aspect): (1) perilunar dislocation of the carpus; (2) periscapholunar dislocation of the carpus; (3) trans-scapho perilunar dislocation of the carpus. (Not illustrated are the rare transcapitate, transtriquetral perilunar dislocations and others.) In the second main group of injuries, the distal row re-aligns with the radius and part of the proximal row is extruded: hence: (4) dislocation of the scaphoid; (5) dislocation of the lunate; (6) dislocation of the lunate and scaphoid; (7) dislocation of the lunate and part of the scaphoid. (Note the correspondence between 1 and 5, 2 and 6, 3 and 7.)

98. **Dislocation of the lunate:** This is the commonest of all the carpal dislocations, and generally results from a fall on the outstretched hand. It is frequently overlooked, and this is nearly always due to failure in interpretation of the radiographs. Note in the normal radiographs of the carpus (Illus.) that the pisiform bone stands out to a varying degree from the rest of the volar surface.

99. **Dislocation of the lunate:** The *shape* of the dislocated lunate is quite different from the ovoid/quadrilateral mass of the pisiform. The *concave surface* in which the capitate usually sits is *rotated* anteriorly, and the crescent moon shape of the bone (and hence its name) is rendered obvious. The articular surfaces of the scaphoid and triquetral remain aligned with the radius while the lunate is *displaced* anteriorly. In the AP projection, the lunate is sector shaped (resembling a foil-wrapped cheese segment). *Diagnosis:* This is established on the basis of a history of injury, local tenderness and the radiographs. Evidence of median nerve involvement is very suggestive (may result from direct pressure of the displaced bone on the nerve).

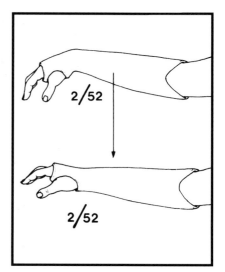

**100. Treatment (1):** Reduction can generally be achieved by closed methods under general anaesthesia. (1) Apply traction to the supinated wrist. (2) Extend the wrist, maintaining traction, (3) Apply pressure with the thumb over the lunate. (4) Flex the wrist as soon as you feel the lunate slip into position.

**101. Treatment (2):** Alternatively, if an assistant is available, he should apply traction in supination and extension as before (1) while you use both thumbs to push the lunate posteriorly and distally (2). When it is felt to reduce, the wrist is once again flexed. The reduction should be checked with radiographs before the anaesthetic is discontinued. (Failure is an indication for open reduction.)

**102. Treatment (3):** (a) The wrist is encased in plaster in a position of moderate flexion for 1–2 weeks. (b) The plaster is then changed for one with the wrist in the neutral position for a further 2 weeks. (c) Physiotherapy may then be required, depending on the degree of residual stiffness. Swelling may be a problem initially, and the usual precautions should be taken (e.g. generous padding, elevation, sling, etc.).

**103. Complications (1): Late diagnosis:** If there is delay in making the diagnosis, manipulative reduction becomes increasingly difficult, and after a week may not be possible. Open reduction is then necessary, and carries with it the greatly increased risk of avascular necrosis. Surgery should be performed through an anterior incision, and every effort made to reduce the bone without disturbing any of its ligamentous attachments (evidence suggests the major blood supply enters anteriorly) or further damaging the median nerve.

**(2) Median nerve palsy:** Prompt reduction of the dislocation is usually followed by early complete recovery. After late reduction recovery may be incomplete, but seldom requires separate treatment.

**(3) Sudeck's atrophy:** This is a common complication and is treated along previously described lines (178, 46).

**104. Complications (4): Avascular necrosis:** This leads to collapse of the lunate and secondary osteo-arthritis which advances with great rapidity. *All cases of dislocated lunate should have monthly radiographs for 6 months* to allow early detection of this complication. If detected early, excision with or without prosthetic replacement may prevent progressive osteo-arthritis. In many cases, and certainly at the later stages, arthrodesis of the wrist is preferable.

Note that repeated trauma to the wrist without frank dislocation of the lunate may lead to similar radiographic appearances (Kienbock's disease); this condition is found particularly in manual workers such as carpenters, cobblers and pneumatic drill operators, etc.

**105. Dislocation and subluxation of the scaphoid (see also Carpal Instability and Scapholunate Dissociation):** These uncommon injuries are diagnosed radiologically and, if suspected, AP projections in both radial and ulnar deviation may be helpful. The most striking feature is the widening of the space between the scaphoid and lunate.

*Treatment:* (a) If the displacement is anterior and complete as shown, manipulate as for dislocation of the lunate. (b) In many cases, dislocation is incomplete, with the proximal pole being tilted posteriorly and the distal pole anteriorly. Such injuries have often a toggle-like instability within the dorsiflexion/palmar flexion range (and the stable position within this phase must be found by trial and error during reduction).

**106. (b) *ctd:*** Reduction may be achieved by pressure over the proximal pole. If possible, an image intensifier should be used to check the reduction and stability. If a stable position is found, the wrist should be put up in plaster in that position, with some added radial deviation; the plaster should be retained for 6 weeks, with frequent radiographs to check the position. If instability is not easily controlled, then the scaphoid should be fixed with Kirschner wires.

**107. Dislocation of the lunate and half the scaphoid:** They may be treated initially by closed reduction in the same way as an uncomplicated dislocation of the lunate. Thereafter, however, the scaphoid fracture dominates the picture, and the treatment should follow the lines described for that injury. If after reduction there is gross carpal instability, internal fixation of the scaphoid should be considered.

**108. Trans-scapho perilunar dislocation of the carpus:** This injury corresponds to dislocation of the lunate and half the scaphoid just described. It is the commonest of the first group of carpal dislocations. In some cases there may be associated fractures of the styloid process of the radius and the ulna. Treatment: reduction by traction is usually easy. Thereafter the management is that of fracture of the scaphoid. If, however, the scaphoid reduction is poor or if the wrist is very unstable, internal fixation of the scaphoid must be considered.

**109. Other carpal injuries (1): Perilunar dislocation of the carpus:** This corresponds to isolated dislocation of the lunate.

*Treatment:* (a) Reduce by traction.
(b) Apply plaster with the wrist in flexion and retain for 1–2 weeks before (c) changing the plaster to one with the wrist in the neutral position. This should be retained for a further 2 weeks.
(d) Thereafter physiotherapy may be required to mobilise the wrist.

**110. Other carpal injuries** *ctd* **(2): Dislocation of both the lunate and scaphoid:** This should be treated as for dislocation of the lunate (187, 98). **(3) Periscapholunar dislocation of the carpus:** This should be treated in the same way as perilunar dislocation of the carpus (190, 109). **(4) Dislocation of the trapezium, trapezoid or hamate** are rare. Closed reduction should always be attempted, but open reduction is frequently required. In the face of instability, transfixion by Kirshner wires may be helpful. **(5) Fractures through the bodies of any of the carpal bones other than the scaphoid** are rare, and should be treated symptomatically by 6 weeks' fixation in a Colles or scaphoid plaster (depending on the injury). Fractures of the hamate and pisiform may be complicated by ulnar nerve palsy, which should be treated expectantly. **(6) Small chip fractures of the carpus** are common and generally result from hyperflexion or hyperextension injuries of the wrist. Direct violence is sometimes responsible. The bone of origin is often in doubt. Rest of the wrist in plaster for 3 weeks is all that is required, and full recovery of function is the rule.

**111. Other carpal injuries** *ctd* **(7): Fracture of the hook of the hamate:** This injury is seen most often as a result of a heavy golf or tennis swing, but may follow a fall, or a direct blow in the palm. There is local pain and tenderness. The fracture is best shown by CAT scan of both wrists in the praying position (1), or by carpal tunnel films (2). The best treatment is to excise the hamate fragment. (h = hamate; c = capitate; t = trapezium; S = scaphoid; P = pisiform; Q = triquetral; L = lunate)

**112. Carpal instabilities:** A carpal instability is a condition in which there is a loss of normal carpal alignment which develops at an early or late stage after an injury. There are a number of clinical patterns, but the anatomical details, the complex dynamics of the region, and continuing controversy over pathomechanics make this a difficult area of study. There are two main types of carpal instability: static and dynamic.

In *static carpal instabilities* there is an abnormal carpal alignment which can be seen by careful study of standard AP and lateral radiographs of the wrist. In *dorsiflexion instability* the lunate is rotated into dorsiflexion; in *palmar flexion instability* the lunate is rotated into palmar flexion; in *ulnar translocation* the whole carpus is displaced in an ulnar direction. (This pattern of deformity is common in rheumatoid arthritis); and in *dorsal subluxation* the carpus in displaced in a dorsal direction. (This is seen most often in mal-united Colles fractures where there is loss of the normal palmar tilt of the articular surface of the radius.)

In *dynamic carpal instabilities* routine radiographs are normal. The patient is usually able to toggle his carpal alignment from normal to abnormal and back, or manipulation of the scaphoid by the examiner may reproduce the sensation of instability of which the patient usually complains. The commonest instability occurs between the *scaphoid and lunate*. Less common are instabilities between the *lunate and triquetral* or at the *midcarpal joint*. To establish the diagnosis, place lead markers on the skin over points of local tenderness, and take radiographs in both stable and unstable positions. In the case of scapholunate instability, AP views of the supinated wrist in both radial and ulnar deviation are usually diagnostic. Examination of the wrist in motion using an image intensifier may also be helpful. Other investigations: (a) a radio-isotope bone scan may be carried out. If this is negative, either the diagnosis is incorrect, or local inflammatory changes are of such a minor degree that no more than conservative managements should be considered (b) arthrography may be helpful in detecting the presence and location of (intercarpal) ligament tears.

**113. Carpal instabilities (2): Scapholunate dissociation** (Illus.) if untreated may be followed by osteoarthritis. *Treatment:* (a) In the acute case: manipulative reduction using the image intensifier, followed by closed pinning; *or* open repair of the torn ligaments. (b) In chronic cases reattachment of the avulsed scapholunate ligament may be carried out, but where there are arthritic changes and subluxation, silastic replacement of the scaphoid and a midcarpal arthrodesis may be considered.

**114. Injuries to the metacarpals and phalanges: general principles:** In assessing how best to treat a specific injury, begin by making sure there is no significant soft-tissue involvement such as nerve or tendon injury, or substantial skin loss (see later for further details). Next, from the radiographs, assess whether the bony alignment can be judged as being acceptable. (Illus: acceptable undisplaced fractures of the shafts of the middle and ring metacarpals.)

**115. Assessing position** *ctd:* Generally speaking, the position of a metacarpal or phalangeal fracture can be considered acceptable (a) if angulation does not exceed 10° in either the lateral or AP projections (1): but in the lateral, 20° may be accepted in the metaphysis (2) and 45° in the neck of the fifth metacarpal (3); (b) if there is at least 50% bony contact (4); (c) if there is no rotational deformity (5).

**116. Assessing position** *ctd:* Rotational deformity may not always be obvious on the radiographs, or clinically when a finger is in the extended position. Note, however, that when the fingers are individually flexed that they all touch the palm close to the scaphoid. Check that this is the case. (The same precaution should be taken when the quality of a reduction is being assessed or when splintage is being applied.)

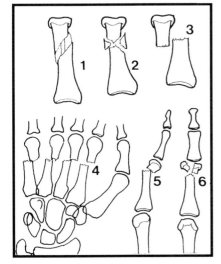

**117. Assessing stability:** Now go on and make an assessment of the *stability* of the fracture. Undisplaced transverse and longitudinal fractures are generally *stable*, but the following are usually *unstable:* (1) rotated spiral and some oblique fractures; (2) multifragmentary fractures; (3) severely displaced fractures; (4) multiple fractures; (5) fractures through the neck of a proximal phalanx; (6) displaced articular fractures.

**118. Assessing stability** *ctd:* If there is some remaining doubt, assess the *functional stability* of the fracture. This is done by asking the patient to flex the injured finger (without assistance) and assessing the range of movements in the joints on either side of the fracture. If the fracture is functionally stable the range obtained should reach 30% of the normal range. (i.e. MP = 27° (N = 90°); PIP = 30° (N = 100°); DIP = 24° (N = 80°).)

**119. Treatment (1):** (a) If there is no significant soft-tissue injury, if the fracture is in an acceptable position, and if it is clinically and radiologically stable, treatment should be directed at controlling the initial pain and swelling. Elevation of the arm in a sling may be helpful, *provided the sling is applied in such a way that the hand is not dependent.* Any pressure dressing should be applied in such a way that it avoids any local constriction. Mobilise early.

120. **Treatment (2):** (b) If the position is unsatisfactory, the fracture should be manipulated. If a good stable position can be obtained, treat as above. (c) If the position is acceptable, or an acceptable position has been obtained by manipulation, but the fracture is unstable, splintage will be required. For the less severe injuries garter strapping to an adjacent finger with interdigital felt padding provides the ideal combination of stability while retaining movement.

121. **Treatment (3):** If the injury is more severe, and a more restricting cast or bandaging is necessary, close attention must be paid to the position of the fingers. The MP joints should *never* be splinted in extension. When recovery of movements is hoped for, the MP joints should be flexed to 90°, the IP joints extended, and the thumb abducted. In practice this is often difficult to achieve, but MP joint extension should be studiously avoided.

122. **Treatment (4):** The previously described position, where return of function is expected, reduces the effects of fibrosis in the collateral ligaments, and places the finger joints in a favourable position for mobilisation. It must be carefully differentiated from the position of *fixation* where no return of function is anticipated (e.g. the position a joint is placed in for fusion). In the latter case, the MP and IP joints are put up in mid-flexion.

123. **Treatment (5):** (d) If the fracture cannot be reduced or held with simple splintage in acceptable position, then open reduction and/or stabilisation with some form of internal fixation (or an external fixator) should be considered. Other indications for this approach include: (1) The presence of a significant soft tissue injury; (2) the presence of multiple fractures; (3) fractures involving or disrupting joint surface. (Illus.: open unstable fracture of proximal phalanx in an unacceptable position.)

124. **Methods of internal fixation.** The aim is to achieve a rigidity of fixation that will allow early mobilisation, thereby greatly enhancing the chances of recovery. Unfortunately the bones of the hand are small and the soft tissue cover seldom generous. These factors, along with the proximity of the gliding structures, and the risks of tendon and joint adhesions have led to modification of methods used elsewhere, and to the development of alternative techniques: these include: **Type A Intraosseous wiring (1).** This is suitable for transverse fractures, and employs a single loop of 26G monofilament stainless steel wire and a Kirschner wire.

125. **Type A Intraosseous wiring *ctd:* Technique:** The fracture may be approached through a mid-line dorsal incision (except in the case of the distal phalanx, when an H incision is used). Two transverse holes, situated marginally towards the dorsal surfaces and 3–4 mm from the bone ends, are drilled using a trocar pointed 0.035″ (0.89 mm) Kirschner wire (or equivalent drill) (1). Through these holes the wire is threaded, using if required, a 20G needle as a carrier (2). A Kirschner wire is then inserted obliquely through the distal fragment (3).

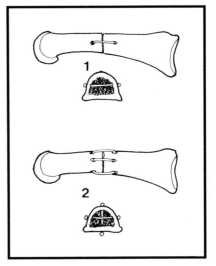

**126. Type A intraosseous wiring *ctd:*** The K-wire is partially withdrawn (4), the fracture reduced, and the K-wire driven through the opposite cortex (5). The wire is twisted (6), and the ends cropped and tucked into a hole drilled in the cortex (7). External splintage (e.g. bandages, sling, POP backshell) may be used for comfort, but this should be discarded by the seventh day. A biodegradable bone peg may be used instead of the K-wire. This form of wiring is not recommended for metacarpal shaft fractures.

**127. Type B intraosseous wiring (2):** This is suitable for small articular fragments. *Technique.* The fracture is reduced, and a hole drilled at right angles to the fracture line (1). Leave the drill (0.035″ K-wire) in position, and with a second drill make a hole parallel to the first (2). Insert the wire, using a hypodermic needle as a carrier, tighten, crop and bury as before (3). If the fragment is too small to drill, it may be snared by passing the wire next to bone (e.g. through the collateral ligament attachment) (4).

**128. 90–90 intraosseous wiring (3):** This resembles Type A wiring, but instead of a single wire (1), two wires are used at right angles to one another (2). It is a strong method of holding transverse fractures of the metacarpals and phalanges, and is useful for fusions and replants. It should not be used if there is osteoporosis or fragmentation. *Technique.* The bone ends are trimmed if necessary to provide flat contiguous surfaces, and holes drilled with careful attention to orientation.

**129. 90–90 intraosseous wiring *ctd:*** A 20G needle may be used as a carrier, flexing the finger at the fracture site as required for placing the vertical wire (1 and 2). When both wires have been inserted (3), the fracture is reduced and the wires tightened by twisting. The ends should be buried to avoid interference with the gliding structures. After closure, additional external splintage may be employed for patient comfort; this should be discarded and mobilisation commenced within 7 days.

**130. Tension band wiring (4):** This can give very strong fixation, and is useful for unstable fractures of the phalanges and metacarpals, especially when there is a degree of fragmentation. *Technique.* The fractures are reduced and held with single or paired Kirschner wires; the wires are cropped so that the amount protruding from the bone is just enough to give anchorage for tension band wires. These are looped round the *dorsal* surface of the bone before tightening.

**131. Percutaneous Kirschner wires (5):** This is used most often to stabilise phalangeal (1), and metacarpal fractures at all levels (2). In many cases the wires can be inserted without exposing the fracture. The quality of fixation is seldom perfect, and additional external splintage is often required. Although there can be problems with loosening, migration, infection, distraction and non-union, it is a valuable technique. Best results are obtained when trocar pointed wires are inserted with slow drilling speeds.

**132. Compression screws (6):** These may be used to reconstruct articular fractures, or to hold unstable fractures of the metacarpals or phalanges. The bone fragments are often small and friable, and secure fixation without risk of devascularisation or fragment fracture requires careful case selection. As a general rule, any fragment should be at least three times the diameter of the screw intended to be used. (2.7 mm screws may be used in metacarpal fractures; 2.0 and 1.5 mm screws are used in phalangeal fractures.)

**133. Plate fixation (7):** Plates must be carefully placed to avoid interference with the gliding structures. They are of value in comminuted fractures (1), fractures with bone loss, T- and Y- (2) and other intra-articular and periarticular fractures. The AO Group recommend lateral incisions for the phalanges. Plates available include 1/4 tubular, DCP, T-shaped condylar, and Mennen (3). In the latter (used for metacarpal fractures) the prongs are crimped round the bone after the fracture has been reduced.

**134. Rigid mini external fixators (8):** Small external fixators may be used for multifragmentary fractures, fractures with bone loss and/or severe soft-tissue involvement, infected fractures, and fracture dislocations of the PIP joint. Traction (e.g. for joint disruptions) or compression techniques may be employed. Unilateral, bilateral, and combination systems (Illus.) can be used. Their application can be difficult, the pin tracks are susceptible to infection, and the pins may interfere with the gliding structures.

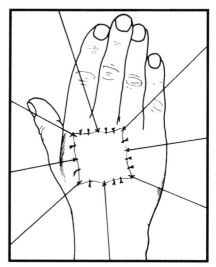

**135. Flexible mini external fixators (9):** The Stockport Serpentine Spring System (S-Quatro) is useful for displaced fracture–dislocations, giving distraction and some joint movement. A pin is inserted in the middle phalanx distal to the central slip, and a second through a small incision through the tendon; the pins should diverge if traction is required, and the degree is adjusted by selecting the spring notches and their position along the grooved pins. The springs are cemented to the pins, and retained for 3–6 weeks.

**136. Soft-tissue management (1):** Where there is necrotic or foreign material, a thorough debridement should be performed under a tourniquet to minimise the risks of infection. There is little tissue to spare in the hand, and wide excision of wounds is to be avoided. (2) The tourniquet should be released prior to closure to secure bleeding points and reduce wound haematoma.

**137. Soft-tissue management _ctd_ (3):** Where there is skin loss, every attempt should be made to ensure that healing will be achieved as quickly as possible to permit early mobilisation. The exposure of fractures, joints and bones should be avoided, and if the situation permits a primary skin grafting procedure or plastic repair should be carried out.

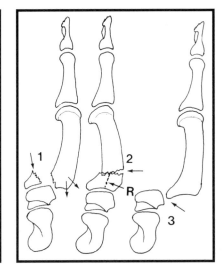

**138. Soft-tissue management *ctd* (4):** If there is division of both neurovascular bundles to a finger, amputation should be advised unless facilities for microsurgery are available and the particular circumstances (e.g. employment, hobbies, etc.) make an attempt at preservation particularly desirable. In all cases, the maximum length of thumb must be preserved.

**139. Soft-tissue management *ctd* (5):** If there is appreciable risk of infection (e.g. ragged wound, dirty causal instrument) primary suture of nerves and also of tendons in the 'no man's area' of the tendon sheaths should not be undertaken. Where, however, the circumstances are ideal; the experienced surgeon may achieve the best results by primary repair.

**140. Injuries to the thumb: The base:** The commonest injuries involving the base of the thumb are (1) Bennett's fracture (or Bennett's fracture–dislocation as it may be more aptly called), (2) fractures of the base of the thumb metacarpal; when there is a vertical extension into the joint, converting it into a T- or Y-fracture, the prognosis is less good (Rolando fracture); (3) carpometacarpal dislocation of the thumb.

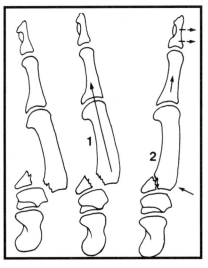

**141. Diagnosis:** Injuries of the base usually result from force being applied along the long axis of the thumb—e.g. from a fall or blow on the clenched fist (1)—or from forced abduction of the thumb (2). Any of these may be mistaken for scaphoid fracture, but tenderness is maximal distal to the snuff box (and deformity may be obvious).

**142. Bennett's fracture:** Note the distinctive features of this fracture: (1) a small medial fragment of bone which may tilt, but maintains its relationship with the trapezium, (2) the (vertical) fracture line involves the joint between the thumb metacarpal and the trapezium (trapezometacarpal joint), (3) most important, the proximal and lateral subluxation of the thumb metacarpal.

**143. Treatment (1):** The principle of reduction is straightforward: traction is applied to the thumb (1) and reduction completed by abducting it and applying pressure to the lateral aspect of the base (2). A general anaesthetic or Bier block is usually necessary. Maintaining reduction can be troublesome, and careful attention must be paid to the details of plaster fixation.

**144. Treatment (2):** (a) Begin by applying stockingette to the arm (1) and the thumb (2). Bony prominences should be protected as required with wool roll (3). (b) A small felt pad is placed over the base of the thumb metacarpal (4). (*Note:* adhesive felt should not be applied directly to the skin in this situation if a pustular rash is to be avoided.)

**145. Treatment (3):** (c) An assistant applies traction to the thumb and steadies the lateral three fingers (1). (d) Two to three 15 cm (6″) POP bandages (with or without an anterior slab) are applied to the *forearm* (2). (e) Two 10 cm (4″) POP bandages are then quickly applied to the wrist and up to the IP joint of the thumb (3).

**146. Treatment (4):** The surgeon now takes the thumb (the plaster being set on the forearm while the distal part remains soft). He must apply traction (1), abduct the thumb (2), maintain pressure over the base of the first metacarpal (3), and mould the plaster well into the MP joint on its flexor aspect (4).

**147. After care:** (a) Check radiographs are taken to confirm that reduction has been achieved. (b) The arm may require elevating with a sling for the first few days. (c) The patient should be seen at weekly intervals for the first 2–3 weeks and the thumb X-rayed. If the plaster appears slack at any stage it must be changed. If there is evidence of slipping of the fracture a new plaster should also be applied (no anaesthetic is generally required). During the setting of the plaster, light traction should be applied to the thumb while the plaster is well moulded round the base (in the position described for the initial reduction). (d) Plaster fixation should be maintained for 6 weeks.

**148. Alternative methods of treatment:** A good result is the rule following reduction and plaster fixation, but alternative methods of holding this fracture are practised. These include: (1) screw fixation (e.g. using the AO small fragment set and (2) the use of two Kirschner wires to stabilise the thumb metacarpal.

**149. Fractures near the base of the thumb metacarpal:** Greenstick fractures of this type are common in children. Angulation is usually slight or moderate, and should be accepted; gross angulations should be manipulated, using the technique described for Bennett's fracture. Plaster fixation for about 5 weeks is desirable. Rolando fractures require careful reduction, and good results are claimed for stabilisation with an external fixator, the pins being placed in the metacarpal and the trapezium.

**150. Carpometacarpal dislocation of the thumb:** The thumb may dislocate at the joint between the metacarpal base and the trapezium, or the whole of the first ray may be involved, the trapezium remaining with the thumb metacarpal, with the dislocation taking place between the trapezium and the scaphoid (Illus.). Both these injuries result from forcible abduction of the thumb. *Treatment*: Reduce by applying traction to thumb and local pressure over the base. Thereafter apply a well-padded plaster of scaphoid type for 3 weeks. Elevation of the limb for the first few days is desirable. Physiotherapy is seldom required.

**151. Injuries at the MP joint of the thumb: Posterior dislocation (1):** This injury generally results from forcible hyperextension of the thumb. It is common in children. In a number of cases there is 'button holing' of the capsule by the metacarpal head and closed methods of reduction will fail. Nevertheless, manipulation should be tried first in all cases.

**152. Posterior dislocation (2):** Manipulative reduction may often be attempted without anaesthesia (by the quick confident application of traction to the thumb with simultaneous pressure over the metacarpal head). When open reduction is required this should be performed through a lateral incision under a tourniquet. In all cases a light plaster splint should be worn for 2–3 weeks after reduction.

**153. Rupture of the ulnar collateral ligament (Gamekeeper's thumb) (1):** This injury is caused by forcible abduction (1). If unrecognised and untreated, there may be progressive MP subluxation (2) with interference with grasp, causing significant permanent disability. (a) *Suspect* this injury when there is complaint of pain in this region. (b) *Look for tenderness* on the medial side of the MP joint.

**154. Ulnar collateral ligament (2):** (c) Extend the MP joint fully and apply stress to the ulnar collateral ligament by abducting the proximal phalanx. Repeat with the thumb flexed at the MP joint. Note the presence of any 'give'. Carefully compare one side with the other. If in doubt, stress radiographs should be taken.

**155. Ulnar collateral ligament (3):** (d)
Study radiographs of the joint: (i) Subluxation may or may not be apparent in the unstressed films. (ii) An avulsion fracture (Illus.) may betray this type of injury. If a fracture is present, note its position. (Marked displacement, or rotation so that its articular surface is pointing distally, are indications for surgery.)

**156. Ulnar collateral ligament (4):**
*Treatment:* (a) Slight laxity (incomplete tear) or minimally displaced avulsion fracture: scaphoid cast for 6 weeks (1); (b) Rotated fragment: reduction and internal fixation, e.g. with Type B wiring. (c) Gross laxity (complete tear): conservative treatment (a) may give a good result, but many prefer primary surgical repair (d). (d) Late diagnosed complete tear: repair of the capsulo-ligamentous complex with a palmaris longus free tendon graft; or as salvage procedure, MP joint fusion (2).

**157. Fracture of the proximal phalanx:**
The severely angled fracture (1) should be reduced by traction and local pressure. Hold with a dorsal (or volar) slab (2) to which is added a girdered extension (3), held on with bandages. If the position cannot be readily held, internal fixation (e.g. by one of the wiring methods) is indicated. The minimally angled fracture (4) or the splinter fracture (5) may be protected by a local slab (similar to 3) bandaged in position. Elevation may be required.

**158. IP joint dislocation of the thumb:**
Reduce by traction as described for MP joint dislocations (197, 152). Only occasionally is anaesthesia required (ring or Bier block). Thereafter splint for 2–3 weeks with a local plaster slab. *Fractures of the terminal phalanx:* Crushing injuries are the usual cause, and any soft-tissue damage takes priority in management. A light local splint (e.g. of plaster) will prevent pain from stubbing.

**159. Injuries to the fifth metacarpal:** The commonest fractures involving the metacarpal of the little finger are: (1) fractures of the neck, (2) spiral fractures of the shaft, usually undisplaced (3) transverse fractures of the shaft, often angulated, (4) fractures of the base, (5) fractures of the head. (b = base, h = head.)

**160. Fractures of the neck of the fifth metacarpal (1):** These are nearly always caused by the clenched fist meeting resistance—for example, as a result of a fight (1). Angulation and impaction are common (2). When angulation is slight (3) or moderate (4) it should be accepted, and the fracture supported for 3–4 weeks until local pain settles.

**161. Neck of fifth metacarpal (2):** A simple dorsal slab (1), completed after a few days, may be quite satisfactory. Better fixation is achieved by the addition of a finger extension (2) to the basic slab. Still more support is provided by the use of garter strapping (3) and the inclusion of the ring and little fingers in the extension (4) (securing bandages omitted in Illus. for clarity).

**162. Neck of fifth metacarpal (3):** If angulation is gross (more than 45°), an attempt may be made to correct it. The MP joint is flexed; pressure is then applied to the head via the proximal phalanx, using the thumb. The fingers apply counter-pressure to the shaft. Reduction is generally easy. The position may be maintained using a Kirschner wire or with a plaster cast.

**163. Neck of fifth metacarpal (4):** The following technique may be employed. Stockingette is applied to the arm (1) and to the little finger (2). A thin strip of felt (3) is placed over the finger (4). A substantial dorsal slab is applied (5). The finger should be flexed into the palm and the striking point checked (191, 116).

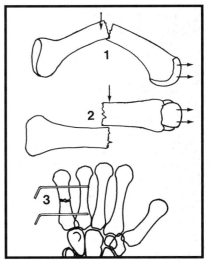

**164. Neck of fifth metacarpal (5):** A finger slab, made from a thrice-folded slab formed from three layers or so of 10 cm (4″) plaster bandage (6) is applied from wrist to finger tip (7). Pressure is maintained while the slab is setting (or with one hand as in 199, 163). Meanwhile an assistant can be securing the slabs with a wet gauze bandage (8). Complete in 2–3 days and retain for 4–5 weeks only.

**165. Injuries of the fifth metacarpal** *ctd:* Spiral fractures of the shaft (2), transverse fractures of the shaft with slight or moderate angulation or displacement (3) and fractures of the base (4) may be treated quite adequately by the application of a Colles plaster for 3–4 weeks.

**166. Injuries of the fifth metacarpal** *ctd:* Marked angulation of a shaft fracture should be treated by traction and local pressure prior to plaster fixation (1). Displaced fractures may be similarly reduced (2) but soft tissue between the bone ends may render reduction possible only by open methods. If that is required, reduction may be maintained by percutaneous (3) or intramedullary Kirschner wiring 90–90 intraosseous wiring or plating.

**169. Injuries to the index, middle and ring metacarpals** *ctd:* Severely displaced fractures of the index metacarpal should be managed along the lines described for fractures of the fifth metacarpal. In particular, badly displaced fractures should be reduced, and if necessary secured by some form of internal fixation. If Kirschner wires are used they should be retained for 3 weeks; plaster fixation may be needed for a further 2 weeks.

When the AP radiographs show the presence of an isolated off-ended fracture of the middle or ring metacarpals, or moderate angulation or shortening, the position can generally be accepted. The striking point of the finger should be checked, a dorsal slab applied and the limb elevated to counteract swelling. If off-ending or angulation is conspicuous in the *lateral projection*, reduction should be carried out, either by manipulation or by an open procedure.

**167. Injuries of the fifth metacarpal** *ctd:* (4) Fractures of the *head* of the fifth metacarpal (198, 159(5)) may be treated by garter strapping and early mobilisation; if symptoms are marked a dorsal slab may also be used for the first 1–2 weeks. If the fragment is substantial and displaced, internal fixation using a screw or Type B intraosseous wiring may be considered. (5) *Dislocation of the base* of the metacarpal (Illus.) is usually easily reduced with traction, but may need Kirschner wire stabilisation.

**168. Injuries to the index, middle and ring metacarpals:** The commonest fracture is a spiral fracture of the shaft (especially of the ring metacarpal), but fractures involving the base and neck are frequent, as are transverse fractures of the shaft (Illus.). Undisplaced fractures may be supported by a Colles type slab, but be on guard for swelling which can be severe, especially in multiple fractures.

**170. Fractures of the proximal and middle phalanges (1):** Undisplaced, simple fractures—e.g. of the shaft (1), base (2), neck (3), intercondylar region (4) or epiphyseal injuries (5)—seldom present any problem. Garter strapping (6) for 3–4 weeks may give adequate support, but if symptoms are marked this may be supplemented by the use of a volar or dorsal slab, with finger extension.

**171. Proximal and middle phalanges (2):** There is a tendency for angulation to occur due to intrinsic muscle pull; if more than 10° this should be corrected under general anaesthesia by gentle traction, using the thumb as a fulcrum. Generally these fractures are stable in flexion, and the affected finger may require to be fixed initially in this position.

**172. Proximal and middle phalanges (3):** There are various methods of fixation: these include: (a) foam-plastic-covered malleable aluminium splinting. Although this may hold the finger well, there may be difficulty in strapping it securely to the hand, and incorporation in a dorsal slab may be helpful. Great care must be taken to check the strike point and avoid undue local pressure which may lead to skin sloughing.

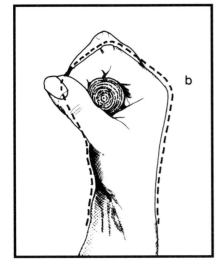

**173. Proximal and middle phalanges (4):** (b) If a rolled bandage can be held in the palm, this may be used as a fulcrum, the injured finger being flexed over it and secured with adhesive tape. Additional encircling bandaging is required for security, but even so dislodging may occur. Some surgeons use a (wetted) POP bandage in the palm.

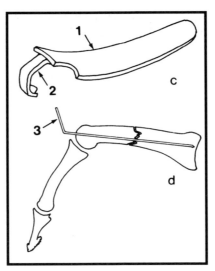

**174. Proximal and middle phalanges (5):** (c) A volar POP slab (1) with a substantial finger extension (2) may be used, moulding the fracture while this is setting; thereafter, the plaster is secured with wet open-weave bandages. If this arrangement appears too flimsy, it may be reinforced with a dorsal slab and dorsal finger extension. Where the fracture is unstable in any position, some form of internal fixation is advisable (d) (e.g. by intraosseous wiring, tension band wiring, or a percutaneous Kirschner wire (3)).

**176. Fractures of the terminal phalanx:** Fractures of the terminal tuft (often comminuted) (1), of the neck (2), and the base (3) are painful but relatively unimportant injuries. Treatment of any associated soft tissue injury takes precedence (e.g. debridement and suture of pulp lacerations).

Nevertheless, strapping the finger to a spatula or use of a plastic finger splint may relieve pain and prevent any painful stubbing incidents.

**175. After care:** In all cases: (a) uninjured fingers should be left free and exercised, (b) rigid fixation should be discarded as soon as possible. In many situations garter strapping may be substituted after 2 weeks, and often all support after 4. *In no instance should the MP joints be fixed in extension.*

*Complications:* (a) *Finger stiffness* is the commonest and most disabling complication, and is due to joint adhesions, fibrosis in the adjacent flexor tendon sheaths and collateral ligament shortening. Infection in open fractures may be a major contributory factor. Stiffness may be minimised by the procedures described (e.g. elevation, correct splinting, early mobilisation) and by intensive physiotherapy and occupational therapy. Physiotherapy and occupational therapy should be continued with vigour until the range of movements and finger power become static. This implies careful recording, at frequent intervals, of these parameters. In this respect it is helpful to note the *total active range of motion* (TAM) in each digit; this overall movement can be assessed by a single goniometer measurement; it is a little less than the sum of the normal maxima of flexion of the individual joints, the normal value of TAM being taken to be 250°.

Early return to work should be encouraged to foster re-adaptation. Inability to work and a static response to physiotherapy requires most careful assessment of the following: (a) possibility of redeployment, (b) possibility of improvement from further surgery (e.g. tenolysis), (c) amputation.

*Amputation* as primary treatment must be raised in open phalangeal fractures when they are associated with flexor tendon division. Division of one or both neurovascular bundles, skin loss or severe crushing are additional factors weighing favour of this procedure (in contrast to attempted repair where treatment is likely to be prolonged and the final result uncertain). With these factors must be considered the patient's age, sex and occupation. (b) *Mal-union:* Problems may arise from: (i) recurrence of deformity, (ii) failure to correct initial deformity, (iii) torsional deformity. In some cases (iv) epiphyseal displacement may have escaped attention. In the latter case remodelling may lead to correction, and in the others trick movements and postural adaptations may remove the patient's initial strong desire for corrective surgery. It is wise not to offer surgical correction until at least 6 months have passed since the injury.

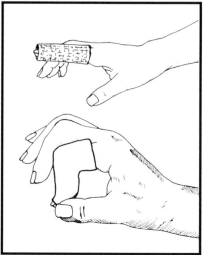

**177. Mallet finger (1):** This is caused by forcible flexion of an extended finger. The distal extensor tendon slip is torn at its attachment to bone (Type I injury) or avulses a fragment of bone (Type II). The patient is unable to extend the DIP joint fully; drooping of the finger tip may be slight (a) or severe (b). In late cases there may be hyperextension of the PIP joint (c) In Type III injuries, more than 20% of the articular surface of the distal phalanx is involved, sometimes with anterior subluxation of the phalanx.

**178. Mallet finger (2):** *Treatment:* All these injuries excepting Type IIIs with subluxation may be treated by splinting the distal joint in extension. A Stack or Abuna splint (Illus.) may be used. Choose the size with care to lessen the risks of skin ulceration. It is strapped to the finger and worn for 6 weeks constantly, and then for a further two at night only. It may be removed for skin hygiene if extension is preserved. Alternatively, support the distal joint with a short length of padded spatula strapped to the volar surface.

**179. Mallet finger (3):** Where the patient's cooperation is in doubt, a Smillie plaster may be used for 6–8 weeks, although it can cause some stiffness. Form a 4-layer tube of 7.5 cm (3″) dry POP bandage round the finger. Dip the hand momentarily in water, asking the patient to flex the PIP joint and extend the DIP joint against the thumb while the POP is smoothed. *Note:* In any case there may be some recurrence on removal of splintage, but disability is seldom more than slight, and spontaneous improvement may occur up to a year after the injury.

**180. Mallet finger (4):** If there is subluxation, see if reduction can be achieved in either flexion or extension, and splint accordingly. If not, consider repair: through a C-shaped incision a pull-out wire may be inserted under the tendon, through bone, and out through the pulp; stabilise the joint with a K-wire. *Late diagnosed mallet finger:* Extension splintage may be successful even as late as 6 months. If there is a swan-neck deformity, an oblique retinacular ligament reconstruction has been advocated.

**181. MP and interphalangeal joint dislocations:** These may be simple or multiple (Illus.) and as they result from hyperextension are almost always posterior dislocations. Reduce as described for the thumb (197, 152). Thereafter garter strapping should be applied for 2 weeks unless there is any evidence of instability—when plaster of Paris splintage may be required for a slightly longer period.

**182. Fracture dislocation:** It is essential that the joint surface is correctly relocated, and important that mobilisation is commenced as soon as possible. Open reduction is usually required, and fixation may be achieved with intraosseous wiring, small fragment set screws, or plating. This should be removed after 2–3 weeks and mobilisation commenced using garter strapping for the first week or so until the fracture becomes more stable.

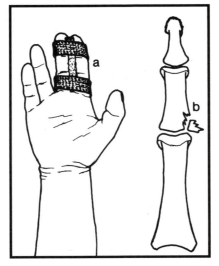

**183. 'Sprains' and lateral subluxations (1):** These are usually caused by falls in which the side of a finger strikes some resistant object. There is avulsion or tearing of a collateral ligament. Spontaneous reduction is the rule. *Diagnosis:* The injury should be suspected on the basis of the history and the presence of local tenderness. Confirmation is obtained by noting instability on stressing the collateral ligament.

**184. Sprains and lateral subluxations (2):** Radiographs may show a tell-tale avulsion fracture. If doubt remains, stress films may be taken. Treatment: (a) Garter strapping for 5 weeks should be adequate. (b) If an avulsion fracture is present and has rotated, it should be replaced. *Complications:* Fusiform swellings of the finger may persist for many months even in the treated injury.

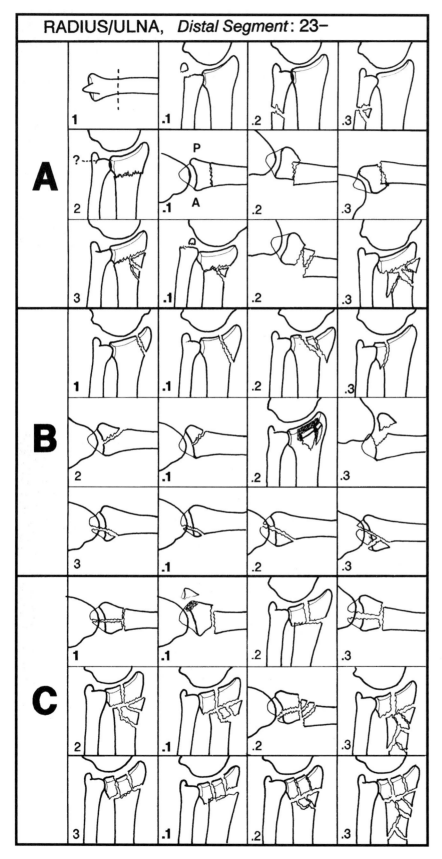

**RADIUS/ULNA,** *Distal Segment* : 23–

**185. AO Classification of Fractures of the Radius/Ulna, Distal Segment (23–):**

**Type A** fractures are extra-articular.
A1 = Fracture of the ulna only: .1 styloid process; .2 simple, of the metaphysis; .3 multifragmentary of the metaphysis.
A2 = Simple impacted fracture of the radius: .1 undisplaced; .2 with dorsal tilting (Colles pattern); .3 with anterior tilting (Smith pattern).
A3 = Multifragmentary fracture of the radius: .1 with axial impaction and shortening; .2 with a wedge; .3 complex.

**Type B** fractures are partial articular fractures of the radius.
B1 = Partial articular fracture of radius in the sagittal plane: .1 simple lateral; .2 multifragmentary lateral; .3 medial.
B2 = Partial articular fracture of the radius with involvement of the posterior lip (dorsal rim) (Barton's fracture): .1 simple; .2 with an additional lateral sagittal fracture; .3 with dorsal dislocation of the carpus (fracture dislocation of the wrist).
B3 = Partial articular fracture of the radius with involvement of the anterior lip (volar rim) (Reverse Barton's fracture): .1 simple with a small fragment; .2 simple with a large fragment; .3 multifragmentary.

**Type C** fractures are complete articular fractures.
C1 = Both the metaphyseal and articular elements are simple; .1 with a posteromedial articular fragment; .2 with the articular fracture line in the sagittal plane; .3 with articular fracture line in the frontal plane.
C2 = The articular fracture is simple, but the metaphyseal fracture is multifragmentary: .1 the articular fracture line is in the sagittal plane; .2 the articular fracture line is in the frontal plane; .3 the metaphyseal fracture extends into the diaphysis.
C3 = The articular fracture is multifragmentary: .1 metaphyseal simple; .2 the metaphyseal fracture is also multifragmentary; .3 multifragmentary metaphyseal fracture extending into the diaphysis.

186. Describe this AP radiograph of the wrist; the history is of pain and marked swelling following a fall on the outstretched hand.

187. History of deformity of the wrist persisting after an injury some years previously: diagnosis?

188. History of a crushing injury of the hand and fingers. Describe the radiograph.

189. The complaint is of pain and deformity of the hand following an injury in which the fingers were forced backwards. What does the radiograph show?

190. Describe this injury sustained by a child in a fall.

191. Describe the radiographic appearances. The history is of a fall on the outstretched hand.

192. What does this radiograph show?

193. What injury is being treated here?

194. What is the injury? How would you treat it?

195. What is this injury: What special precaution would you take if attempting treatment by closed methods?

196. What is this injury, and how is it being treated?

197. What does this radiograph show? What functional restriction would you expect?

198.  What is this injury? How would you treat it?

199.  What is this injury? How would you treat it?

200.  What fracture complication is shown on this radiograph?

201.  What does this lateral radiograph show?

202.  What type of fracture is present? What is the prognosis? How might it be treated?

203.  What is this injury? How would you treat it?

186. Fracture of the distal radius; the distal fragment is fragmented, with the fracture line involving the radiocarpal joint; fracture of the ulnar styloid. AO 23–C1.2.

187. Mal-union of a Smith's fracture. AO 23–C1.2.

188. (1) There is a transverse fracture of the base of the proximal phalanx of the ring finger; the single film suggests that there is no significant angulation or displacement. (2) There is a fracture of the base of the proximal phalanx of the middle finger, with vertical splinter fractures running into the proximal IP joint. There is angulation of the fracture. The single oblique view suggests that this is mainly anterior angulation.

189. Posterior dislocation of all the fingers at the MP joints. The thumb is not affected.

190. Greenstick fractures of the radius and ulna just proximal to the epiphyseal lines. There is slight subluxation of the distal ulna whose angulation is less than that of the radius. The deformity corresponds to that found in a Smith's fracture, and the combination of fracture of the radius with ulnar subluxation has some of the feature of the Galeazzi lesion.

191. (1) There is a highly comminuted fracture of the distal radius with the radial displacement, ulnar angulation and impaction usually associated with a comminuted Colles fracture with involvement of the radiocarpal joint. A lateral projection would be required to differentiate it with certainty from a Smith's fracture. (2) There is a fracture through the waist of the scaphoid. AO 23–C3.1.

192. Long-standing non-union of the scaphoid, with early secondary osteo-arthritic changes in the wrist joint.

193. Bennet's fracture of the thumb being held with fine crossed Kirschner wires.

194. This is a slipped distal radial epiphysis, uncommonly associated with a greenstick fracture of the ulna in its distal third. This should reduce easily by manipulation; subsequent treatment would be by plaster fixation.

195. MP dislocation of the thumb in a child; theatre facilities should be available (for an open reduction) should manipulation under general anaesthesia fail.

196. Unstable fracture of the distal radius with an associated injury to the ulnar styloid (Colles type fracture); this is being treated by an external fixator. Injuries of this pattern would normally be treated conservatively unless open and accompanied by much soft-tissue damage.

197. Mal-union of a fracture of a middle phalanx. There would be inevitable loss of flexion in the distal IP joint.

198. Mallet finger, with a small avulsion fracture of the base of the distal phalanx; there is no joint subluxation, and the injury should respond well to 6 weeks' splintage in extension.

199. Dislocation of the proximal IP joint of the ring finger. Treat by manipulative reduction followed by garter strapping splintage.

200. Avascular necrosis of the scaphoid.

201. Slipped distal radial epiphysis.

202. Displaced and possibly slightly comminuted fracture of the waist of the scaphoid. This injury has a bad prognosis, and primary internal fixation might be desirable.

203. Carpometacarpal dislocation of the thumb, with a small associated fracture, possibly of the metacarpal base. Manipulative reduction followed by plaster fixation.

# 10.  The spine

1. **General principles: (1) The main concern** in any spinal injury is not with the spine itself, but with the closely related neurological elements (the spinal cord, issuing nerve roots and cauda equina).

**(2) If there is no neurological complication** risks of later neurological involvement must be assessed; if there is some risk of this, *precautions must be taken to see that this is avoided at all stages.*

**(3) If there is an incomplete paraplegia** complicating the injury *great care must be taken to see that no deterioration is allowed to occur.*

**(4) If paraplegia is present and complete,** the prognosis regarding potential recovery must be firmly established as early as possible. Only if this is pronounced *total and permanent* can vigilance in the handling of the spinal injury be relaxed.

2. **Anatomical features (after Kapandji) (1):** The components of a typical vertebra have a complex relationship, and can be illustrated with an exploded diagram. The elements comprise the vertebral body (1) composed of cancellous bone covered with an outer shell of cortical bone, the horseshoe-shaped neural arch (2), two articular masses or processes which take part in the facet (interarticular) joints (3) and the transverse (4) and spinous (5) processes.

3. **Anatomical features (2):** When these components are brought together they form a protective bony covering for the cord (6) and the issuing nerve roots (7) The neural arch (2) is divided by the articular processes (3) into pedicles (8) and laminae (9).

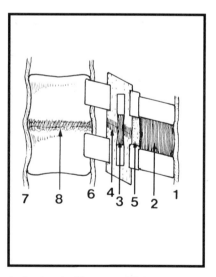

4. **Anatomical features (3):** The vertebrae are bound together by the following structures: The supraspinous (1), interspinous (2), intertransverse (3) and capsular ligaments (4), and the ligamentum flavum (5): together these form the so-called posterior ligament complex. Playing a less powerful but nevertheless important role are the posterior (6) and anterior (7) longitudinal ligaments and the annular ligaments (8). Trauma may result in damage to any of the bony or ligamentous structures of the spine, either in isolation or in combination.

5. **Assessment of spinal injuries (1):** In managing any case of spinal injury it is important to determine which structures have been involved and the extent of the damage they have suffered; with this information an assessment may be made of the risks of complication. Note (a) the history may direct you to the type of injury to suspect; (b) the clinical examination may be a valuable guide to the extent of bony and ligamentous injury, and any neurological complication; (c) investigation by X-ray and CAT scan is likely to provide the most information. It is important to make an early assessment of the stability of the spine—i.e. to assess whether it is able to withstand stress without progressive deformity or further neurological damage. *Instability may be purely mechanical* (e.g. in some compression fractures where further kyphotic deformity may occur). *Instability may be neurological* (e.g. where shifting or further extrusion of bone fragments within the spinal canal may lead to neurological deterioration). *Combined mechanical and neurological instability* may be present. *In assessing instability it may be helpful to regard the spine as having three main elements or columns.*

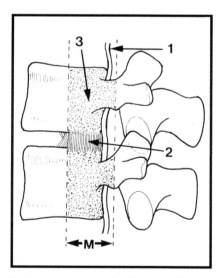

6. **Assessment of spinal injuries (2):** The *middle column* (M) consists of the posterior longitudinal ligament (1), the posterior part of the annular ligament (2), and the posterior wall of the vertebral column (3). Unstable injuries occur when damage to the middle column is combined with damage to either the anterior column or damage to the posterior column.

**7. Assessment of spinal injuries (3):** The *posterior column* (P) comprises the neural arch, the pedicles, the spinous process, and the post. ligt. complex. The *anterior column* (A) is formed by the ant. long. ligament, the anterior part of the annular ligt., and the anterior part of the vertebral body. Note that the concern is the integrity of these columns, and that failure in their role as supports can be due to *either* bone *or* ligamentous involvement (or a combination). Denis classifies four categories of spinal injury:

**8. Classification of spinal injuries: Compression fractures (1):** Simple compression fractures are common stable injuries involving the anterior column only. Hyperflexion of the spine round an axis passing through the disc space leads to mechanical failure of bone with either anterior (Illus.) or lateral wedging. The height of the posterior part of the vertebral body is maintained. (Note that *severe* wedging—e.g. more than 15–20°—often indicates damage to the other columns and a burst fracture or fracture dislocation.)

**9. Burst fractures (2):** Axial loading of the spine may cause failure of the anterior and middle columns. One or both vertebral body end plates may be involved, and bone fragments may be extruded into the spinal canal, compromising the neurological structures and causing neurological instability. Radiographs may show the vertebral body fracture, loss of vertebral height, and in the AP, laminar fractures and separation of the pedicles. A CAT scan is invaluable in showing bony extrusion; myelography is also sometimes of help.

**10. Seat belt type injuries (3):** Rapid deceleration causes the spine to jack-knife round an axis brought forward by a lap type seatbelt, and *tension* forces lead to failure of the posterior and middle columns. The spine is unstable in flexion. Failure may occur entirely through bone (Chance fracture) (1), or ligaments (2), or a combination (3), involving either one (1 & 2) or two (3) levels of the spine. Injuries of this pattern may be seen in situations outside road traffic accidents, but the essential element is tension failure.

**11. Fracture dislocations (4):** All 3 columns fail, and there is loss of the normal constraints, so that dislocation or subluxation may occur. Suspect if: (i) there are multiple rib or transverse process fractures; (ii) there is a slight increase in the height of a disc or a fracture of an articular process. *Types:* (a) *Flexion–rotation fracture–dislocation.* There is often a fracture of an articular process on one side (F), or a slicing fracture through a vertebral body, leading to rotation and subluxation of the spine.

**12. (4 *ctd*):** (b) *Shear types of fracture–dislocation:* In the posteroanterior type the upper segment is sheared forwards, often with fracture of the posterior arch at 1 or 2 levels (1). In the anteroposterior type there is complete ligamentous disruption, but often no fracture (2). (c) *Flexion–distraction type of fracture–dislocation:* This is a tension type of injury as in the seatbelt lesion, but there is an anterior annular tear with stripping of the anterior long. ligt. allowing anterior subluxation (3).

13. **Diagnosis:** Suspect involvement of the cervical spine where the patient: (a) complains of neck, occipital or shoulder pain after trauma, (b) has a torticollis (Illus.), complains of restriction of neck movements or supports the head with the hands, or (c) is found unconscious after a head injury, especially in road traffic accidents. In all cases, further investigation by radiographs is essential.

14. **Initial management (1):** If you suspect that the cervical spine has been injured, your first move should be to safeguard the cord by controlling neck movements. The simplest and best way of doing this is by applying a cervical collar. (Illus.: commercially available collar adjustable in depth and girth.) At the roadside, an adequate collar may be fashioned from rolled newspapers pushed into a nylon stocking and wrapped round the neck.

15. **Initial management (2):** Alternatively, if the patient is on a trolley, the head may be supported by sandbags. *Do not allow the head to flex forwards, and do not hyperextend.* Keep the head in a neutral position wherever possible, and in the conscious patient quickly check that there is active movement in all limbs.

16. **Initial management (3):** Especially if there is some evidence of neurological involvement, *do not* check the range of movements in the cervical spine. Accompany the patient to the X-ray department, supporting the head during the positioning of the tube and making sure that the spine is not forced in to flexion. For initial screening an AP, lateral and a through-the-mouth projection of C1 and C2 should be taken.

17. **Initial management (4):** If these films appear normal, you may proceed in reasonable safety to (i) further examination of the neck for localising tenderness, restriction of active movements and protective spasm, and (ii) a more thorough neurological examination. If these show no departure from normal, the patient may be treated with a cervical collar, with a follow-up review in 1 week.

18. **Initial management (5):** If there is, however, persistent material limitation of movements or evidence of neurological disturbance further investigation is necessary. The following additional radiographs should be taken: (a) two more lateral projections, one in flexion and one in extension; these again should be supervised; (b) right and left oblique projections of the cervical spine. The commonest difficulty is the technical one of visualising the lower cervical vertebrae in the stocky patient. The upper border of T1 *must* be seen. *Accept* that detail may be poor. *Do not accept* that the spine cannot be shown in sufficient detail to exclude dislocation of one vertebra over another. If necessary, assist the radiographer by arranging for traction to be applied to the arms—one in adduction and the other in abduction; slight angulation of the tube and increase in exposure may be helpful. Computer-assisted tomography, if available, may provide valuable information. Apart from confirming the presence of fractures (especially of the neural arches and facet joints), which may be poorly visualised on normal films, it can give useful additional information on any encroachment on the neural canal, especially in the case of bursting fractures.

In some cases screening of the cervical spine movements may be useful.

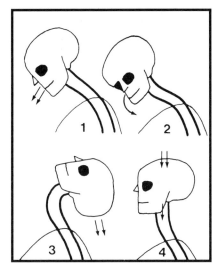

19. **Classification of cervical spine injuries:** Injuries of the cervical spine may be grouped according to the mechanism of injury:
(A) flexion injuries, 1;
(B) flexion and rotation injuries, 2;
(C) extension injuries, 3;
(D) compression injuries, 4.

20. **Causes of flexion and flexion/rotation injuries:** These may result from: (a) falls on the back of the head leading to flexion of the neck—e.g. in motor cycle spills, diving in shallow water, pole vaulting and rugby football, (b) blows on the back of the head from falling objects (e.g. in the building and mining industries), (c) rapid deceleration in head-on car accidents.

21. **(A) Flexion injuries: Stable anterior wedge fracture (1):** The vertebral body is wedged anteriorly, while the posterior part is generally intact. Before the injury can be declared stable, there must be (1) no evidence of injury to the posterior ligament complex—no separation or avulsion of the vertebral spines, or clinical evidence of ligament tear (see 228, 98)—(2) no damage to the neural arches or facets. (3) In addition, flexion and extension laterals must be taken, and must show no vertebral instability.

22. **Stable anterior wedge fracture (2):** Assuming these criteria are satisfied, neurological disturbance is rare and the prognosis excellent. Treat with a cervical collar for 6 weeks. Rarely when there is a degree of lateral wedging there may be troublesome nerve root involvement usually with (mainly) sensory disturbance in the corresponding dermatome. *If instability is at all suspected, treat as a cervical dislocation* (see 217, 45).

23. **(B) Flexion/rotation injuries: (a) Unilateral dislocation with a locked facet joint (1):** One facet joint dislocates, so that in the lateral projection of the cervical spine one vertebral body is seen to overlap the one below by about a third. The AP view may not be helpful, or it may show malalignment of spinous processes. There is often little difference between laterals taken in flexion and extension.

24. **Unilateral dislocation (2):** Oblique projections will, however, confirm the diagnosis. On one side the columnar arrangement of bodies, foramina and facet joints will be regular (Illus.), while on the other it will be broken. Damage to the posterior ligament complex is variable, and *after reduction* these injuries may be quite stable **but note**: if there is an associated fracture involving a facet joint the injury is **most certainly unstable** and fusion will be required after reduction.

25. **Unilateral dislocation (3):** On clinical examination of the patient with a unilateral dislocation, the head is slightly rotated and inclined to the side (1) away from the locked facet (2). There is often great pain with radiation (3) due to pressure on the nerve root at the level of the affected joint, and there may be cord involvement. Proceed to treatment if there is no neurological defect: *otherwise see 217, 45.*

26. **Treatment (1):** The initial aim in treatment is to reduce the dislocation, and the secret of this is well-controlled traction. (A) The patient is given a general anaesthetic; the head must be well supported during induction, the administration of any muscle relaxant and intubation (which must be carried out without undue extension of the neck). (B) X-ray facilities should be available (preferably an image intensifier).

27. **Treatment (2):** (C) The surgeon must have freedom to manipulate the head, and may do this with the patient fully on the table, or pulled up till the head is supported in the lap of the surgeon seated at the top end of the table. Place the thumbs under the jaw, clasp the fingers behind the occiput, and apply firm traction in *lateral flexion* away from the side of the locked facet, i.e. in the direction the head is usually inclined.

28. **Treatment (3):** (D) Maintaining traction, bring the head into the midline position, correcting the rotation element *before* lateral flexion. Release the traction, support the head (e.g. with foam plastic blocks) while check radiographs are taken. If reduction has not been achieved, repeat the manoeuvre with greater anaesthetic relaxation. Screening may be used. (If reduction fails (rare), or if preferred use skull traction as at 216, 39 et seq.)

29. **Treatment (4):** (E) Once reduction has been achieved, a cervical collar should be applied, and worn continuously for 6 weeks. (F) Fortnightly radiographs of the neck should be taken, and flexion and extension laterals at the end of the 6 weeks' fixation. *If there is any evidence of late subluxation* (Illus.) the patient should be admitted for local cervical fusion.

30. **(B) Flexion/rotation injuries:** (b) **Unstable injuries:** The commonest injury of this type is one where there is a pure cervical dislocation without fracture. Displacement may be severe, and there is frequently locking of both facets (Illus.). Damage to the posterior ligament complex is always present, and is generally obvious from the degree of vertebral displacement.

**31. Unstable injuries (2):** There may be other evidence of instability associated with disruption of the posterior ligament complex, e.g. (1) avulsion fracture(s) of a spinous process, (2) widening of the gap between two spinous processes or (3) *evidence of forward slip on the flexion lateral of the spine compared with the extension lateral.* Proceed to treatment if there is no neurological defect: *otherwise see 217, 45.*

**32. Unstable injuries (3): Treatment (1):** Unstable injuries without fracture require fusion; skull traction will be required to achieve and maintain reduction and should be applied without delay. Several types of calliper are available, and the following description applies to those of Cone's pattern (but see 215, 36).
(a) Shave the skin round the proposed insertion points (approximately 6–7 cm above the external auditory meati) and infiltrate the areas deeply on both sides with local anaesthetic.

**33. Treatment (2):** (b) Make a small incision (about 1 cm in length) on each side down to bone. Bleeding is usually brisk, but generally controllable by firm local pressure applied for a few moments; if not, secure and tie off any remaining bleeding points. (c) Now insinuate one point holder through the temporalis muscle fibres until it is in contact with the skull.

**34. Treatment (3):** (d) Keep the point holder pressed firmly against the skull; straighten out the calliper, and close it with the turnbuckle spanner. (e) Guide the second point holder through the skin wound; oscillate the calliper slightly to allow its tapered end to part the temporalis fibres on the second side. Close the calliper until both point holders are in firm but not hard contact with the skull.

**35. Treatment (4):** (f) Now screw the points in (you should check that their protrusion is limited to about 3 mm) to penetrate the outer cortex only; tighten them with a key. If the points fail to enter, either they are blunt or the bone unduly hard. In these circumstances, a small awl may be used as a starter, taking great care to avoid penetration of the inner cortex. Now seal the wound with strips of gauze soaked in Nobecutane® or a similar preparation.

**36. Other traction devices:** (2) *Blackburn callipers* are designed to hook into the diplöe of the skull, and a trephine is used to remove a tiny lid of outer cortex. Occasionally no diplöe is present, and the points must hook under the full thickness of the skull, and come in contact with the dura. (3) *Crutchfield traction tongs* are inserted nearer the vertex than the other two devices.

**37. Reduction (1):** If reduction is required, many surgeons prefer to do this manually under general anaesthesia with good relaxation. X-ray facilities are essential, and great care must be taken during induction and throughout the procedure to avoid uncontrolled movements of the head. When all is ready, the head is supported and the end of the table dropped; firm traction is applied in the neutral position or slight flexion (1) to unlock the facets (2).

**38. Reduction (2):** Maintaining firm traction the neck is slowly extended (3). The hand supporting the occiput may be moved in anticipation down the neck to act as a fulcrum (4). The traction is then slowly reduced, the table end raised and, whilst maintaining a little controlling traction, the position is checked with radiographs.

**39. Reduction (3): Alternative techniques:** Continuous (weight) traction may be used to overcome muscle tension and unlock overriding facets. The *direction* of traction may be controlled by altering the position of the traction pulley, or by the use of pads under the head or shoulders. The *amount* of traction can be adjusted by the weights. The duration of maximal traction is monitored by radiographs.

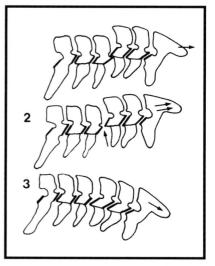

**40. Reduction (4):** A better arrangement is for traction to be applied with the patient in a sitting-up position. Traction is more efficient, being countered by the body weight: the patient can see what is going on and, if paraplegic, breathing is easier as the diaphragm is unobstructed. A framework of slotted angle (e.g. Dexion®) (1) may be attached to the mattress frame if the hospital bed has not this facility, and the frame may be racked up and down (2) while pressure points are being attended to. The weight required (3) will be found to vary from about 7 kg (15 lb) for a light adult woman to 14 kg (30 lb) + for a heavy man. The line of traction should start in the neutral position or slight flexion (4). The patient should be sedated, *and in the recently injured patient radiographs to check progress should be taken every 15 minutes.*

**41. Reduction (5):** As soon as the neck has been stretched sufficiently to allow the locked facets just to clear one another (2), the neck should be extended to complete the reduction (3). If the injury is long standing (say 1–3 weeks) progress will be much slower, and in extreme cases can extend to days.

**42. Reduction (6):** As soon as check radiographs confirm the reduction (illus.: reduction of case shown in 215, 31) the traction should be reduced to about 2.5 kg (6 lb). *On no account should the neck be allowed to over distract.*

**43. Reduction (7): Alternative techniques: Sillar's method:** The patient is anaesthetised and placed on the theatre table with the break at shoulder level. Shoulder rests are fitted (1) and traction cord stretched between the skull callipers (2) and some theatre fixture (3). The cord is tightened with a windlass (4) and when sufficient tension is present the end of the table can be dropped (5). Thereafter the spine should be visualised with image intensifier screening or serial radiographs. The windlass is tightened until the facets unlock. Thereafter the cervical spine may be extended by tilting the table (6), and the traction slackened off. The advantage of this method is that reduction is rapid and that there is fine *linear* control of the spine (as opposed to the trial and error method of weight adjustment over an indefinite time).

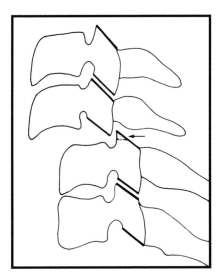

**44. Reduction failure:** Failure to obtain reduction is unusual in recent injuries, but there may be difficulty after 3–4 weeks. Assuming that there is not complete paraplegia, open reduction should be attempted by local trimming of those parts of the facets which are blocking reduction (facetectomy). Note that in very long-standing dislocations, spinal stability is more important than accurate reduction, and the spine may be fused in the dislocated position if reduction cannot be obtained.

**45. Treatment of fracture dislocations where there is a neurological defect on admission:** In about 10% of cervical spine dislocations posterior extrusion of intervertebral disc material can compromise the cord, and there is a risk that the situation can be aggravated if reduction is undertaken without prior decompression. A thorough neurological examination should be carried out on admission, and if there is evidence of neurological involvement (particularly of the cord) then further investigation of the state of the relevant intervertebral disc should be undertaken. This is best done by a carefully supervised MRI scan; failing this myelography with a postmyelography CAT scan should be carried out. If there is evidence of cord compression, then a decompression by the anterior route *before* reduction is advocated.

**Post reduction after care:** In the common situation where there is dislocation of the cervical spine without fracture, the posterior ligament complex never regains its former strength irrespective of the method of reduction or duration of subsequent traction. Spontaneous recurrence of the displacement is inevitable unless posterior fusion is carried out. The decision about surgery depends on your assessment of the neurological picture, and may be deferred until this is reasonably clear. In the interval traction should be maintained. The following situations are common: (a) If there is no neurological disturbance, spinal fusion should be carried out; it is reasonable to do this as a carefully planned procedure after a few days. (b) If there is an incomplete paraplegia, there may be a reasonable delay of 1–2 weeks. (c) If paraplegia is complete, fusion is not required. Traction may be discontinued and a collar substituted after 4–6 weeks. (d) Where the injury is accompanied by fracture, and union in this fracture may result in stability (e.g. fracture of the *base* of a spinous process) traction either in bed or by means of a head rest may be continued until union occurs (say after 8 weeks). The final stability of the spine should nevertheless always be checked by flexion and extension laterals.

**46. Cervical fusion (1):** Under the circumstances of a posterior ligament complex rupture, anterior cervical fusion is unreliable, and a posterior fusion is advocated. *Note:* (a) Traction is maintained during the procedure (1). (b) After carefully controlled intubation, the patient is turned to the prone position, with the head supported in a head ring (2). (c) The cervical spines are exposed through a midline incision (3).

**47. Cervical fusion (2):** (d) The ruptured posterior ligament is identified and the adjacent spinous processes, laminae and facet joints rawed. (e) The spines are wired together (Illus.). (f) Two iliac bone grafts are placed (and sometimes wired together) on either side of the spines, bridging them. (g) Cancellous bone chips are packed into the area before closure. (h) Traction is continued for 6–8 weeks and a collar substituted when there is evidence of graft incorporation. As an

alternative to wiring, hook plates, similar in concept to Zuelzer plates, may be used, one on each side of the spinous processes. In practice each is bent so that its hook portion can slip under the inferior edge of a lamina, suitably notched to receive it and to prevent it from drifting; its upper end is held with a single screw into the articular mass. Bone grafts are then applied. The AO Group recommend an H graft technique.

**48. (C) Extension injuries: Mechanisms:** Commonly: (a) as a result of a fall downstairs, striking the forehead against the ground; (b) in front impact car accidents where the forehead strikes the car roof, fascia or bonnet (3rd, 4th and 5th phases of injury); (c) in rear impact car accidents in which the neck extends due to the inertia of the head.

**Pathology:** These injuries are particularly common in the middle aged and elderly who suffer from cervical spondylosis. Osteoarthritic rigidity in the spine may lead to excessive concentration of violence at any area of the spine retaining mobility. A similar predisposition is found in those suffering from ankylosing spondylitis, severe rheumatoid arthritis, or congenital deformity of the spine with localised areas of fusion (e.g. Klippel–Feil syndrome).

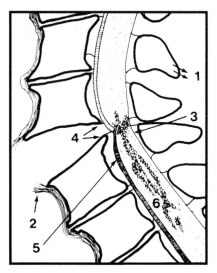

**49. Pathology *ctd:*** The neck hyperextends (1) leading to tearing or avulsion of the anterior longitudinal ligament (2). During the period of extension the cord may be stretched at the level of the vertebral lesion (3). At the same time, or when the vertebrae snap together again, the cord may be nipped by backward projecting osteophytes (4) (in the patient with advanced spondylosis). Stretching and kinking of spinal vessels may lead to extensive spreading thrombosis (5). The cord damage is

often diffuse and may not correspond exactly with the level of injury (6). Spread of thrombosis may lead to a deteriorating neurological picture. As far as the cord is concerned sole involvement of the central area is rare, but when it occurs the effect is: (a) Motor loss, if present, tends to be greater in the arms than in the legs. (b) Temperature and pain conduction are more likely to be affected than proprioception and light touch, which are frequently spared.

*Diagnosis: (1)* The history of injury, pain in the neck and complaint of weakness in the arms are suggestive. (2) Where the causal force is anterior (218, 48, a, b,) bruising or laceration of the forehead is an invaluable sign.

**50. Radiographs:** Spontaneous reduction is the rule, so that the radiographs *may be quite normal.* Nevertheless, plane films may show (1) avulsion of the ant. long. ligament from its attachment to the vertebral body (Illus.) or an osteophyte; (2) anterior displacement of the pharyngeal shadow secondary to haemorrhage; (3) rarely there may be fractures of the laminae or spinous processes, or (4) tearing open of a vertebral body. MRI imaging is of great value in showing ant. long. ligament ruptures in doubtful cases.

**51. Treatment:** Extension injuries of the spine are stable. *Local treatment* consists of the judicious use of a collar till local pain and cervical muscle spasm settle. *The general treatment* is that of the accompanying neurological problem which may be minor or profound.

*(D) Compression fractures of the cervical spine: Mechanisms:* These injuries may be caused by: (a) heavy objects falling on the head, (b) the vertex striking the ground as in falls, diving and other athletic accidents, (c) the head striking the roof in head-on car accidents (phase 2).

*Diagnosis:* (a) The history of injury may be suggestive. (b) There may be tell-tale lacerations on the crown of the head.(c) Complaint of pain in the neck should lead to the taking of the radiographs which will clarify the diagnosis.

**52. Radiographs (1):** The appearances are dependent on the degree of causal violence. When the forces are moderate, a fissure fracture of the vertebral body may be produced, most obvious in the AP projection (Illus.: vertical fracture through the body of C5, with a similar but less marked fracture of C6). Where the deformity is greater, lateral displacement of the pedicles may be obvious.

**53. Radiographs (2):** In more severe injuries the vertebral body may be comminuted and flattened. Fragments of the vertebral body may be extruded in any direction; when this occurs the cord may be endangered. (Illus.: compression fracture of C5; note the encroachment on the neural canal by the posterior part of the body.) *CAT scanning is of particular value in clarifying the extent of fractures of this type.*

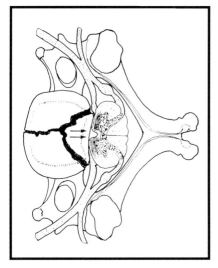

**54. Neurological involvement:** The most vulnerable part of the cord lies anteriorly, affecting firstly the motor supply of the upper limbs *before* the motor pathways to the lower limbs: hence paralysis tends to be maximal in the upper limbs. Next to be involved are the spinothalamic tracts carrying pain and temperature, and lastly the posterior columns (proprioception and light touch).

**55. Neurological assessment:** On admission, a complete neurological examination should be carried out: this should involve testing: (1) all the main muscle groups in the upper and lower limbs, (2) the skin and tendon reflexes, (3) sensation to pin prick and light touch, (4) proprioception. If the paralysis is bilateral, symmetrical and complete, testing should be repeated meticulously at 6 hours, 12 hours, and 24 hours post injury. No recovery after 24 hours in injuries at cervical level almost certainly indicates a hopeless prognosis. *Be careful to note, however, that a profound neurological loss cannot be declared complete unless proprioception and light touch have been most carefully assessed.* Many apparent recoveries in lesions first described as complete may well have been due to failure in carrying out a careful examination of these modalities of sensation.

*Treatment:* (1) The posterior ligament complex is intact, and once these fractures have healed there is no tendency to subsequent displacement. They are generally best treated by cervical traction for 6 weeks until cancellous union has occurred. Traction also minimises the chances of backward displacement of bone fragments.
(2) Removal of backward projecting bone fragments which are interfering with cord

function may be carried out through an anterior approach. This is indicated in the face of the following criteria: (i) an incomplete cord lesion, (ii) a deteriorating neurological picture, (iii) a local block on myelography, (iv) confirmatory evidence on CAT or MRI scan of spinal encroachment. The indications are less clear when the neurological condition is static, and even less so when it is complete. Where on exploration there is evidence of marked spinal instability, internal fixation is advisable. For this purpose cervical spine locking plates (e.g. by Synthes®) have been developed to avoid having to have screws engaging the posterior cortex of the vertebral bodies. The coarse threaded cancellous screws employed are locked to shallow profile plates by separate set screws which expand their upper ends (Illus.).

**56. The upper two cervical vertebrae: (A) Atlanto-occipital subluxations and dislocations:** Traumatic lesions at this level are usually fatal, but a few survive. Subluxations from rheumatoid arthritis and spinal infections (Illus: cervical tuberculosis: atlanto-occipital subluxation and retropharyngeal abscess) are seen more frequently. Cervical fusion (occiput to C1 and C2) with a period of halo traction (see 222, 67) is generally advocated.

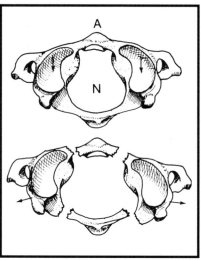

**57. (B) Fractures of atlas (1):** The usual pattern of fracture is *quadripartite*, and is produced as a result of severe downward pressure of the occipital condyles on the atlas. Such force may result from: (a) a weight falling on the head (e.g. in the construction industry), (b) the head striking the roof of a car in a road traffic accident, (c) from a fall from a height on to the heels.

**58. Fracture of the atlas (2):** Clinically, if the patient is conscious he may resent sitting up and may support the head with the hands. There may be complaint of severe occipital pain due to local pressure on the great occipital nerve. About 50% of patients survive this injury without significant neurological involvement.

**59. Radiographs (1):** The *lateral* radiograph may show the fracture of the posterior arch. The plain AP view is generally unhelpful. A through-the-mouth projection is generally most valuable and should reveal the lateral displacement of the lateral masses. Nevertheless pain and resistance to all movement may lead to failure; if this is the case, an oblique lateral centred on C3, AP and lateral tomography and CAT scanning may be useful.

**60. Radiographs (2):** Congenital absence of part of the posterior arch may cause confusion, but in itself is of no significance, being a stable condition. *Treatment of arch fractures:* These cannot be reduced; with *slight* displacement a well-fitting collar for 6 weeks with observation in hospital for 2–3 weeks *at least* is desirable. With more severe displacements, 6 weeks' skull traction is advisable.

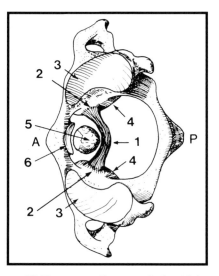

**61. (C) Transverse ligament lesions (1):** The transverse ligament (1) runs between two bony tubercles (2) which lie between the joint surfaces (3) which articulate with the occiput and those which articulate below with the axis (4). The odontoid process (5) articulates with the anterior arch (6) and the transverse ligament restrains its backward travel.

shift in an arthritic spine.) (ii) There is generally a degree of rotatory deformity, and a through-the-mouth view may show an asymmetrical location of the odontoid peg relative to the lateral masses of the atlas. (iii) If there is remaining doubt, flexion and extension laterals should be taken under close supervision. An abnormal excursion of the odontoid peg in relation to the anterior arch of the atlas is diagnostic. If available, CAT scanning may be used to clarify the relationship between the odontoid peg and the anterior arch of the atlas.

**62. Transverse ligament (2):** The ligament may be torn in sudden flexion injuries; it may become attenuated or rupture in rheumatoid arthritis (or in soft-tissue infections of the neck in children). In either case the risk to the cord is great as it becomes pinched between the posterior arch of the atlas and the odontoid peg (as shown here diagrammatically).

**63. Transverse ligament (3): Diagnosis:** The condition may be suspected from the history, by pain in the neck *and the head*, and by the presence of marked cervical spasm. *Radiographs:* The diagnosis is established by radiographs. (i) Plain lateral films should be examined and the gap between the posterior face of the anterior arch and the odontoid carefully measured. In the adult, the upper limit of normal is 4 mm, and measurements in excess of this are pathological. (Illus.: gross

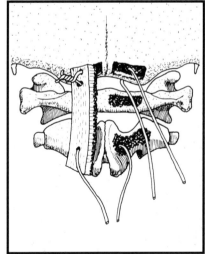

**64. Treatment (1):** As an initial measure, skull traction of about 3 kg (6–7 lb) in extension should be set up. In children, a period of 6 weeks' traction alone may suffice to restore stability to the spine. This is especially so where the pathology has been due primarily to local infection and this has been in addition adequately dealt with.

**65. Treatment (2):** Where the pathology is secondary to rheumatoid arthritis, local cervical fusion is generally advised to prevent subluxation of C1 on C2. The posterior arches of C1 and C2 are rawed (1). Two stout grafts (from tibia or iliac crest) are wired in position (one side only shown) (2). The upper wires (3) pass round the arch while the lower (4) is passed through a hole drilled in the spine of C2. The area is packed with bone chips.

**66. Treatment (3):** If the posterior arch of C1 is very frail, it may be necessary to include the occiput in the grafted region; great care must be taken in passing the fixing wires through holes drilled in the edge of the foramen magnum.

After surgery, traction is maintained for 6 weeks, and a collar is generally worn for a further 2–3 months.

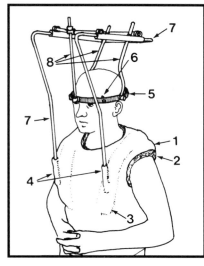

67. **Treatment:** If the dislocation is due to recent trauma, conservative treatment by the use of halo traction over a period of 8 weeks may be successful. The apparatus is cumbersome and the patient must be well motivated. With the *halo vest* the side bars which carry the pillars supporting the halo are incorporated in an off-the-shelf 'vest' which stretches from the shoulders to the pelvis; this is well padded, and can be adjusted with straps

and buckles over both shoulders and round the waist. In default, the halo supports may be incorporated in plaster. A plaster jacket (1) is applied over stockingette and generous wool and felt padding (2) to cushion the weight of the plaster and the apparatus. A rigid metal frame (3) is buried in the plaster. It incorporates tubular sockets (4) to take the main frame. When the plaster has dried, the head is shaved; the skull callipers are removed and replaced with the halo (5). This metal ring is attached to the skull with four diametrically opposed metal points (6) screwed into position in a similar manner to the points in Cone's callipers. Once this is securely in position the cantilever frame (7) shaped like an inverted bent 'U' is attached to the sockets in the plaster. The halo is connected to the cantilever frame by three bars (8) which have adjustable couplings at both ends.

The satisfactory establishment and maintenance of this equipment is not easy; complications have been recorded in over 50% of cases, some serious. (These include osteitis of the skull and intracranial abscess, and are seen most often when the treatment is prolonged.) In a number of patients, plaster fixation (224, 80) may be a viable alternative.

When the device is finally removed, stability must be assessed with flexion and extension laterals; if there is evidence of persisting instability, fusion will be needed.

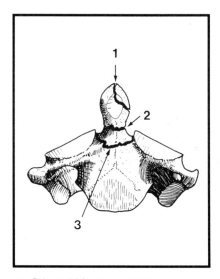

68. **Odontoid fractures (1):** These may be classified as follows: Type I injuries (1) involve the tip of the peg, are generally stable and have a good prognosis; they require symptomatic treatment only with a collar. Type II injuries (2) involve the junction of odontoid peg with the body, and are the commonest of these fractures. In Type III fractures (3), although they run deeply into the body of C2, union fails to occur in about a quarter of cases, so they must be handled as carefully as Type II fractures.

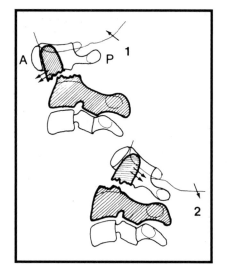

69. **Odontoid fractures (2):** Fracture may result from sudden severe flexion (1) or extension (2) of the neck (flexion and extension fractures). *Diagnosis:* This injury may be suspected from the history and the site of pain and protective muscle spasm. Occasionally the original injury may be ignored, and discovered only on investigation of an advancing ataxia or other neurological disturbance.

70. **Odontoid fractures (3):** The diagnosis may be readily confirmed by routine radiography; the fracture may show clearly in the through-the-mouth AP projection (Illus.: fracture of the base) and/or in the standard lateral view. Only if there is doubt need carefully supervised flexion and extension laterals be taken, or CAT scans or tomography carried out. Confusion can sometimes arise, however, from certain congenital abnormalities.

71. **Congenital abnormalities** of the odontoid include: (1) complete absence (predisposing to dislocation); (2) hypoplasia: (3) non-fusion of the odontoid process (persistent os odontoideum). (The ossification centre for the apex normally appears at 2 years with fusion occurring by 12.) Rounded edges and a separate articulation with the atlas may help to distinguish it from a fracture (even though it may behave as such).

and confinement to bed. A stout well-fitting cervical collar may be used. In the young patient, however, better support will be afforded with a Minerva plaster (see 224, 79) or with halopelvic traction. In all instances, external support should be continued without interruption for 8 weeks.

(3) Stability should then be assessed with flexion and extension laterals. Surgical treatment (fusion of C1 and C2) is indicated: (a) if conservative treatment fails, (b) if the case presents late, (c) if a good reduction cannot be obtained, (d) where the delays and complications of conservative management are thought to present a greater hazard than the risks of primary surgery.

Treat displacements of the os odontoideum conservatively unless the forward slip is extensive or there are severe or progressive neurological signs.

Fractures of the odontoid process in adults may be treated by the experienced surgeon with screw fixation and grafting, using an anteromedial approach.

**72. Flexion injuries:** The atlas and dens displace anteriorly in relation to C2. (Illus.: flexion injury made obvious by flexion and extension laterals.) There may be an associated rotational injury. If the fracture is junctional (222, 68 (2)) the incidence of non-union is about 60%, with risk of progressive subluxation and neurological involvement.

*Treatment:* In spite of the risks of complications these injuries are frequently treated conservatively, especially in children.

*Method:* (1) Reduce by applying traction in extension, using skull callipers (as in ruptures of the transverse ligament, 221, 64). In the older patient a good reduction should be aimed for, in order to lessen the risks of non-union. In the younger patient, persistent displacement can in fact re-model well.

(2) After 1–2 weeks in traction, it may be possible to mobilise the patient; this is, of course, especially desirable in the elderly patient who will not tolerate prolonged traction

**73. Extension injuries:** Fracture with backward displacement of the odontoid fragment is commoner in the elderly, and is a relatively stable lesion.

*Treatment:* (1) If the shift is slight, a collar for 8 weeks should suffice. (2) If marked, apply traction in slight flexion with callipers, but slacken off the weight as soon as reduction has been achieved to avoid distraction. After 2–4 weeks a collar may be substituted.

**74. Fractures of the pedicles of C2 (1):** Fractures of the pedicles of the axis may occur in two distinct ways: (a) Fracture may follow simultaneous extension and distraction of the neck. This is the mechanism of death by hanging. Similar, and not always fatal, injuries occur in cyclists who are caught under the chin by a tree branch or a rope; nevertheless, neurological disturbance is usually profound.

**75. Fractures of the pedicles of C2 (2):** (b) Radiologically identical fractures may be produced by forcible extension of the neck accompanied by compression; this may occur in road traffic accidents if the head strikes the vehicle roof and ricochets into extension. Neurological involvement here is rare. These two types of injury may be distinguished by the history, site of bruising (neck or forehead) and neurological disturbance.

radiographs suggest distraction, or if neurological signs are advancing, traction must be abandoned. There would then be an indication for local fusion.

(b) *Extension injuries with compression:* (i) If the injury appears stable and there is no neurological disturbance, a well-fitting collar should be worn for 6 weeks. (ii) If there is neurological involvement, a 6-week period of cervical (skull) traction should be advised. Thereafter (iii) if there is any evidence of instability, fusion is indicated. Posterior and anterior fusion have both been advocated for C2 fractures.

**76. Fractures of the pedicles of C2 (3):**
The fracture normally shows clearly in lateral radiographs of the cervical spine. Occasionally there is spondylolisthesis of C2 on C3.

*Treatment:* (a) *Extension injuries with distraction:* Skull traction for a period of 4–6 weeks is advocated to maintain position only. There is always the risk in this type of injury of further distraction, and it is therefore important to limit traction to a maximum of 2 kg (5 lb). If

**77. Isolated spinous process fractures:**
Fracture of the spinous process of C7 or T1 (clay shoveller's fracture) may result from sudden muscular contraction (avulsion fracture). This is a stable injury, and symptomatic treatment only is required (e.g. a cervical collar for 2–3 weeks). It must be carefully distinguished from a cervical dislocation with associated fracture. (If in doubt, flexion and extension laterals should be taken.)

**78. Plaster fixation in cervical spine injuries (1):** Plaster fixation is occasionally indicated as a substitute for a well-fitting collar. It may afford a little more support and be helpful in treating the poorly motivated patient who may be tempted to remove the support. Stockingette is applied to the head and trunk (1), and wool padding to pressure areas (2). Felt pads to the chin and occiput are advisable.

**79. Plaster fixation (2):** Four plaster slabs are prepared from 15 cm (6") plaster bandages; two are applied over the shoulders (3), one from midscapular region to the occiput (4) and one over the point of the chin on to the chest (5). The slabs are joined with circular bandages; the stockingette and wool are turned down and trimmed (6). This plaster is best applied with the patient seated on a stool.

**80. The Minerva plaster:** This extensive plaster, although not giving as much support as halopelvic fixation, is sometimes used as an alternative, for the same indications (especially in children).

*Method:* A plaster jacket is applied first (1); this is extended with slabs to form a collar (as in 224, 78–79) (2); additional support is provided with a head band (3) and side struts (4). If to be worn for any length of time, the head should be cropped or shaved (5).

**81. Soft-tissue injuries of the neck (whiplash injuries):** Whiplash injuries of the cervical region occur most frequently in road traffic accidents. In the classical incident the spine is hyperextended following a rear impact collision (1) and then rapidly flexed as the vehicle in which the patient is travelling hits an object in front—usually another car (2). 'Whiplash injury' is a somewhat emotive term and has been considerably abused, being at times chosen with regrettable imprecision to describe virtually any neck injury unaccompanied by fracture.

*Diagnosis:* The commonest symptoms are of pain and stiffness in the neck. In addition there may be radiation of pain and numbness into the shoulder, arm and hand, or to the interscapular region or occiput. In an appreciable number of cases there may be an additional complaint of low back pain.

*Clinically* neck movements are restricted, and widespread cervical tenderness is usual, often with involvement of the anterior cervical muscles. Objective neurological signs are rare.

*Radiographs:* (1) There may be loss of the usual cervical curvature or localised kinking (of greater significance). (2) Occasionally there may be evidence of hyperextension (anterior osteophytic avulsion) or hyperflexion (flake fracture of a spinous process). (3) The presence of pre-existing osteoarthritic changes in the cervical spine predispose to injury (by concentrating local stresses) and worsen the prognosis. There is some evidence that joint space narrowing and other spondylotic changes may appear 1–2 years after the incident and be related to it.

*Treatment:* Treatment is primarily conservative: only in the most severe and persistent case is local fusion ever considered: (a) A cervical collar and analgesics are prescribed initially. (b) If after 6–8 weeks symptoms are not controlled, local heat with or without cervical traction is advised.

*Prognosis:* In this common condition, seen in a third of all road traffic accident cases attending hospital, four degrees of severity have been described. In group A (12% of cases) full recovery occurs within 2 weeks. In group B (48%) a steady state is reached after 2 weeks when there are mild (but long-term) symptoms, insufficient to affect work or leisure. In group C (28%) no or little further improvement occurs after 2 months, and symptoms are intrusive, affecting work and leisure and requiring the use of analgesics, a collar and physiotherapy. In group D (12%), after 3 months, symptoms remain severe, and often lead to job loss, and the need for the continued use of analgesics and a collar.

*Prognostic factors:* Poor prognostic factors include (1) pre-existing spondylotic changes, (2) localised spinal kinking, (3) positive neurological findings.

*Barré–Lieou syndrome:* This may follow a whiplash incident. There is complaint of headache, vertigo, tinnitus, ocular problems and facial pain. It is thought that it may be due to a sympathetic nerve disturbance at the C3–4 level, and in 75% of the cases there is impairment of sensation in the C4 dermatome, with weakness of shoulder and scapular movements. Myelography may show nerve root sleeve disturbances. Good results have been claimed for anterior discectomy combined with local cervical fusion.

**82. Fractures of the thoracic and lumbar spine: Mechanism:** Fractures of the thoracic and lumbar spine occur most frequently as a result of forces which tend to produce flexion of the spine (1). A rotational element is frequently present (2).

*Causes:* The many possible causes of this type of injury include: (a) falls from a height on to the heels, where the normal curvature of the spine results in further flexion, (b) blows across the back and shoulders which cause the spine to jack-knife at the thoracolumbar junction—e.g., injuries in the mining and construction industries, (c) flexion and rotational forces transmitted to the spine from road or vehicle impact in car and motor cycle accidents, (d) heavy lifting, especially in the middle aged and elderly, where there is often the pathological element of osteoporosis or osteomalacia. Less commonly malignancy (especially metastatic deposits) may be a factor, when the causal force may be slight or not even remembered.

**83. Diagnosis:** Suspect on a history of back pain after trauma, especially if there is local spinal tenderness (1), pain on spinal percussion (2), or especially if there is an angular kyphosis (3). Thoracic or abdominal radicular pain may wrongly divert attention to the chest or abdomen, and in the elderly there may be no convincing history of injury; any suspicion merits radiography.

84. **Radiographs (1):** AP and lateral radiographs only should be taken in the first instance. In the obviously seriously injured patient there may be difficulty in obtaining a lateral because of severe pain, or through fear of causing cord damage. In these circumstances, a shoot-through lateral may be taken using a fixed grid or chest bucky. (Illus.: shoot-through lateral; note tacks securing canvas to stretcher poles, but detail sufficient to show a wedge fracture of L3, with anterior subluxation and obvious instability.)

85. **Radiographs (2):** If these measures are unsatisfactory you should *personally* supervise the turning of the patient on his side in order to obtain a lateral projection; in essence you should see that the patient is turned gently and smoothly in such a way that the upper part of the spine with the shoulders is rotated in pace with the pelvis, and that the patient remains well supported (e.g. by pillows) when he is on his side.

86. **Note:** (1) The most important decision to make in any spinal injury is whether it is stable. This profoundly influences treatment. (2) *Most stable fractures* are uncomplicated by damage to the cord or cauda equina, although certain mechanically stable bursting fractures may be neurologically unstable. (3) *Unstable fractures* of the spine may be accompanied by neurological involvement. If this is incomplete, there is always hope of recovery. There is the risk that further displacement at the fracture site may jeopardise this, or convert an uncomplicated injury to a complicated one. Treatment is, therefore, vitally important. (4) The commonest spinal injury *by far* is the wedge compression fracture. (5) In practice, the most frequent problem is to recognise a wedge fracture and decide whether it is stable. (6) Other types of injury are most often unstable.

87. **Stable wedge fractures (1):** Wedge fractures are most commonly observed in the lateral radiographs (anterior wedge fractures) and are caused by pure flexion forces. (Illus.: wedge fracture of D11; note the difference in height between the anterior and posterior margins of the vertebral body.)

88. **Stable wedge fractures (2):** Less commonly, when there is a rotational element added to forward flexion, vertebral wedging may be apparent in the AP projection (lateral wedging). (Illus.: lateral wedging of L3.) This form of wedging is often associated with root compression on the narrowed side, and these injuries have a poorer prognosis regarding ultimate functional recovery and freedom from pain.

**89. Interpreting the radiographs (1):** In the thoracic spine, an anterior wedge fracture of a single vertebra will lead to localised kinking (1) with or without an overlying gibbus (2). Multiple fractures in the thoracic spine, especially when wedging is slight in each of the affected vertebrae, will lead to a more regular kyphosis (3). In either of these circumstances, the increased thoracic curvature will tend to produce an increased lumbar lordosis (4) and/or hyperextension in the hip joints. In the case of the lumbar spine, anterior wedge fractures lead to obliteration or reversal of the normal lumbar lordosis (5). (Compare with the normal profile, N.)

**90. Interpreting the radiographs (2):** In anterior wedge fractures, the anterior border of the vertebra will measure less than the posterior border. The crushing of the anterior portion may be quite regular, or may result in a marginal shearing fracture (generally the anterior superior corner) (Illus.). If the *posterior* margin appears to show a decrease in height (compared with the heights of the vertebrae above and below) this is evidence of greater violence, and raises the possibility of an element of burst fracture, with the risk of bony fragments encroaching the vertebral canal. If this is suspected, a CAT scan to clarify the issue is recommended.

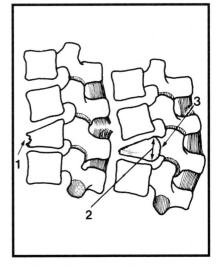

**91. Interpreting the radiographs (3):** Assess the amount of wedging; the fracture is likely to be stable if the height of the anterior margin still amounts to two-thirds or more of the posterior margin or, putting this another way, if the degree of wedging is 15° or less, or if the width of the body divided by the difference in the heights is greater than 3.75:

$$\left(\text{i.e. } x < 15°, \text{ or } \frac{c}{b-a} > 3.75\right).$$

**92. Interpreting the radiographs (4):** In the case of the upper eight thoracic vertebrae, note any associated fractures of the sternum. Each of the upper thoracic vertebrae is linked by ribs to the sternum, and *appreciable* wedging cannot take place without involvement of these structures.

**93. Unstable fractures (1):** Marked wedging (20° or more, or collapse of the anterior margin to less than half the posterior) (1) is likely to denote instability (as it is associated with posterior ligament complex rupture). If the posterior margin is reduced in height (2) a greater degree of wedging is possible without rupture of the posterior ligament complex, but indicates a bursting fracture element (see also 227, 90). Posterior *lumbar* bulging (3) is less serious than in the dorsal spine where the canal is narrow.

**94. Unstable fractures (2):** Look for other evidence of damage to the posterior ligament complex and associated structures fundamental to spinal stability. Note especially avulsion fracture of a spinous process (1), avulsion fracture of the tip of a spinous process (2), wide separation of the vertebral spines at the level of injury (3).

**95. Unstable fractures (3):** Examine the radiographs carefully for evidence of fractures at the level of the facet joints (1) or pedicles (2). A comminuted fracture of a vertebral body (3) with involvement of these structures (Illus.: facet joint fracture, 4) is generally unstable; bilateral pedicle fractures are invariably unstable. If there is any doubt regarding the integrity of the articular processes, CAT scans may give valuable additional information.

**96. Unstable fractures (4):** Look for shift of one vertebra relative to another. This is an invariable sign of instability. Vertebral displacement patterns include the following: (a) Ruptured posterior ligament with unilateral facet joint displacement (1), in the lateral projection, the degree of forward shift is about a third or less (2): (b) Bilateral dislocated facet joints, often with body fracture and a greater degree of displacement (3).

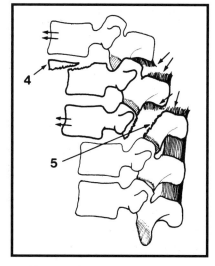

**97. Unstable fractures (5):** (c) Shearing fracture of a vertebral body (4); (d) Bilateral neural arch fractures and traumatic spondylolisthesis (5). *Note in all these injuries there is damage to the posterior ligament complex.* If there is any remaining doubt the following additional radiographs should be taken: (1) oblique projections, (2) a further lateral, *supervised*, in slight flexion. (3) If available, a CAT scan of the area may provide useful additional information.

**98. Unstable fractures (6):** The spinal radiographs may give unequivocal evidence of instability. In other cases where there is the *slightest* suspicion of the posterior ligament complex being involved, that structure must be carefully examined clinically. Press firmly between successive spines, preferably in slight flexion. If the interspinous ligaments are torn, the examining finger will encounter a boggy softness instead of the normal resistance to pressure.

**99. Treatment: Stable fractures:** (1) Admit for complete bed rest in recumbency with one pillow. (2) Analgesics as required. (3) When acute symptoms have settled (say after 1 week) extension exercises should be commenced and vigorously practised (Illus.). (4) The patient can be allowed up and home at 6 weeks. This programme may be compressed if wedging is minimal.

100. **Treatment of unstable fractures, with either no neurological lesion or an incomplete neurological lesion (1):** The aims of treatment are: (a) to reduce any displacement that is present, (b) to prevent any recurrence of displacement (with risks of neurological disasters) until stability is regained.

Stability may be achieved in the following ways: (a) by the occurrence of spontaneous anterior fusion, (b) by healing of the torn posterior ligament complex (very uncertain in its occurrence and something that cannot be relied upon, especially in cases uncomplicated by fracture), (c) by internal fixation and fusion.

Where a fracture is present, as a rule stability returns as the fracture unites. In such circumstances, if an acceptable reduction can be obtained, the injury may be treated conservatively throughout.

Conservative management may also be undertaken in other cases to give the patient time to recover from his injuries (to the spine and elsewhere) and to allow a thorough assessment of the case to be made. Surgical treatment may then be undertaken as an elective procedure.

101. **Treatment (2):** Reduction can generally be achieved by gently extending the spine with a pillow or a sandbag at the level of injury. (If this is unsuccessful, or if there are locked facets, open reduction will be required.) After reduction, further care is dependent on the nature of the injury and the availability of equipment.

102. **Treatment (3):** (a) The patient may be nursed in a Stryker frame. This special bed allows the patient to be rotated from the supine to the prone position with minimal nursing effort. During the manoeuvre, the patient is sandwiched between two mattresses (1, 2) which are locked together, and turned round a pivot at one end (3) and a quadrant (4) at the other. The frame is then locked and the uppermost mattress removed.

103. **Treatment (4):** (b) Alternatively, where instability is minimal _or_ as a follow up to a period in a Stryker frame (e.g. after 6 weeks), a POP jacket may be applied with the spine in extension. The sedated but conscious patient supports himself by the thighs (1) and shoulders (2) between two tables (3) while the plaster is applied over stockingette (4). Felt and wool are used to protect the bony prominences prior to the application of slabs and encircling bandages (5). The patient is lifted on to pillows and the cast trimmed when dry.

104. **Treatment (5):** If the fracture cannot be reduced by simple measures (e.g. if there are locked facets), open reduction will be required; the opportunity may then be taken to internally splint the spine. Meurig Williams plates, connected with set screws passed through the spinous processes, are safe to apply. They do tend to cut out after a few weeks, and the support they offer must be reinforced by other methods (e.g. the use of a Stryker frame, a plaster jacket, or (preferably) the performance of an elective spinal fusion).

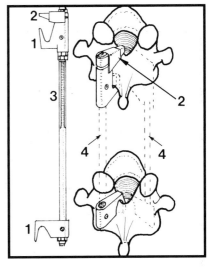

105. **Treatment (6):** More rigid methods of fixation are available; these are generally combined with a fusion (where as a rule the spinous processes and laminae are rawed and the area packed with bone chips. Sometimes bone onlays are wired to the spinous processes). The _locking hook spinal rod system_ may be used between T3 and T10. The hooks (1) snug against the laminae, and can be locked to them as required (2). They are locked to partially threaded rods (3) and can be used in pairs (4)

106. **Treatment (7):** Most other systems obtain a sound anchorage by means of screws passed through the pedicles into the vertebral bodies. The entry point (1) is below the facet close to the upper margin of the transverse process, with the track through the pedicle inclined downwards (2) and medially (3) at an angle which varies with the vertebral level. Great care must be taken (by probing and image intensifier control) to see that the spinal canal is not entered. AO notched plates (4) and 4.5 mm screws may be used from T6 to S1.

107. **Treatment (8):** Paired Schanz screws (1) and *internal* fixators (2) may also be used. After careful introduction, the upper and lower pairs of screws are locked to fixators, one on each side of the spinous processes. One fixator can be linked to the other across the midline. The ends of the pins are cut off (3) so that all can be buried. Angulation can be corrected (4) before the fixator is tightened. Bone chips can be packed into the collapsed vertebra through a small funnel.

108. **Treatment (9):** The Oswestry pedicle screw system can be used from T10 to S1, and employs rigid self-tapping pedicle screws (1). These are inserted after the accuracy of their proposed paths has been confirmed with probing and the use of plain and twisted wire pedicle markers (for side discrimination), using an image intensifier. The pedicle screws are linked with connecting bars (2) which can be bent to suit the local contours, before being locked with square socket grub screws (3) in the threaded ends of the pedicle screws.

109. **Treatment of unstable fractures with a complete, irrecoverable cord lesion:**
If the spine is grossly unstable, internal fixation may be indicated on the following grounds:
(i) to facilitate nursing;
(ii) to prevent or minimise spinal deformity which if marked may compromise respiratory function and the ability to sit up, to use a wheelchair, and complete a satisfactory programme of rehabilitation;
(iii) to permit earlier mobilisation;
(iv) to reduce the risks of chronic back pain from nerve root involvement.
   If the spine is not wildly unstable, and first-class nursing is available, there is less need for internal fixation, and the treatment is then of the accompanying paraplegia.

110. **Other injuries (1):**
**Retrospondylolisthesis** (1) especially at T12–L1 may follow a distally sited blow (2). There may be shearing through the disc (3), the vertebral body (4) or the pedicles (5) so that the articular processes impinge on the vertebral body (6). Any neurological involvement is seldom complete, but as the posterior ligament complex is damaged instability may be present; these injuries should be treated with caution.

111. **Fractured transverse processes.** In the lumbar region these may result from direct trauma or avulsion (from sudden contraction of quadratus lumborum). They may be associated (as is sometimes the case with multiple rib fractures) with fracture dislocation of the spine. Even without spinal instability multiple fractures may be complicated by retroperitoneal haemorrhage, shock, paralytic ileus or renal damage, all of which will require appropriate treatment. No treatment apart from rest is needed for uncomplicated transverse process fractures.

### 112. Neurological assessment

1. Where there is evidence of a deficit, a thorough neurological examination is required on admission. This must include as a minimum:

a. Testing for evidence of muscle activity and its power in all muscle groups below the level of injury.

b. Testing sensation of pin prick and light touch over the entire area affected.

c. Testing proprioception.

d. Testing the reflexes—the tendon reflexes, the plantar responses; the anal reflex (stimulation of the perineum leading to contraction of the external anal sphincter) and the glansbulbar reflex (compression of the glans leading to perineal muscle contraction).

2. If the findings indicate a complete spinal lesion, the examination should be repeated after 6 hours, 12 hours and 24 hours.

### The common lesions:

a. Spinal concussion causes a temporary arrest of conduction within the cord; its effects are patchy and recovery is rapid. If, for example, there is a *complete* spinal lesion on first examination, spinal concussion is an unlikely but possible cause. If after 12 hours the lesion remains complete, spinal concussion is *not* the cause.

b. If there is any evidence of voluntary motor activity, skin sensation or proprioception below the level of the lesion, the cord has not been transected (and further recovery is possible).

c. After an injury to the cord, the reflexes generally disappear for at least some hours, and sometimes for as long as 2 weeks. Return of reflex activity with continued absence of all sensation and voluntary muscle contraction confirms a *transection of the cord*.

d. Where the injury is at a level where there is potential damage to lumbar nerve roots or the cauda equina (e.g. injuries at the thoracolumbar junction) persistent absence of reflexes would confirm such damage.

e. Note that cord transection is irrecoverable, but there is potential recovery where there is involvement of nerve roots and the cauda equina.

113. **Neurological lesion in spinal injuries:** *Note:* (1) The spinal cord ends at L1; any injury distal to this can involve the cauda but not the cord. (2) All the lumbar and sacral segments of the cord lie between D10 and L1 only. (3) Injuries at the thoracolumbar junction produce a great variety of neurological disturbances as: (a) the cord may or may not be transected, (b) the nerve roots may be undamaged, partly divided or completely divided.

114. Cord or root damage is reflected in disturbance of myotomes or dermatomes. **Myotomes (1):** As a rule, motion in each joint is logically controlled by four myotomes in sequence: viz. Hip flexion, L2, 3, extension L4, 5. Knee extension, L3, 4 (including knee jerk), flexion L5, S1. Ankle dorsiflexion L4, 5, plantar flexion S1, S2 (including ankle jerk). (In addition, inversion is controlled by L4 and eversion by L5, S1.)

115. **Myotomes (2):** In the upper limb, the arrangement is less regular: *Shoulder abduction* C5, adduction C6, 7. *Elbow flexion* C5, 6 (including biceps jerk), extension C7, 8 (including triceps jerk). *Wrist flexion and extension;* both C6, 7. *Finger flexion and extension,* C 7, 8. *Pronation and supination* C6 (including supinator jerk). *Hand intrinsic muscles* T1.

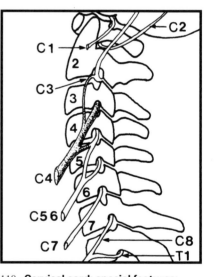

116. **Dermatomes (1):** The lumbar and sacral dermatomes have a complex arrangement which is difficult to commit to memory. Remember by the facts that: (a) the outer border of the foot is supplied by S1, (b) the medial part of the foot and the lateral part of the leg is supplied by L5, (c) the 'stocking top' area is supplied by L2 and (d) the saddle area by S3.

117. **Dermatomes (2):** In the upper limb, the anterior axial line follows the lie of the second rib from the angle of Louis, and continues down the anterior aspect of the arm, splitting near the middle finger which is supplied by C7. The other dermatomes are arranged in a regular fashion on either side of the axial line.

118. **Cervical cord: special features:** *Note:* (a) the phrenic nerve arises from C4, with minor contributions from C3 and C5. Cord section proximal to the phrenic nerve will lead to rapid death from respiratory paralysis. Those with lesions at C4–5, and more distal, are capable of respiration without external support. (b) C2 and C3 supply the vertex and occiput (accounting for pain here in upper cervical lesions). C5–T1 contribute to the brachial plexus. (Drawing is diagrammatic.)

**119. Neurological control of the bladder:** *Note:* (a) Autonomic fibres controlling the detrusor muscle of the bladder and the internal sphincter travel from cord segments S2 and 3 to the bladder via the cauda equina (1). (b) Under normal circumstances bladder sensation and voluntary emptying are mediated through pathways stretching between the brain and the sacral centres (2).

**120. Neurological control of the bladder *ctd:*** (c) If the cord is transected above the S2, 3 segments (e.g. by a thoracic spine fracture) voluntary control is lost, but the potential for co-ordinated contraction of the bladder wall, relaxation of the sphincter and complete emptying remains. (Normally 200–400 ml of urine is passed every 2–4 hours, the reflex activity being triggered by rising bladder pressure or skin stimulation.) (Automatic bladder or cord bladder.)

**121. Neurological control of the bladder *ctd:*** (d) Injuries which damage the sacral centres (1) or the cauda (2) prevent co-ordinated reflex control of bladder activity. Bladder emptying is always incomplete and irregular, and occurs only as a result of distension. Its efficiency varies with the patient's state of health, the presence of urinary infection and muscle spasms. (Autonomous or isolated atonic bladder.)

## 122. Treatment of spinal paralysis

1. The aim of treatment is: (a) maximal physical recovery and mental readjustment with, ideally, (b) complete physical independence and (c) return to full-time employment.
2. These ideals can be most fully realised through the special resources and environment of a paraplegic unit, and no effort should be spared in having the patient transferred to such a unit at the earliest convenience.
3. Pending transfer, and assuming the injury has been dealt with in an appropriate fashion, it is vital that attention is paid to the problems of the skin and bladder.

**(a) The skin:** If pressure is applied to the skin it becomes ischaemic; if pressure is maintained, necrosis from tissue anoxia results. The skin of the elderly is thin, and least able to tolerate pressure. Poorly nourished skin, anaemia, and local skin damage such as abrasions (which increase oxygen demand) are also adverse factors. The most important points, both of which are amenable to treatment, are (i) the duration of ischaemia, (ii) the amount of pressure applied to the skin.

The *duration of pressure* applied to any one area is in practice regulated by regular turning of the patient. During the initial weeks of treatment it is essential that the patient does not lie for longer than 2 hours in one position. If the patient is being nursed on a Stryker frame, then he alternates from the prone to the supine; if he is being nursed in bed, then he alternates between lying on each side and in the supine position. It is important to note that regular turning of the patient should start from the time of injury; irreversible damage may be done on the day of admission when other problems allow this vital aspect of treatment to be overlooked for some hours.

The *amount of pressure* applied to the skin is obviously important: if the body weight is locally concentrated then ischaemia will be complete. If the skin loading is reduced by being spread over a large area, then ischaemia will be less severe and more tolerable. Because of these loading factors, pressure sores tend to commence over bony prominences—the sacrum, the trochanters, the heels, the elbows and the malleoli. Particular attention should be paid to these areas, and local padding over the ankles and elbows may help. To distribute the body weight more evenly, the patient may be nursed on pillows laid across the bed from head to foot. When the patient is lying on his back, additional pillows laid horizontally may be used to support the elbows and arms. Pillows may also be placed under the legs so that the heels are relieved of pressure. When the patient is lying on his side, a pillow may be placed between the legs and the legs positioned in such a way that the malleoli and knees are free from pressure. In some centres, water beds or sand beds are used to help distribute the loads on the skin.

It is important to preserve the tone and general condition of the skin. If it becomes moist it becomes susceptible to bacterial invasion. If it is subjected to friction through contact with rough, unyielding surfaces, local abrasions may occur. Local injury of this nature increases tissue demands and may initiate the production of pressure sores. To prevent this, (i) unstarched, soft bed linen should be used and non-porous surfaces avoided. Nursing the patient on sheepskin is sometimes advocated. (ii) The skin should be protected from incontinence. (iii) Skin hygiene should be maintained by frequent, thorough cleansing with soap and water. After washing, the skin must be thoroughly dried; rubbing with alcohol may help this, and at the same time lead to temporary, local vasodilatation. Talcum powder is also used to help drying and reduce friction between the skin and the bed linen.

If pressure sores occur, preventative measures should be tightened up, and any underlying anaemia corrected. Any local sloughs or sequestra should be removed. If the area involved is small, healing may be achieved with local dressings, going through the stages of granulation and contraction. If a large area is involved, rotational flaps usually afford the best means of closure. If sores persist, they are frequently followed by progressive anaemia, deterioration in general health and well being, and often amyloid disease.

**(b) The bladder:** The effects of spinal paralysis on the bladder are dependent on the level of injury, and have been described. The immediate problem is prevention of overdistension of the bladder while minimising the risks of infection. The methods available include:

*(i) Intermittent suprapubic cystostomy using plastic tubing:* This method is demanding on staff and facilities, and carries the risk of pelvic infection.

*(ii) Intermittent catheterisation:* If properly performed with a full aseptic ritual, the risks of infection are probably lowest with this method, but it is very demanding on staff.

*(iii) Indwelling catheterisation:* This is probably the commonest method

employed, but is almost invariably accompanied by some degree of urinary infection.

Mechanical emptying of the bladder by one of these methods is usually required for 3–4 weeks, after which, in the appropriate lesions, automatic function will be starting to take over. This should be assessed by (i) removing the catheter, (ii) giving copious fluids, (iii) when filling of the bladder is apparent, trying to achieve emptying by stroking the skin in the inner groin area or by applying manual pressure over the bladder.

If these measures fail, recatheterisation will be necessary, and the procedure repeated after a week. Thereafter the efficiency of emptying should be assessed by measuring the residual urine every 3–6 months. Renal function should be reviewed by a yearly intravenous pyelogram, urine culture and estimation of the serum urea. Failure to establish a satisfactory emptying pattern will require skilled urological investigation and management.

*4. Physiotherapy and occupational therapy:* These measures should be commenced without delay, attention being paid to the following aspects of management.

(i)  Chest: The risks and effects of respiratory infection should be minimised by deep-breathing exercises, the development of the accessory muscles of respiration, assisted coughing, percussion and postural drainage.

(ii)  The joints: Mobility should be preserved in the paralysed joints by passive movements. This must be done with caution if there is any spasticity; overstretching must be avoided to minimise the risks of myositis ossificans.

(iii)  The unparalysed muscles: These should be developed for compensatory use—e.g. shoulder girdle exercises to make unaided bed-wheelchair transfers possible. Troublesome muscle spasms may be controlled with diazepam.

Depending on the level of the lesion the patient may require assistance in some or all of the following areas:

(iv)   Regaining balance for sitting or standing.

(v)   Tuition in calliper walking (or gait improvement in partial lesions).

(vi)   Overcoming problems of dressing.

(vii)   Help with alterations and adjustments within the home to permit wheelchair use.

(viii) Industrial retraining or other measures to help return to employment.

123. Describe the lesion shown. Is the injury stable or unstable?

124. Describe this through-the-mouth view of the first two cervical vertebrae.

125. Is there any abnormality showing in this oblique projection of the cervical spine?

126. This lateral radiograph is of an elderly patient complaining of pain in the back after lifting a heavy weight. What do the radiographs show?

127. Describe this fracture; is it likely to be stable or unstable, complicated or uncomplicated?

128. Describe this injury. What treatment would be required?

129. What does this CAT scan of L1 show?

130. This is a further CAT scan of the previous patient made at a different level in the same vertebra. What does it show? What neurological complication is likely?

131. What is this injury? Is it a stable injury?

132. What is this fracture? What is the likely mechanism of injury?

133. What does this AP radiograph show? Which two neurological complications are most likely to be associated with the injury?

123.  Dislocation of C5 on C6 with bilateral locked facets. 50% forward shift is present and the injury is unstable. There is no accompanying fracture.

124.  There is a congenital deformity of the odontoid process (hypoplasia). No fracture is present and there is no evidence of other injury. The shadow lying above the hypoplastic odontoid process is that of one of the incisors.

125.  There is a subluxation of C4 on C5 involving the facet joint on the right side. The articular surfaces are still in contact and the subluxation has not reached the stage of a frank dislocation with locking of the facet joint.

126.  Anterior wedge fractures of L1, L2, L3. Central ballooning of the disc into L4. Gross demineralisation of the spine, probably secondary to osteoporosis or osteomalacia (i.e. pathological fracture).

127.  Gross compression of the body of L4, with posterior displacement of fragments into the spinal canal (burst fracture). In this case there was additional damage to the posterior ligament complex, with spinal instability. There was neurological involvement of the cauda equina.

128.  Anterior dislocation of L5 on the sacrum, with bilateral locked facets, and a fracture of the anterior margin of the first piece of the sacrum. This is a fracture dislocation of the flexion distraction type. Open reduction was required.

129.  This is a vertical fissure fracture through the body of L1.

130.  The scan at this level shows a bursting fracture of the vertebral body, with bone fragments extruded both anteriorly and posteriorly. The large posterior fragment endangers the terminal part of the spinal cord, with the grave risk of paraplegia.

131.  Severe wedging of L4, with a slicing element present. The severity of the deformity would suggest that the injury is unstable.

132.  There is a fracture of the spinous process of C2, almost certainly the result of a severe flexion injury.

133.  There is a burst fracture of L3, with marked wedging, a vertical split through the vertebral body, and separation of the pedicles. The structures most at risk are: (a) the L3 nerve passing through the neural foramen on the wedged side of the spine, (b) the cauda equina within the spinal canal. A CAT scan would help clarify how much bony material has been extruded into the canal; in practice, burst fractures in this region have generally a very good prognosis, even in the face of gross extrusions.

# 11. Fractures of the pelvis, hip and femoral neck

**1. General principles (1):** The two wings of the pelvis are joined to the sacrum behind (1) by the very strong sacro-iliac ligaments. In front they are united by the symphysis pubis (2). This arrangement forms a cylinder of bone, the pelvic ring (3) which protects the pelvic organs and transfers the body weight from the spine to the limbs.

**2. General principles (2):** If the pelvic ring is broken at two levels, the pelvis may be free to open out or displace proximally (1), carrying the limb with it. Isolated (single) injuries of the ring do not have this tendency. This simple concept underlines the main consideration in classifying pelvic fractures, namely to decide whether the injury is *stable or unstable.* Conversely, if there is a major pelvic displacement, the pelvic ring must be broken at two levels even if on first inspection only one is obvious.

**3. Anatomical considerations (1):** If the pelvis is subjected to splaying forces, the weak symphysis tends to give first (1); with greater violence, the sacro-spinous (2), the sacro-tuberous (3), and the anterior sacro-iliac ligaments (4) rupture, so that the halves of the pelvis can externally rotate. If the pelvis is subjected to vertical shear forces, the interosseous (5) and posterior sacro-iliac ligaments (6) are torn, leading to dislocation of the sacro-iliac joint and proximal migration of the hemi-pelvis. In many injuries local fractures replace ligament tears (7).

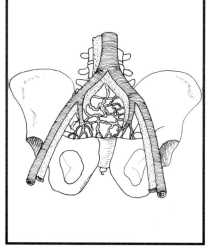

**6. Classification of pelvic fractures:** In both the Tile and the AO Classification three clearly defined Types are recognised: *Stable* fractures are classified as Type A; fractures which are *Rotationally unstable but vertically stable* fall into Type B; and fractures which are both *rotationally and vertically unstable* form Type C. In Tile's widely used classification the subgroups are as follows:

A1: Fractures of the pelvis not involving the pelvic ring

A2: Stable, minimally displaced fractures of the pelvic ring

B1: Antero-posterior compression fractures (open book)

B2: Lateral compression (ipsilateral)

B3: Lateral compression (contralateral)

C1: Unilateral

C2: Bilateral

C3: Associated with acetabular fracture

*Diagnosis:* Fractures of the pelvis commonly occur in falls from a height and from crushing injuries. *Screening films of the pelvis should be taken* in every case of multiple trauma (especially in the unconscious patient), unexplained shock following trauma, blunt abdominal injury, and femoral shaft fractures. Instability is best assessed by pelvic inlet and outlet films and by CAT scan. If the software for 3-D imaging is available, this greatly facilitates interpretation of the exact relationship of the bony elements involved.

**4. Anatomical considerations (2):** The urogenital diaphragm (1) is pierced by the membranous urethra (2), and the bladder lies behind the pubic bones. Fractures of the pelvis, especially in the region of the symphysis and pubic rami, are often associated with damage to the urethra or bladder: rarely there may be involvement of the rectum.

**5. Anatomical considerations (3):** The pelvis is richly supplied with blood vessels which are frequently damaged by fractures. *Internal haemorrhage is often severe, leading to shock which can be rapidly fatal.* NB: Shock should be *anticipated* in pelvic fractures and merits *first consideration* (see 244, 22). In the region of the sacro-iliac joint the lumbo-sacral trunk, the sacral nerves are also susceptible to injury.

**7. Stable fractures not involving the ring: Avulsion fracture (A1): (1):** Sudden muscle contraction, especially in athletes, may avulse the anterior superior spine (sartorius) (1), the anterior inferior spine (rectus femoris) (2), the ischial tuberosity (hamstrings) (3), the posterior spine (erector spinae) (4), and the crest (abdominal muscles) (5). The crest and blade (6) may also be fractured by direct violence. In all cases there is localised tenderness, and symptomatic treatment is all that is usually required.

**8. Avulsion fractures (2):** In the case of the ischial tuberosity, non-union is an appreciable risk, and if this occurs there may be problems with chronic pain and disability. To prevent this, open reduction and internal fixation have been advocated, and this is especially indicated if there is much separation of the fragments (2 cm or more).

**9. Stable fractures of the pelvic ring (1):** These like many other pelvic fractures may result from a fall on the side (1), force being transmitted through the trochanter or iliac crest, or from crushing accidents (e.g. from reversing vehicles (2), rock falls etc.), or through violence transmitted along the femoral shaft (e.g. road accidents, falls from a height etc.). Other stable injuries may follow anterior compression forces.

**10. Stable fractures of the pelvic ring (2):** By far the commonest fracture is one involving the superior pubic ramus. This is seen frequently in the elderly patient following a fall on the side. Osteoporosis or osteomalacia are frequently contributory factors. *This injury is often missed* and should always be suspected if there is difficulty in walking after a fall, and a femoral neck fracture has been excluded. Clinically there will be tenderness over the superior ramus, and pain on side-to-side compression of the pelvis; movements of the hips may be relatively pain-free. Radiographs of the hip may fail to visualise the area and full pelvic films are required. Treatment is by bed rest for 2–3 weeks until the pain settles and mobilisation can be commenced.

**11. Stable fractures of the pelvic ring (3):** Other fractures of this type include: (1) fractures of two rami on one side; (2) fracture of the ilium running into the sciatic notch; (3) fracture of the ilium or sacrum involving the sacro-iliac joint. The nature of these injuries often suggests at least momentary involvement elsewhere in the ring: nevertheless, assuming that they are uncomplicated, they may be treated as in the previous frame.

**12. Stable fractures of the pelvic ring (4):** Many quadripartite (butterfly) fractures (1) of the pelvis, and double fractures of the rami with involvement of the symphysis (2) are stable injuries. They usually result from AP compression of the pelvis which is insufficient to disrupt the anterior sacro-iliac ligaments: the posterior part of the pelvic ring remains intact and rigid, while the loose anterior fragment is only slightly displaced. *Anticipate shock and damage to the urethra*, but otherwise treat with 6 weeks' recumbency.

**13. Rotationally unstable, vertically stable fractures: Type B1: Anteroposterior compression fractures (1):** These injuries frequently result from run-over incidents where the wheel of a motor vehicle forces the anterior superior iliac spines backwards and outwards (1); they may also occur when the pelvis is compressed by falling rock or masonry which pins the patient to the ground. The ring fails *anteriorly* (e.g. at the symphysis or through two rami) (2), *and posteriorly* (3). The pelvis opens out (hence the term *open-book fractures*).

**14. Anteroposterior compression fractures (2):** As the pelvis opens out the sacro-spinous and sacro-tuberous ligaments are torn, and CAT scans may show the resulting anterior widening of the sacro-iliac joints. The posterior sacro-iliac ligaments remain intact, so that there is no vertical instability.
*Treatment:* (a) Where the posterior damage is minimal and the anterior gap does not exceed 2.5 cm: treat by bed rest until the pain settles; monitor the symphyseal separation by repeated radiographs. (b) Where the separation exceeds 2.5 cm, more active treatment is required.

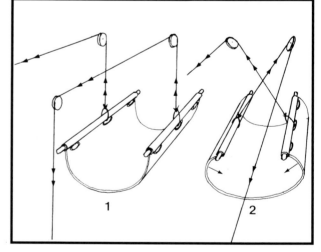

**15. Treatment (2):** The symphyseal gap may be narrowed by manipulation and held with an external fixator. These devices differ in the rigidity and placement of the fixing pins. The Orthofix® system is applied formally under general anaesthesia using an image intensifier to check the pins and the fracture. The pelvic rims are exposed anteriorly, and the paired threaded fixing pins (1) are inserted while the pelvic wall on both sides is palpated (2) to guide their direction and avoid broaching. The wounds are closed and the pin tracks sealed. The pins are connected with a pelvic fixator, articulated to give room for the abdomen (3). The pelvis is compressed from side to side (e.g. by turning the patient on his side), the device is tightened, and check radiographs are taken.

**16. Treatment (3):** These injuries may also be treated conservatively using a canvas pelvic sling. The upper edges of the sling are reinforced with steel rods and eyelets, and it may be padded with wool prior to being positioned under the pelvis. Weights in the order of 4–8 kg are applied through pulleys in a balkan beam (1), resulting in an inward thrust on the sides of the pelvis. If check radiographs show the reduction is incomplete, the weights may be increased or the traction cords crossed (2). The treatment should be continued for 6 weeks, taking the usual precautions over skin care; weight bearing can generally be allowed after 8 weeks.

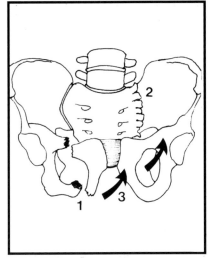

**17. Treatment (4):** If an abdominal exploration is required, the opportunity may be taken to consider internal fixation. This procedure can be followed by a disabling osteitis of the symphysis, and is contraindicated if there is faecal or urinary contamination. The separation is reduced and held with spiked forceps while a semitubular plate (1) is used to bridge the symphysis. (If there is any instability in the vertical plane) a second plate must be applied anteriorly (2) if no other fixation is being used.)

**18. Ipsilateral lateral compression injuries (B1):** Violence to the side of the pelvis (1) may cause fracture of the rami (2) or overlapping of the pubic bones; the posterior sacro-iliac ligts. remain intact (3), and the hemi-pelvis hinges round them, often with crushing of the anterior margin of the sacro-iliac joint (4). If tissue elasticity leads to spontaneous reduction, no fixation is needed; otherwise an external fixator may be used to control any instability. (Open reduction is required in the rare tilt fracture where bone protrudes in the perineum.)

**19. Contralateral compression injuries (bucket handle fractures) (B3):** Two rami fracture (1) opposite the posterior injury (2) (or there is a butterfly fracture). The hemi-pelvis rotates (3), causing leg shortening without vertical migration. The majority are stable, and best accepted; only if the deformity is gross, the leg shortening in excess of 1.5 cm, and the risks of intervention discussed, should more active treatment be considered. Reduction of the rotational deformity may be tried using pins inserted in the pelvis followed with a fixator.

**20. Rotationally and vertically unstable injuries (C1, 2 & 3):** The pelvic ring is completely disrupted at two levels or more. *Anteriorly*, in the *unilateral (C1)* injury the symphysis is disrupted (1) or the rami fractured (2). *Posteriorly*, there is total loss of continuity between the sacrum and pelvis. This may result from complete ligamentous rupture and dislocation of the sacro-iliac joint (3); or it may involve fractures of the posterior iliac spines (4), the ilium at other levels, or the sacrum. *In bilateral (C2)* injuries (5), there is extensive disruption (often with an anterior butterfly fracture (6)) involving both sides of the pelvis, so that both are free to migrate proximally.

**21. Rotationally and vertically unstable injuries (2):** On the radiographs the most obvious sign of vertical instability is the proximal migration of a hemipelvis. In addition, there may be avulsion of the transverse process of L5, and avulsion of the tip of the ischial spine. In the CAT scan, posterior displacement of a hemipelvis by more than 1 cm is diagnostic. Note in the above radiograph gross vertical instability on the left, with fracture of both rami and dislocation of the sacro-iliac joint. There is in addition disruption of the symphysis pubis and a fracture through the sacrum on the right (most noticeable at the inferior margin of the sacro-iliac joint). Although not clearly shown, the transverse processes of L5 are fractured on both sides. This is a C2 (bilateral) fracture.

**22. Rotationally and vertically unstable injuries (2): Treatment (1):** These serious injuries are those most frequently associated with life-threatening internal haemorrhage, other complications, and permanent disability. Prompt application of an external fixator avoiding a formal procedure may be performed using angled percutaneous pins (1) (at the ASS and iliac tubercle) connected by a frame; this may help control blood loss. For the conservative management of these injuries the rotational instability is best controlled with an external fixator, but a canvas sling may also be used (2). Proximal migration of the hemipelvis must also be dealt with, using traction (up to 20 kg) applied through a supracondylar (3) or tibial (4) Steinman pin.

**23. Treatment (2):** Surgery should be avoided if possible because of the high morbidity which includes uncontrollable intraoperative haemorrhage, break down of posterior wounds, neurological damage, and infection. Open reduction and internal fixation should be considered if advantage can be taken of existing wounds in the affected region (but not the perineum) or if there is an irreduceable sacro-iliac joint dislocation (which carries the highest risk of permanent disability): but only if the surgeon has the vital experience and skills. An *anterior approach* may be used to reduce, curette, graft, fuse and plate a dislocated sacro-iliac joint (1); to apply reconstruction plates to the ilium (2); and to plate the symphysis or rami (3).

**24. Treatment (3):** A *posterior approach* may be used to apply sacral bars, a safe and effective procedure for stabilising and compressing sacral fractures (1). The sacro-iliac joint may be stabilised by screws passed into the lateral mass of the sacrum (2). If the sacrum is fractured, fixing screws must engage the body of the sacrum (3) and there is very considerable risk in this procedure of entering the canal (4) or pelvis (5). *Note: In Type C3 injuries the acetabular injury takes priority: see 245, 32 et seq.*

**25. Fracture of the sacrum (1):** *The ala of the sacrum* (1) may be fractured as a result of either side-to-side or anteroposterior compression of the pelvis. *Transverse fractures of the sacrum* usually result from falls from a height on to hard surfaces. These fractures may be undisplaced (2), or they may be associated with some lateral (3) or anterior displacement (4).

**26. Fractures of the sacrum (2):** In some cases there may be involvement of sacral nerve roots, leading to sensory disturbance, weakness in the leg(s) or saddle anaesthesia and incontinence. Treatment of the sacral fractures is symptomatic with 2–3 weeks' bed rest. In the majority of cases the neurological disturbances is transitory (lesion in continuity) but if there is failure to improve (usually in gross displacements only) laminectomy may be advised.

**29. Diagnosis:** (1) Clinically, there is local tenderness. (2) When there is anterior subluxation, the prominent sharp edge of the sacrum may be obvious on palpation (S). (3) The displacement may be detected on rectal examination. The diagnosis is confirmed by localised radiographs of the region, although film quality may be poor in the obese patient.

*Treatment:* (a) Sitting on hard surfaces should be avoided, and initially the patient should use an inflatable rubber ring cushion. The patient should not be allowed to become constipated. (b) If symptoms become chronic, local short-wave diathermy or ultrasound may be tried: alternatively the painful area may be injected with a long acting local anaesthetic—e.g. 10 ml of 0.5% Bupivaine Hydrochloride (Marcaine®). (c) If all conservative measures fail, excision of the coccyx should be considered.

**27. Coccygeal injuries (A):** The coccyx is usually injured by a fall in a seated position against a hard surface—e.g. the edge of a step. There is local pain and tenderness, and sometimes pain on defaecation. Sitting on hard surfaces is always painful. (Note that coccygeal pain may also be caused by lumbar disc prolapse, pelvic inflammatory disease, chordoma and other tumours of the sacrum.)

**28. Coccygeal injuries (B):** The main patterns of injury are: (1) fracture of the coccyx, with a varying degree of anteversion, (2) anterior subluxation of the coccyx, (3) anterior displacement of the coccyx secondary to fracture of the end piece of the sacrum, (4) rarely, posterior subluxation of the coccyx.

**32. Diagnosis (2):** When the hip joint is seriously disorganised, open reduction and internal fixation of the fragments can give good results. Nevertheless, it is clear that a very careful analysis of these fractures is necessary to select the few cases suitable for this type of treatment. The first screening procedures should be: (1) a standard AP projection of the *pelvis* showing both hips on the one film, along with (2) a lateral projection of the hip. If there is any significant displacement of the fragments of the femoral head, further films will be required to answer the questions posed in the following frames.

**30. Central dislocation of the hip/ fracture of the acetabulum:** In this group of injuries the pelvis is fractured as a result of force transmitted through the femoral head. This may occur from a blow or fall on the side (1) or when force is transmitted up the limb (2) via the foot, as in a fall from a height or through the knee as in a car dashboard injury.

**31. Diagnosis (1):** The fracture is easily diagnosed by routine radiographs which reveal characteristic disturbance of the acetabulum. There are, however, many patterns of injury due to variations in the amount and direction of the causal force. Pending full assessment, the patient should be treated for any accompanying shock, and skin traction (*c.*4 kg) applied to the limb.

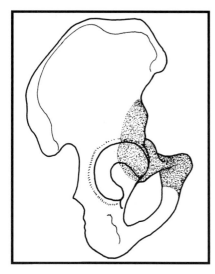

**33. (a) Is the anterior column intact?**
**(1):** The anterior column is the name given to the mass of bone which stretches downwards from the anterior inferior iliac spine, and includes the pubis and the anterior part of the acetabular floor. To help clarify this, a three-quarter internal oblique view of the hip should be obtained.

**34. (a) Is the anterior column intact? (2):** Foam wedges are placed under the buttock on the *affected* side until the pelvis is tilted at 45° (1). The rotation of the pelvis from the AP plane (3) to the oblique position (4) places the blade of the ilium in profile (5) to the central ray (2). The radiographic appearances are complex, especially if the fracture is badly displaced, but note on the films the state of the shaded portion (6) which represents the anterior column. Note also the easily identified posterior margin of the acetabulum (7), its less obvious anterior margin (8) and its floor (9). (10 and 11 are the anterior superior iliac spine and the iliac crest.) *Isolated fractures of the anterior column are uncommon, but are important to recognise as they require an anterior surgical approach for reduction.*

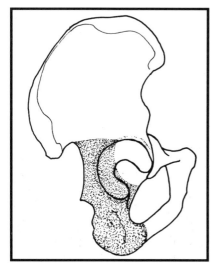

**35. (b) Is the posterior column intact?**
**(1):** The posterior column stretches upwards from the ischial tuberosity to the sciatic notch, and includes the posterior part of the acetabular floor. To clarify this a second oblique projection is often helpful (three-quarter external oblique projection).

**36. (b) Is the posterior column intact? (2):** The pelvis is tilted 45° towards the injured side by sandbags under the good side (1). This rotation of the pelvis from the normal position (2) to the oblique (3) throws the area of the posterior column (4) away from the rest of the pelvis. Note on the radiographs the area of the posterior column (shaded), the ischial spine (5), and the anterior lip of the acetabulum (6). Careful study of the AP, lateral and two 45° obliques may allow you to assess the state of the columns, but if there is still some doubt a CAT scan (especially if there is the facility for 3-D imaging) will usually reveal the main elements involved and any displacement of the femoral head with great clarity; it should be used without hesitation if available. If not, stereoradiography or intensifier screening may be of further help.

**37. (c) Is the floor of the acetabulum fragmented?** (If this is the case, the chances of restoring the articular surface of the acetabulum by surgery so that it is once again congruous with the femoral head are poor: so that in this particular group of fractures, conservative treatment is normally advised — see 247, 41.) Having assessed the state of the columns and the acetabular floor you may find it helpful to relate your findings to the AO Classification of acetabular fractures.

**38. AO Classification of acetabular fractures: Type A:** In Type A fractures one column only is involved, the other remaining intact.
A1: fractures of the posterior wall and certain variations; these injuries may be associated with posterior dislocation of the hip (see 253, 48).
A2: fractures of the posterior column and variations.
A3: fractures of the anterior column and variations.

**39. AO Classification of acetabular fractures: Type B:** In Type B fractures the main fracture line lies transversely. Part of the acetabular roof always remains in continuity with the ilium.
B1: transverse fracture with or without involvement of the posterior acetabular wall.
B2: a vertical fracture added to the transverse fracture forms a T-fracture, of which there are several variations.
B3: a vertical fracture added to the transverse fracture involves the anterior column.

**40. AO Classification of acetabular fractures: Type C:** In Type C fractures both columns are involved, and no part of the acetabulum remains in continuity with the ilium.
C1: the portion of the fracture involving the anterior column extends to the iliac crest.
C2: the portion of the fracture involving the anterior column extends to the anterior border of the ilium.
C3: the fracture involves the sacro-iliac joint.

**41. Treatment (1):** *Is the displacement of the fracture minimal* or *is the acetabular floor highly fragmented?:* If so, treat the injury conservatively with traction (e.g, Hamilton–Russell of 3 kg) for 6 weeks, with active hip movements during this period; weight bearing may be permitted after a further 3 weeks. Some loss of hip movements is inevitable, but overall function is often very good. Further treatment will only be required if secondary osteo-arthritis supervenes.

**42. Treatment (2):** *Is the main weight-carrying part of the acetabulum intact* but *the femoral head displaced? Is the disruption of the acetabulum such that reduction and fixation of three or less main fragments is likely to be technically feasible and will allow its reasonable restoration?* If so, such cases should be considered for surgery. (Illus: fracture of both columns, with an associated fracture of the femoral shaft which has been treated by intramedullary nailing.)

43. **Treatment (3):** Open reduction of acetabular fractures is seldom easy. An extensive exposure is always required, and attendant haemorrhage is a common problem. There is often great difficulty in obtaining a substantial improvement in the position of the bone fragments and in subsequently holding them, so that operating time can be very long, increasing the risks of infection and other complications. Such surgery is contraindicated in the elderly or the unfit. As these fractures are of highly vascular cancellous bone, the vigorous processes of repair may render reduction impossible if surgery is delayed for much longer than a week or so.

Assuming the patient is considered fit and suitable for surgery, that substantial blood replacement facilities are available, and that the surgeon has the necessary skills and familiarity with the region, the choice of surgical exposure depends on which columns and which parts of the acetabulum have been involved. The most frequent requirement is access to the posterior column, and for this a posterior approach such as that of Moore or Kocher may be used. *In the Moore approach* (see upper Illus.) a sandbag (1) is placed under the hip. The skin incision starts well lateral the posterior superior iliac spine, bisects the tip of the greater trochanter in the mid-line (2) and extends 7.5 cm (3″) down the lateral aspect of the femur (3). The incision is deepened over the trochanter to expose the extensive subtrochanteric bursa (4). The opening is extended proximally by splitting the fibres of gluteus maximus (5) or the ilio-tibial tract (6) at their attachment. The sciatic nerve (7) is identified, and if required taped with saline-soaked ribbon gauze and safely positioned without traction. The short rotators (8) are divided close to the femur to expose the acetabulum from the sciatic notch to the ischium.

Where the anterior column is mainly involved, a modified *Smith–Petersen or ilio-femoral approach,* exposing both lateral and medial surfaces of the ilium may be used (see lower illustration). A sandbag (1) is placed under the buttock and the skin incision (2) made along the crest of the anterior spine and downwards about 10 cm (4″) in the direction of the lateral patellar margin. The interval (3) between the sartorius (4) and tensor fascia lata (5) is opened up; gluteus medius (6) and the tensor are reflected to expose the lateral lip of the acetabulum (A). The anterior margin is visualised by dissecting rectus femoris (7) medially. Dissection close to bone on the medial side of the ilium (8) will expose the pelvic side of the anterior column by reflection

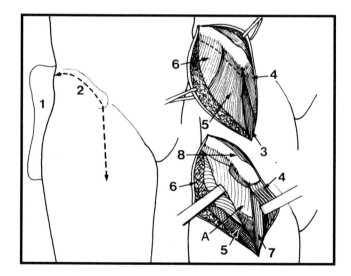

of iliacus. A lateral approach with detachment of the greater trochanter gives access to the posterior column, the roof of the acetabulum, and most of the lateral aspect of the ilium. Wide access to both columns is given by the the very extensive Carnesale approach, or by that of Reinert *et al.* (Their lateral approach through a T-shaped incision exposes the lateral side of the acetabulum by detaching the greater trochanter and elevating the gluteus medius; access to the medial side is obtained by osteotomy and reflection of the ilium.)

Once the fracture has been exposed, reduction may be facilitated by traction applied in the line of the femoral neck or inclined in a more distal direction. For this purpose a threaded screw may be passed into the femoral head or an AO femoral distractor applied between the iliac crest and the lateral aspect of the femur.

Once a reduction has been obtained the fragments may be held by the most appropriate methods which include cancellous screws and reconstruction plates.

### 44. Complications of pelvic fractures

### 1. Haemorrhage

a. Substantial internal haemorrhage is common, particularly where there is disruption of the pelvic ring and proximal migration of the hemi-pelvis (Tile Type C injuries). Shock must be anticipated in all but the most minor of fractures by (i) routine blood grouping and cross-matching, (ii) setting up a good intravenous line, (iii) monitoring the pulse rate, blood pressure and, where applicable, the urinary output. Replacement requirements are frequently substantial (transfusion in excess of 5 litres of whole blood not being uncommon) and additional measures for monitoring response (such as measuring central venous pressure) may be required. The effects of massive transfusion must be kept in mind and appropriate precautions taken (e.g. blood warming, addition of calcium, etc.). There is a growing body of evidence to suggest that internal haemorrhage may be greatly reduced by the prompt stabilisation of the pelvic fracture by application of an external fixator as an emergency procedure. The use of an anti-shock pneumatic garment has also been advocated.

   b. Bruising appearing in the scrotum or buttock, or spreading diffusely along the line of the inguinal ligament are indicative of a major internal haemorrhage. In the abdomen a large retroperitoneal haemorrhage may be felt as a discrete mass on palpation. If the peritoneum on the posterior abdominal wall has been broached, blood may escape into the abdominal cavity. Intraperitoneal haemorrhage may also result (rarely) from the tearing of mesenteric vessels. This is a serious complication and may be suspected by loss of bowel sounds, abdominal guarding, a progressive increase in abdominal girth, and a blood-stained peritoneal tap; it is an indication for abdominal exploration. Where haemorrhage is extraperitoneal, exploration is generally unprofitable and likely to aggravate blood loss; treatment should be by replacement only in the first instance.

   c. Ischaemia in one leg is a grave sign and may be due to rupture or intimal damage to an iliac artery. If the patient's condition will permit, exploration of this vessel is indicated.

   d. In the uncommon case of a severe retroperitoneal haemorrhage, where in spite of a massive transfusion programme losses continue to gain over replacement, small-bore arterial bleeding may sometimes be brought under control by selective embolisation using image intensifier angiography. Exploration may also be reconsidered. It is seldom that a single bleeding source can be found, the haemorrhage generally arising from massive disruption of the pelvic venous plexus. Occasionally successful results have been claimed in these circumstances from ligation of one or both internal iliac arteries.

### 2. Damage to the urethra and bladder

   **Incidence:** Out of every hundred fractures of the pelvis, roughly five are likely to have a urinary tract complication; more than two-thirds involve the urethra. Butterfly fractures are the main cause of urethral damage, whilst displaced fractures of the hemipelvis are generally responsible for the sharp edge of a superior pubic ramus rupturing the bladder.

**Types of injury:** *a. Rupture of the membranous urethra:* the majority of cases are partial ruptures, with an intact portion of the urethral wall still connected to the bladder. Less commonly there is complete rupture with the bladder losing all continuity with the urethra; the bladder often displaces upwards.

*b. Extraperitoneal rupture of the bladder:* This is usually caused by a sharp spike of bone penetrating the anterior wall.

*c. Intraperitoneal rupture of the bladder:* This may result from the same mechanism, but only occurs if the bladder is full at the time of injury.

*d. Rupture of the penile urethra:* Injuries of this type generally follow a fall astride a bar or similar object.

**Diagnosis:** (1) Suspicion should be particularly aroused if the radiographs show either of the fractures described.

(2)  The presence of perineal bruising is highly suggestive.

(3)  The presence of blood at the tip of the penis is diagnostic.

(4)  If there is no penile blood, and damage to the bladder or urethra thought possible but not probable, the patient should be asked to attempt to pass urine. (The dangers of urinary extravasation have been exaggerated in the past and are no longer considered to be of import.) If clear urine is passed, no further investigation or treatment is required. A positive chemical test for blood in the presence of macroscopically clear urine should in these circumstances be ignored. If after several tries the patient fails to pass urine, the patient should be re-assessed. The palpability of the bladder should be determined and catheterisation considered.

(5)  Catheterisation carries the risk of converting a partial urethral tear into a complete one, and of introducing infection. A diagnostic catheterisation should be approached with caution: a full aseptic regimen should be followed, and a fine catheter employed. The procedure should be quickly abandoned if the catheter cannot be introduced with ease. If the tap is dry, this suggests intraperitoneal rupture of the bladder; if blood-stained urine is obtained, this suggests an extraperitoneal tear of the bladder or a partial tear of the urethra; if blood only is obtained, this suggests a major tear of the posterior urethra.

(6)  If there are strong grounds for suggesting significant damage to the bladder or urethra (e.g. penile blood) a urethrogram should be performed in preference to catheterisation. The end of a syringe containing 20 ml of 45% Hypaque® is introduced into the urethra and injected; the penis is closed off with the fingers and radiographs taken. The volume injected may be doubled if required. The following are common findings: (a) The bladder shadow is clearly outlined without spillage: *no significant abnormality is likely to be present*. (b) The bladder is partly filled and there is extravasation of the radio-opaque dye to the side: this suggests *extraperitoneal rupture of the bladder*. (c) The bladder fails to fill, and there is extravasation of the dye into the pelvic floor: there is *rupture of the membranous urethra*. (d) The bladder fails to fill, and there is extravasation of dye beneath the pelvic floor: there is *rupture of the penile urethra*.

**Treatment of injuries to the urethra and bladder:**
*(1) Intraperitoneal rupture of the bladder:* The bladder is explored and the tear located and sutured. The bladder is drained subsequently with a Foley catheter.

*(2) Extraperitoneal rupture of the bladder:* The bladder is explored and the diagnosis confirmed. The rupture is repaired and drained by by-pass (suprapubic) catheterisation.

*(3) Incomplete tear of the urethra:* If there is evidence of tearing of the membranous urethra, but the bladder is undisplaced, it is likely that some urethral tissue remains in continuity; a suprapubic drain is inserted and the urethrogram repeated after 10 days. If the circumstances are favourable, a Foley catheter may be introduced at this stage and the suprapubic catheter withdrawn. Later serial bouginage may be required.

*(4) Complete rupture of the urethra:* If the bladder is floating free it must be drawn down to position. This may be achieved by opening the bladder and rail-roading a Foley catheter downwards. After the balloon has been inflated, the catheter may be used for applying gentle traction. The bladder is drained by a suprapubic catheter which is kept in position for several days. The retropubic space may require separate drainage.

*(5) Rupture of the penile urethra:* An incision is made over the tip of a catheter passed to the level of the obstruction. The catheter is then passed into the bladder through the other end of the urethra. If this cannot be located, the bladder will require opening and the distal end of the urethra identified by instrumentation from above. The urethra is then repaired, using the catheter as a stent.

### 3. Injury to the bowel

The rectum may be torn in open fractures with perineal involvement, and rarely in closed injuries of the central dislocation of the hip type. Injury to the small bowel (mesenteric tears or shearing injuries of the wall leading to infarction or perforation) may be produced by crushing injuries of the pelvis. Bowel involvement may be suspected in the closed injury by abdominal rigidity, loss of bowel sounds, loss of liver dullness and distension. Exploration and a defunctioning colostomy are essential.

### 4. Rupture of the diaphragm

Routine radiography of the chest should be performed in all major fractures of the pelvis and the standard AP projection should eliminate this often-missed complication. If a rupture is confirmed, a thoraco-abdominal repair through the bed of the eighth rib should be undertaken as soon as the patient's general condition will permit.

### 5. Paralytic ileus

This complication may result from disturbance of the autonomic outflow to the bowel due to the accumulation of a retroperitoneal haematoma. Treatment by nasogastric suction and intravenous fluids usually bring rapid resolution within 2–3 days.

### 6. Limb shortening

Shortening of one leg may result from persistent proximal displacement of the hemipelvis (Type C injuries) or from rotation of the hemipelvis in contralateral lateral compression fractures (Type B3 injuries). Clinical measurement of the amount of shortening is difficult: leg length as measured from the anterior superior spine to the medial malleolus is unaffected, heel-blocking techniques are rather unsatisfactory and the measurement of the distance from the umbilicus or xiphisternum to the medial malleolus somewhat inaccurate. The amount of shortening may be judged with greatest accuracy from the radiographs by noting any discrepancy between the level of the iliac crests on the AP film (after making a little allowance for film magnification effects). A correction (raise) should be made to the footwear if there is shortening of over 1.25 cm (½″).

### 7. Neurological damage

Neurological damage may involve (a) the lumbosacral trunk at the triangle of Marcille where there are fractures involving displacement of the hemipelvis, (b) isolated sacral nerves in fractures of the sacrum, (c) the sciatic nerve itself as it passes behind the hip.

Lesions in continuity predominate, and exploration is seldom indicated although some persistent disability is the rule. Impotence occurs in about a sixth of major pelvic fractures, and in about half of those cases in which there is rupture of the urethra. It is frequently permanent.

### 8. Obstetrical difficulties

Even in the case of quite marked postfracture pelvic distortion, natural childbirth is rarely affected to a degree requiring caesarian section. Where there has been a symphyseal disruption, this may recur, persist, and warrant surgery.

### 9. Persistent sacro-iliac joint pain

Sacro-iliac pain is a common complication of pelvic fractures, especially where there has been clear involvement of a sacro-iliac joint (e.g. in open book fractures, Type B1) and may be permanent. Where there has been a sacro-iliac joint dislocation, the risks of severe, disabling pain are particularly high and are related to the degree of persisting displacement. In some cases consideration of local fusion is merited.

### 10. Persistent symphyseal instability

This is a rare complication and an indication for internal fixation; screening may be of help in confirming the diagnosis.

### 11. Osteo-arthritis of the hip

Central dislocation of the hip is not infrequently followed by this complication. It is dealt with along routine lines. Many cases may come to and are suitable for total hip replacement, and prior reduction of a major displacement will render this easier.

### 12. Myositis ossificans

Myositis ossificans is seen most frequently after operative intervention or where there is an accompanying head injury. The treatment is along the lines previously indicated.

**45. Traumatic dislocation of the hip:**
The hip may dislocate as a result of force being transmitted up the femoral shaft. This most commonly occurs as a result of dashboard impact in road traffic accidents (1). Note that this mechanism may be responsible for simultaneous fracture of the patella (2) or of the femoral shaft (3). Force transmitted up the limbs from falls on the foot, force applied to the lumbar region (e.g. in roof falls on

kneeling miners) and rarely force applied directly to the trochanter may also cause the hip to dislocate. If the leg is flexed at the hip and adducted (4) at the time of impact, the femur dislocates posteriorly (5), internally rotating at the same time (6). In some cases, the posterior lip of the acetabulum is fractured (7). If the hip is widely abducted, anterior dislocation may occur—even without any

axial transmission of force (8). The femur externally rotates (9). Note that, if the femur is in some other part of the abduction/adduction range, these mechanisms may be responsible for central dislocation type fractures of the pelvis (10). A congenital reduction in the normal degree of anteversion of the hip is a common finding in those who suffer posterior dislocations of the hip.

**46. Posterior dislocation of the hip:**
**Diagnosis:** In a typical posterior dislocation, the hip is held slightly flexed, adducted and internally rotated (1). The leg appears short (2). Few other injuries are associated with the agony accompanying posterior dislocation, and this is almost as diagnostic as the deformity. Pain is less severe if the acetabulum is fractured, and the deformity may be concealed if there is an associated femoral fracture (3).

**47. Radiographs (1):** The diagnosis is confirmed by radiographs of the hip; the deformity is usually obvious on the AP projection, but dislocation cannot be *excluded* with one view (cf. dislocation of the shoulder); a lateral projection is helpful in confirming the distinction between an anterior and posterior dislocation, and *essential* if no abnormality is obvious on the AP film (Illus.: Obvious posterior dislocation).

**48. Radiographs (2):** Acetabular rim fractures may be produced by the shearing force of the backward travelling femoral head (253, 45, 47). The fragment may be small (Illus.) when it is seldom of consequence. It may be large or comminuted, in which case there is increased risk of sciatic nerve palsy, instability in reduction and later osteo-arthritis.

49. **Sciatic nerve involvement:** The presence or absence of damage to the sciatic nerve should be sought in every case, and particularly where an acetabular rim fracture is present. Enquire about numbness or burning sensations in the limb and, as a minimal screening, test the power of dorsiflexion in the foot (1) and appreciation of pin-prick sensation in the leg below the knee (2).

50. **Reduction (1):** Reduction should be carried out as soon as a general anaesthetic can be arranged. The complication rate is lowest in those treated within the first 6 hours of the injury. The key to success is *complete* muscle relaxation; the anaesthetist should be reminded of this and of the need to transfer the patient on a stretcher canvas on to the floor to allow the hip to be manipulated (1). An assistant should kneel at the side of the patient and steady the pelvis (2).

51. **Reduction (2):** When the patient is fully relaxed (and the administration of suxamethonium chloride (Scoline®) just prior to manipulation is often invaluable) the knee (1) and hip (2) are flexed gently to a right angle, at the same time gently correcting the adduction and internal rotation deformities (3). (*Note:* the assistant's hands, vital to the reduction, have been omitted from this and subsequent drawings for clarity.)

52. **Reduction (3):** The head of the femur should now be lying directly behind the acetabulum and just requires to be lifted forwards. The force required is variable, but great leverage can be obtained by gripping the leg between the knees (1) resting your forearms on your thighs (2) and flexing your knees (3). The assistant keeps the pelvis from lifting by downward pressure (4). Reduction usually occurs with an obvious 'clunk'.

53. **Reduction (4):** Reduction is often less striking when there is a rim fracture, and when a rim fracture is present (shown by the radiographs) the stability of the reduction should always be checked by downward pressure on the femur. Gross instability is an indication for open reduction and internal fixation of the rim fracture.

54. **Reduction (5):** Check radiographs should be taken in two planes, and some advocate routine post manipulation CAT scans. The following possibilities arise: (a) The dislocation has been fully reduced. (b) The dislocation and a rim fracture have both been reduced, and the hip is stable clinically: *In both (a) and (b) further treatment is conservative.* (c) Although the femoral head is concentric with the acetabulum, the joint space is increased. This should be elucidated further (with a CAT scan or by tomography). Persistent displacement of this type may be due to a trapped bone (rim) fragment or infolding of the labrum. A trapped bone fragment should be removed by surgery, as if left it will lead to rapid onset osteo-arthritis. Excision of a trapped labrum is advocated but the grounds for this are less clear; there would seem some justification for a 'wait-and-see' approach.

55. **Check radiographs** *ctd:* (d) There is persistent displacement of a fracture of the rim and the hip is unstable (Illus.: note rim fragment situated near upper lip of the acetabulum). (e) There is a displaced fracture of the rim with a persisting sciatic palsy. Operative reduction and internal (screw) fixation of the fragment are indicated in (d) and (e).

56. **After care:** The hip should be kept at rest for some time to reduce the risks of complications. A common regimen is fixed (skin) traction in a Thomas splint for 4 weeks and bed mobilisation for a further 2 weeks before weight bearing. (Many however advocate much shorter periods of recumbency, e.g. of 1 week.). If there is a rim fracture, weight bearing should be deferred until about 8 weeks' post injury. In some centres, skin traction alone is used.

57. **Alternative methods of reduction: Bigelow's method:** Failure to reduce a posterior dislocation of the hip by the method described is uncommon and generally due to insufficient muscle relaxation; nevertheless, if failure occurs, Bigelow's method may be tried. In essence, the hip is reduced by a continuous movement of circumduction which may be broken down into five stages; (1) the hip is fully flexed and then (2) abducted.

58. **Bigelow's method** *ctd:* After flexing and abducting the hip, the joint is smoothly externally rotated (3) and then gradually extended (4).

59. **Bigelow's method** *ctd:* As extension of the hip progresses, the external rotated limb is turned into the neutral position (5).

  *Stimson's method:* This is occasionally attempted when a general anaesthetic must be withheld or where there is an associated femoral fracture. The patient is turned into the prone position (1). The end section of the theatre table is removed and the unaffected leg held by an assistant (2). The pelvis is supported by the end of the table (3).

60. **Stimson's method** *ctd:* The leg is flexed at the knee and held at the ankle in the neutral position (4). The hip may be reduced by direct pressure over the head of the femur (5) or, if the femur is intact, by downward pressure on the upper calf (6). This may be done manually or by the stockinged foot; the latter procedure allows simultaneous application of pressure over the head of the femur as at (5).

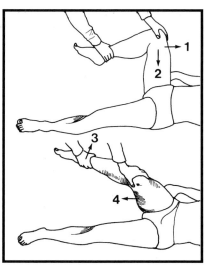

**61. Anterior dislocation of the hip:**
Anterior dislocation of the hip is less common than posterior dislocation. The leg is usually held abducted and in external rotation. There may be swelling and later bruising in the groin. Anterior dislocation may be complicated by femoral vein compression (with the risks of thrombosis and embolism), by femoral nerve paralysis or femoral artery compression. (Persistent absence of the peripheral pulses after reduction is an indication for exploration.)

**62. Reduction:** Proceed as for posterior dislocation, with the well-anaesthetised patient on the floor, and an assistant steadying the pelvis. Flexing the hip (1) and correcting the abduction and external rotation (2) convert an anterior dislocation into a posterior dislocation. At the end of this procedure the head of the femur is lifted up as before into the acetabulum. (Subsequent management is as 255, 56.)

**63. Reduction: Bigelow's method:** This method is less reliable for routine use, but may be tried in the difficult case.
Circumduction of the hip is again carried out in the following order of movements: (1) fully flex, (2) adduct the hip, (3) internally rotate, (4) extend, (5) bring into the neutral position.

**64. Complications of dislocation of the hip:**
*1. Irreducible dislocation:* This may result from in-turning of the labrum or by bony fragments trapped in the acetabulum. Open reduction is necessary, *but be certain* that the patient has been *completely* relaxed during the attempts at closed reduction.

*2. Fracture of the femoral head:* Osteochondral fractures of the femoral head may remain displaced after reduction of the hip. Small fragments should be excised, but large fragments (Illus.) should be replaced and secured with a cancellous screw or other device. Late osteo-arthritis is common.

*3. Intracapsular fracture of the femoral neck:* The risks of avascular necrosis are extremely high, and the following treatment should be considered: (i) In the elderly, excision of the femoral head, and replacement with a Thomson or similar prosthesis. (ii) In the middle-aged, total hip replacement. (iii) In the young, open reduction and internal fixation through a posterolateral approach.

*4. Slipped upper femoral epiphysis complicating hip dislocation:* Treat as *3* (iii).

*5. Extracapsular fracture of the femoral neck:* (a) The fracture should be dealt with first by open reduction and the insertion of a pin and plate or similar device. This can be taxing due to difficulty in interpreting control films in unfamiliar planes of rotation. (b) The dislocation may then be reduced, usually with ease, by closed manipulation.

*6. Fracture of the femoral shaft:* (a) It is sometimes possible to treat both injuries conservatively, reducing the hip dislocation by Stimson's method and treating the femoral fracture in a Thomas splint. (b) If Stimson's method fails, it may be possible to apply sufficient traction to the upper fragment by a substantial threaded screw inserted into the greater trochanter percutaneously. (c) It is more satisfactory to expose the femoral shaft and reduce the dislocation by means of a heavy duty bone clamp applied directly to the upper fragment (temporarily insert a large diameter Küntscher nail into the proximal fragment to prevent the bone being crushed with the clamp, and use the linear aspera for orientation). Thereafter the femoral shaft may be internally fixed (e.g. by plating: this may carry less risk of being complicated by myositis ossificans than intramedullary nailing in this particular situation).

*7. Fracture of the patella and other knee injuries:* The dislocation should be reduced by any of the methods described and the knee injury treated as if isolated (e.g. a comminuted fracture of the patella should be excised).

*8. Sciatic nerve palsy:* This complicates about 10% of dislocations of the hip. Fortunately three out of four are incomplete, and about half recover completely.

If no improvement follows reduction of the hip, exploration is indicated within the first 24 hours of injury *only* if there is a large or comminuted rim fracture which may possibly be causing persistent local pressure on the nerve. Otherwise this complication should be managed conservatively; if the patient is being treated in a Thomas splint, this should be fitted with a foot piece to hold the ankle in the neutral position. When the patient is mobilised, a drop foot splint may be required and precautions must be taken to avoid trophic ulceration in the foot.

*9. Avascular necrosis:* The inevitable tearing of the hip joint capsule accompanying dislocation of the hip may disturb the blood supply to the femoral head; in about 10% of cases this may lead to avascular necrosis. Radiographic changes are usually, but not always, seen within 12 months of injury. Clinically, persistent discomfort in the groin and restriction and pain on internal rotation are suggestive of this complication. Avascular necrosis of the head of the femur leads to secondary osteo-arthritis of the hip.

*10. Secondary osteo-arthritis of the hip:* This is the inevitable sequel to avascular necrosis, but may also occur when dislocation of the hip is accompanied by a fracture involving the articular surfaces. It is also seen as a late complication, sometimes as long as 5–10 years after injury; the cause then is less clear, but may possibly arise from articular cartilage damage concurrent with the initial injury. (An MRI scan at an early stage may sometimes confirm potentially harmful articular cartilage damage.). The incidence of secondary osteo-arthritis rises to nearly 40% in manual workers who continue with their former occupation. In the young patient hip fusion may be considered, but generally total hip replacement is the treatment of choice.

*11. Recurrent dislocation:* This complication is rare; operative fixation of a large acetabular rim fragment in the hip which is demonstrated to be unstable clinically may largely avoid it. Otherwise a bone-block type of repair may have to be considered.

*12. Myositis ossificans:* This is seen most frequently following exploration of the hip, or when the dislocation is accompanied by head injury. It may lead to virtual fusion of the hip. The risk of this complication ensuing may be minimised in the following ways: (a) Avoid surgery if possible. (b) Splint the hip following reduction. (c) Avoid passive movements of the hip in the head injury case with limb spasticity. Late excision (say after 1 year) of a discrete bone mass may restore function, but the recurrence rate in other circumstances is high.

*13. Late diagnosed dislocation:* This is a euphemism for missed dislocation. Always suspect dislocation of the hip as a possible accompaniment of fracture of the patella or femur. (a) If discovered within a week of injury manipulation may be attempted. (b) After a week and up to several months good results have been claimed by heavy (up to 18 kg) skeletal traction for up to 3 weeks under sedation. When radiographs show the femoral head level with or a little beyond the acetabulum, the leg is placed in abduction and the traction decreased; this is generally successful in restoring the head to the acetabulum. If this fails, open reduction may be attempted; in either case pessimism regarding the eventual outcome is often unjustified, many cases achieving a good result without avascular necrosis ensuing. (c) After a year open reduction is unlikely to be feasible and an upper femoral (Schanz) osteotomy may be considered.

65. **Slipped upper femoral epiphysis:**
This condition occurs in adolescence; the term is to some extent a misnomer as in fact it is the femoral shaft which moves proximally (1) and externally rotates (2) on the epiphysis. Only occasionally in advanced cases is there movement of the epiphysis relative to the acetabulum (3). There is never any juxta-epiphyseal fracture (i.e. it is a Salter–Harris Type I lesion).

66. **Aetiology:** Hormonal factors (suspected, but not confirmed) may play an important part in the aetiology for (1) it is commoner in males, (2) it occurs at adolescence, (3) those affected are often adipose and sexually immature, showing features of the Frohlich's syndrome, or are very tall and thin, suggesting increased production of growth hormone, (4) some cases are associated with juvenile hypothyroidism (with lowered thyroxine and thyroid-stimulating hormones), (5) it is often bilateral, and (6) in less than 30% is there a history of injury.

67. **Diagnosis (1):** The condition should be *suspected* in any adolescent with a history of limp and occasional groin or knee pain, especially if belonging to one of the body types described. On clinical examination the leg is usually held externally rotated at the hip, and movements of internal rotation are restricted.

68. **Diagnosis (2):** The diagnosis is confirmed by radiographic examination; and a lateral projection is essential as the earliest signs are more obvious there than in the AP. A line drawn up the centre of the neck should normally bisect the epiphyseal base of the head; if it fails to do so, slip is present, and the percentage slip should be noted. (Illus. 15–20% slip.)

69. **Diagnosis (3):** In the AP view slip is less obvious, but nevertheless may be detected with experience. Radiographs of both hips should be taken to allow comparison and detect early silent slip on the other side. In the normal hip (1) a tangent to the neck should cut through a portion of the epiphysis. When slip is present (2) this is no longer the case.

70. **Diagnosis (4):** Look for radiographic evidence of new bone formation (buttressing) at the inferior and posterior aspects of the neck, i.e. look for evidence of chronicity.

The history, clinical findings and radiographs should allow the case to be diagnosed as: (1) an acute slip, (2) an acute slip superimposed on a degree of long-standing slip, (3) a chronic slip.

**71. Diagnosis (5):** (1) In an acute slip, the history is short (less than 3 weeks) and the radiographs show slipping without buttressing (Illus.). (2) Where an acute slip is superimposed on a degree of chronic slip, there is often a history of intermittent limp and discomfort for several weeks, with recent, sudden deterioration; any buttressing is slight. (3) With a chronic slip, the history is of many weeks' duration, and buttressing is a feature.

**72. Treatment (1):** In all cases further slipping should be prevented, and in the first two groups this is done by pinning (which is often followed by rapid epiphyseal closure). As the epiphysis in the child is very dense, Smith–Petersen or similar nails are unsuitable; instead a Nystrum nail Illus.), two or more Moore pins, or Garden, Howse or AO screws may be used.

**73. Treatment (2): Reduction?** (1) If the slip is less than 30% (e.g. as in 259, 72) *the position should be accepted and pinned without manipulation.* (2) If there is an acute slip, or an acute-on-chronic greater than 30%, *gentle* manipulation may be attempted under general anaesthesia by applying *light* traction in the mid abduction/adduction range and turning the leg into internal rotation: thereafter, if the slip is reduced to 30% or less, pin in that position.

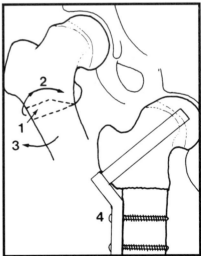

**74. Treatment (3): Reduction?** (3) If under the previous circumstances gentle manipulation fails to reduce an acute slip, or an acute-on-chronic slip, to less than 30%, operative reduction should be considered (but only by the experienced): a lateral approach is used (1). The greater trochanter (2) with its abductor insertion is detached and turned upwards (3). The capsule is opened through a T-shaped incision (4) and the vascular bundle to the head (5) teased from the superior and posterior aspects of the neck. The femoral neck is shortened (6) to allow reduction without tension on the bundle (7). Alternatively, it may be possible by excising any buttress (8) to obtain reduction without tension (9). The hip is then pinned and the trochanter re-attached with a screw. (Thereafter, skin traction for 4 weeks and non-weight bearing with crutches till union (3–6 months).)

**75. Treatment (4):** Where there is chronic slipping, manipulation should be attempted only with caution and slips of under 30% pinned in situ (neck remodelling may make assessment difficult). Where the epiphysis has closed with considerable deformity, functional improvement may be obtained by subtrochanteric osteotomy, with the base of the wedge to be removed placed anteriorly and laterally (1); this allows correction of rotation (2), adduction (3) and extension. The osteotomy may be fixed with a plate (4) or spica till united.

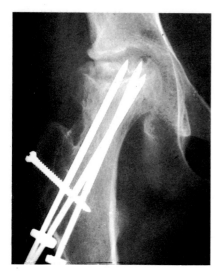

76. **Complications (1): Avascular necrosis:** (Illus.) This is a serious complication in the adolescent, and every attempt must be made to avoid it by: (a) prompt diagnosis, (b) rejection of any attempt to reduce the deformity by forcible manipulation, (c) meticulous handling of the epiphysis and its vascular supply during any operative intervention, (d) avoidance of unsuitable internal fixation devices. Treatment

of the established case is difficult: a choice may have to be made between: (i) the uncertain results of osteotomy, (ii) the difficulty of hip arthrodesis and the risks of late secondary osteo-arthritis in the knee, other hip and spine, (iii) the risks and long-term uncertainties of total hip replacement.

(2) **Involvement of other hip:** In keeping with the aetiology, the other hip may be affected at any time. This is particularly liable to be missed when the patient is being rested in bed during treatment of the primary complaint. Routine radiograph of both hips is advised, particularly in the recumbent patient. If the second hip is involved, treatment is pursued along the lines already described.

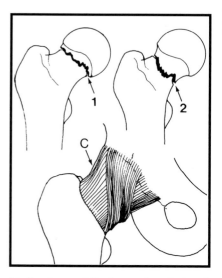

77. **Fractures of the femoral neck: Level of fracture (1):** Four sites of fracture are well recognised, the most important being: (1) subcapital and (2) transcervical. The distinction between these two is rather blurred, as rotation in the plane of the X-rays may be misleading. Both, however, lie clearly within the joint capsule (C) and are well described as *intracapsular fractures*.

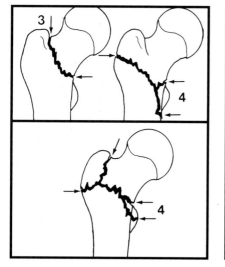

78. **Level of fracture (2):** The other common sites of fracture are *extracapsular*. (3) In the *intertrochanteric* or *basal fracture* the fracture line runs along the base of the femoral neck between the *trochanters*. (4) In *pertrochanteric fractures* the fracture line involves the trochanters, one or both of which may be fractured or separated, so that in effect this is often a comminuted fracture.

79. **Incidence:** The *Y*-axis of the graph represents the yearly incidence per 1000 population and shows that below the age of 60 the fracture occurs most frequently in men, generally from industrial trauma. The incidence increases with age and in later life is three times commoner in women, where hormone-dependent osteoporosis and a degree of osteomalacia are contributory factors. The fracture is seen from time to time in children.

80. **Diagnosis (1):** Inability to bear weight after a fall, particularly in an elderly patient, with or without pain in the hip, is most likely to be due to this common fracture which must be excluded in every case by radiographic examination; fractures of the pubic rami or distal limb fractures are less common causes of this primary complaint. External rotation of the limb, sometimes with a little shortening, is a valuable (but not invariable) sign.

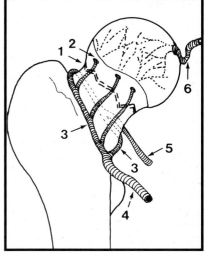

81. **Diagnosis (2):** *Tenderness* will be found over the femoral neck anteriorly (1) and in extracapsular fractures over the greater trochanter. *Pain* is produced by rotation of the hip (2). *Bruising* (3) is a *late* sign in extracapsular fractures, and is absent in acute injuries and in intracapsular fractures. Rarely, with an undisplaced fracture, the patient may be able to bear weight.

82. **Diagnosis (3):** An AP radiograph of the pelvis with a lateral of the affected hip are best for screening of this area. Generally the fracture line is obvious but if not, look for asymmetry in Shenton's lines (1) and in the lateral, angulation of the head with respect to the neck (2) or fragmentation (3). If there is any remaining doubt, a localised AP view should be taken; if this appears negative, re-examine by bone scan after 48 hours, or repeat the plain films after 1–2 weeks.

83. **Intracapsular fractures:** These are prone to complications for two clear reasons: (a) The blood supply to the femoral head may be disturbed by intracapsular fractures (1), leading to *avascular necrosis*. The main supply penetrates the head close to the cartilage margin (2) and arises from an arterial ring (3) fed from the lateral and medial femoral circumflex arteries (4 and 5). A small portion of the head is inconstantly supplied via the ligamentum teres (6).

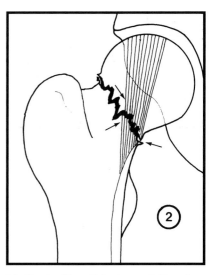

84. **Complications *ctd:*** (b) The head fragment is often a shell containing fragile cancellous bone, and affords poor anchorage for any fixation device. Inadequate fixation may lead to *non-union*. Note that any connection between non-union and avascularity is tenuous—the head is often viable in non-union, and avascular necrosis is seen most frequently in united fractures.

85. **Complications *ctd:*** It follows that complications are most frequent in proximally situated and displaced fractures. Any displacement should be assessed along the lines laid down by Garden which amongst other things take into account disturbance of the weight-carrying trabeculae radiating from the calcar femorale. *In Garden Type 1 fractures,* the inferior cortex is not completely broken, but the trabeculae are angulated (abduction fracture).

86. **Garden Type 2 fractures:** In Type 2 injuries the fracture line is complete; the inferior cortex is clearly broken. The trabecular lines are interrupted but are not angulated. In both Type I and Type 2 fractures there is no obvious displacement of the fragments relative to one another.

**87. Garden Type 3 fractures:** Here the fracture line is obviously complete. There is rotation of the femoral head in the acetabulum; i.e. the proximal fragment is abducted and internally rotated. This may be apparent from the disturbance in the trabecular pattern. The fracture is *slightly displaced*. (Garden Type 2 injury is included for comparison.)

**88. Garden Type 4 fracture:** The fracture here is fully displaced, and the femoral head tends to lie in the neutral position in the acetabulum. (Type 2 injury is included for comparison.)

Garden Type 3 and 4 fractures of the femoral neck carry the worst prognosis.

**89. Garden classification *ctd:*** The radiograph shows a typical subcapital Garden Type 4 fracture. The femoral head is lying in the acetabulum in the neutral position.

**Treatment (1): General principles:**
Intracapsular fractures may be treated by: (i) reduction and internal fixation; (ii) by primary replacement of the femoral head (hemiarthroplasty); (iii) total hip replacement; (iv) conservative measures.

In the case of young and middle aged adults, most centres advocate closed reduction and internal fixation of all grades of intracapsular fracture. (For the management of fractures of the femoral neck *in children* see 267, 113)

In elderly patients Type 2 fractures are also usually treated by closed reduction and internal fixation. Type 1 fractures are generally treated in the same way in order to avoid the risks of disimpaction, but in a very few centres are managed conservatively. In the elderly fit patient internal fixation is usually extended to include fractures of Types 3, and often Type 4, the view being that if the complications of avascular necrosis or non-union supervene, that the patient will be able to tolerate a secondary procedure (usually a total hip replacement). Where the risks of either of these complications are considered in the otherwise fit elderly patient to be particularly high (e.g. a badly displaced, proximally situated Type 4 fracture) then a primary total hip replacement procedure may be considered. Where the patient is less fit, with a life expectancy of perhaps a few but not many years, and the risks of complication are also thought to be high, a hemi-arthroplasty may be considered.

**(2) Investigations:** A few days' delay prior to fixation of the fracture seems to have only a marginal effect on the prognosis, and this interval may be employed profitably to bring the patient into the optimal medical state. The following investigations may prove invaluable in assessment and are performed routinely in many centres: (i) chest radiograph and, if there is a productive cough, a sputum film and culture; (ii) electrocardiograph; (iii) full blood count, with at some stage grouping and cross matching of blood for surgery; (iv) estimation of the serum urea and electrolytes; (v) routine charting of fluid input and output.

**(3) General treatment:** (i) *Preliminary skin traction* (3–4 kg) may help to relieve initial pain and minimise further displacement of the fracture. (ii) *Analgesics, tranquilisers and hypnotics* appropriate to the patient's pain, age and mental state should be prescribed. (iii) In many units, *intravenous fluids* are given routinely (with caution where there are concurrent respiratory and cardiovascular problems) to combat dehydration and minimise the risks of anaemia. (A raised serum urea is clearly associated with a poor prognosis in femoral neck fractures.) Whole blood or packed cells may be required if the patient is markedly anaemic. The type and quantity of replacement are determined by the urinary output, the urea, electrolyte and haemoglobin levels, and the respiratory and cardiac state. Oral fluids are encouraged. (iv) *The physiotherapist* may give valuable assistance

in the management of the moist chest. (v) *Nursing* of the highest standard is required if in particular pressure sores are to be avoided, particularly in the heavy patient who is afraid to move because of pain. (vi) *Antibiotics* may be prescribed where there is a heavy purulent spit or frank urinary tract infection; although treatment may be started immediately, bacteriological confirmation must be sought.

**Internal fixation devices:** A large number of systems have been developed for the internal fixation of intracapsular fracture. None meet all criteria that are desirable in this exacting situation: some have advantages under particular conditions and circumstances, and some in others. Most of the design problems relate to the softness of the bone and restricted size of the proximal fragment; it is often difficult to grip it in a manner that will not further imperil its dubious blood supply, while at the same time holding the fragments in close, reliable and continuing proximity, without penetration of the femoral head or extrusion of the device.

**The AO dynamic hip screw** addresses most of the difficulties encountered in this exacting area, and it and its variations are in widespread use for the treatment of most femoral neck fractures. It is inserted like the majority of devices used here as a *blind procedure* — i.e. the fracture site is not exposed (although the fracture, its reduction, and the placement of the device are visualised with the use of an image intensifier).

90. **The lateral approach for blind nailing procedures:** The patient is placed on an orthopaedic table and the feet secured, either with 10 cm calico bandages to the foot platforms (1) or by the use of foot cases (2). If the fracture is displaced it is reduced by applying traction (3) and internal rotation (in the case of most intracapsular fractures) (4). The position is checked in two planes by an image intensifier (5). If there is difficulty in abducting the sound leg to give sufficient access for the intensifier head for the lateral, some improvement may be gained by slightly

dropping the injured leg (i.e. by extending the hip) and raising the other. Alternatively the sound leg may be positioned clear of the intensifier head by flexing it at the knee and hip (6); traction in this position is, however, less effective as pelvic tilting is unopposed. Failure to achieve reduction may be regarded as an indication for a replacement procedure.

The incision is made in the line of the femur, commencing between the tip of the greater trochanter (7) and the trochanteric ridge (8); its length is dependent on the build of the patient and the size of any plate; small

can always be extended. The incision is deepened through the vastus lateralis; this is reflected with a rugine, and the bone exposed using spike retractors (9) which help control any bleeding.

The next stage is to insert a carefully positioned guide wire which is used to guide the definitive fixation device. Ideally it should lie either centrally or slightly towards the inferior and posterior parts of the femoral neck, and pass through the centre of the femoral head (10).

91. **Insertion of AO dynamic hip screw (1):** An angle guide (1) is used to position the guide wire at an angle to the femoral shaft which corresponds with the geometry of the device. The outer bone cortex is drilled and the guide wire (2) is inserted; its position is checked in two planes with the intensifier. A second guide wire (3) may be inserted well out of the way above the first, in order to steady the head and avoid losing the reduction during the insertion of the device.

92. **DHS insertion (2):** A device (1) which measures the protrusion of the guide wire is used to gauge the length of the screw required (usually 10 mm less than the distance between the shaft and the head margin). The DHS triple reamer (2) is adjusted to the size of the screw, and used to cut a tapping hole for the screw, a hole for the plate sleeve, and a bevel for its shoulder. If the bone of the head is dense, it may be tapped for the screw.

93. **DHS insertion (3):** The screw (1) is inserted with a guide (3) and its position checked; its stem has flats (2) sliding in keyways in the plate sleeve to prevent rotation; these must be aligned. The guide wire is removed and the plate driven home with an impactor (4). It is screwed to the shaft (5) with AO cortical screws. A compression screw (6) which threads into the stem of the DHS screw and abuts on a shoulder (7) in the sleeve may be used to draw the fragments together.

**94. After care:** One of the aims of internal fixation is rapid mobilisation, and in most cases the patient can be allowed out of bed to sit the day following surgery. Early (i.e. within the first week) weight bearing does not seem to affect the union of intracapsular fractures in a material way, and should therefore be encouraged as soon as the patient's general condition will permit. After the wound has healed, the patient may often be allowed home, depending on her mobility and social circumstances. A domiciliary domestic assessment by an occupational therapist is often invaluable in making a decision in this respect.

Out-patient attendances, with check radiographs every 4–6 weeks, should be arranged until the patient is independent; thereafter, she should be seen at intervals of 6 months to 1 year for a total of 3 years to allow detection of avascular necrosis which may be late in declaring itself.

**Complications (1): Avascular necrosis:** In most cases, the cause is disruption of the blood supply by the fracture, and the fate of the femoral head is sealed at the time of injury. It seems possible that on occasion a bulky internal fixation device may further disrupt a tenuous blood supply leading to bone necrosis. It is commonest in Grade 3 and 4 fractures.

 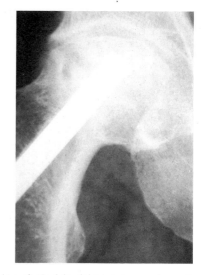

**95. Avascular necrosis (2):** There is complaint of increasing pain (particularly in the groin), a limp, and deteriorating function. In some cases there may be a good period of several months after the initial surgery before the condition declares itself. *Radiological changes:* These are usually present within the first year, but on occasion may not show for as long as 3 years. The whole femoral head may be involved (above left—the fixation device has been removed), with increased density,

loss of sphericity, joint space narrowing and secondary OA lipping. Changes may show only in the weight bearing portion of the head ('superior segmental necrosis') where there is a characteristic double break in the contour of the femoral head (see above right). *Treatment:* Mild symptoms may be controlled with analgesics. In severe cases in the young patient a MacMurray osteotomy should be considered; in the older patient a total hip replacement is usually advised.

**98. Alternative treatments of intracapsular fractures (1): Non-operative management:** All impacted fractures (Garden 1 and some Garden 2) may be treated conservatively, and this is an important consideration, especially where in an ageing population these fractures are on the increase, and where surgical time is in heavy demand. Overall a lowen mortality rate has been claimed in those treated conservatively as opposed to surgically. *Method:* (1) The leg is rested in a gutter splint until pain settles (usually after about a week). (2) Partial weight bearing with crutches is then commenced, and continued for 8 weeks, after which full unsupported weight bearing may be allowed. (3) Check radiographs are taken 2 days after the start of mobilisation, and thereafter every 2 weeks until the eighth week. (4) If the fracture disimpacts and becomes unstable (a 14% incidence only is claimed) then active treatment becomes necessary, when a hemi- or total arthroplasty may be performed. Disimpaction is seen most often in those over 70 especially those in poor general health, or in the younger patient with a low life expectancy. The problems of prolonged recumbency in the elderly may nevertheless follow this line of treatment.

**96. Complications (2): Non-union (1):** This if most frequently seen in Grade 3 and 4 fractures, especially if missed or where the quality of fixation has been poor. In the younger patient bone grafting may be considered, and in some quarters *primary* treatment with pinning and grafting is recommended for high-risk fractures. Techniques vary, but the fracture may be held with a dynamic hip screw, and a segment of fibula, trimmed until it is roughly circular in cross-section, is driven as a graft into a hole drilled to take it.

**97. Non-union (2):** In the older patient, especially in the untreated fracture where the fracture has come seriously adrift (Illus), or where there is pronounced rounding of the bone ends, sclerosis, or marked cystic changes in the neck, prosthetic replacement of the femoral head (hemi-arthroplasty), or total hip replacement are the treatments of choice. A Pauwel's osteotomy is a useful procedure both in the young and in the old (up to the age of 70) for whom a total hip replacement is a fall-back procedure.

**99. Alternative treatments (2):** A Thompson prosthesis (Illus) may be used with or without cement, especially in the elderly patient who has a fracture with a high risk of non-union or avascular necrosis. The mortality rate is influenced by the surgical approach, and Hardinge's is particularly recommended. With a hemi-arthroplasty there is a tendency to late, slow erosion of the acetabulum, so that the procedure is best reserved for the patient who is not likely to have a long or very active life.

**100. Alternative treatments (3):** A successful total hip replacement procedure affords the patient the greatest chance of returning to her prefracture state. The most important consideration is the patient's fitness for this more major procedure; it is fully justified in the adverse conditions described if the patient is in good health, physically and mentally active, and the unit's mortality and morbidity figures are low.

**101. Alternative treatments (4):** There are many other methods described for fixing these notoriously difficult fractures; these include: (1) Moore or Knowles pins (a minimum of 3) are of value in children as they have the least effect on the blood supply of the head; (2) 3 or 4 self-tapping cannulated screws (e.g. MAGNA-Fx™, AO) control any tendency to rotation of the head and may reduce operating time; (3) Trifin nails also control rotation, but have a tendency to back out and are now seldom used.

**104. Intertrochanteric basal neck fractures (3): After care:** (a) The patient can usually be allowed to sit out of bed by the second day. (b) Stitches are removed about the 10th day. (c) If, as is usual, good fixation of the fracture has been obtained, the patient can be gradually mobilised during the first week. Full weight bearing is often achieved within the first 3 weeks. (d) The patient is discharged home as soon as a satisfactory level of independence has been regained. (e) Thereafter the patient attends as an out-patient at intervals of 4–6 weeks. (f) As soon as check radiographs show sound union of the fracture, the patient may be discharged from further attendance (again assuming a good functional result). The fixation device is not removed unless the patient is young (e.g. under the age of 45) or the device is giving rise to symptoms.

**102. Intertrochanteric basal neck fractures (1):** Fractures of this type occurring at the base of the neck have the following points in their favour (a) They are extracapsular, and in the adult are not associated with avascular necrosis. (b) Because of the size of the neck and head fragments, good internal fixation can usually be achieved; non-union is extremely rare, and early weight bearing after internal fixation is usually possible.

**103. Intertrochanteric basal neck fractures (2): Operative treatment:** The patient is placed on the orthopaedic table, and if the fracture is displaced, traction in the neutral position will generally achieve reduction. The proximal femur is exposed as previously described, and the fracture secured either with a dynamic hip screw and a long (e.g. 7-holed) plate, or a one-piece blade or nail plate.

**105. Pertrochanteric fractures (1):** These lie distal to the intertrochanteric line, and several patterns are common (see AO Classification, p. 268 for fuller details). The fracture line may pass through the mass of the greater trochanter and run to the lesser trochanter with (2) or without (1) its separation. It is often highly fragmented, with separation of the greater and usually the lesser trochanter (3). It may be continuous with a spiral fracture of the proximal femoral shaft (4).

**106. Pertrochanteric fractures (2): Treatment (1):** Where there is little or no fragmentation (as in 1 & 2 in 266, 105), stability is not a problem, and a dynamic hip screw with a long plate will give adequate fixation. If the fracture requires preliminary reduction, analysis of the radiographs will indicate whether the limb should be internally rotated, externally rotated, or placed in the neutral position.

**107. Treatment (2):** In the unstable fracture (266, 105, 3 and Illus.), it is difficult to obtain strong reliable fixation. The stresses on any fixation device are high, and mechanical failure is common. A dynamic hip screw with a long plate is nevertheless often successful, and this may also be used in fractures involving the proximal femur, especially in conjunction with neutralising screws.

**108. Treatment (3): Alternative fixation devices (1):** The Gamma nail (or Richards intramedullary hip screw, Illus.) is suitable for many pertrochanteric and proximal subtrochanteric fractures. It uses an IM nail (1), angled (2) to suit the proximal femoral canal, and a lag screw (3). A sleeve (4) with keyways for the lag screw is held with a set screw (5). Rotation of the IM nail is prevented with distal locking screws (5) located with a jig, and the fragments can be compressed with a compression screw (6).

**109. Alternative fixation devices (2):** Where more of the proximal femoral shaft is involved, a blade plate (1) may be used as an alternative to a dynamic hip screw with a long plate. With further involvement of the shaft, a Russel–Taylor reconstruction (locking) nail (2) offers considerable versatility. This has slots distally for 6.4 mm locking screws (3). The proximal end accepts 6.4 mm (4) and 8 mm (5) cancellous screws. A locking screw (6) is available.

**110. Alternative fixation devices (3):** Schanz screws (1) in combination with an external fixator (2) are of particular value in the management of open injuries in this region. This treatment is also advocated in many closed fractures, especially where resources are low. Surgical trauma and blood loss are minimal; the technique is straightforward, quick and inexpensive, and mobilisation on crutches, non-weight bearing, can usually be started after 48 hours. The average time to union is 16 weeks.

**111. Conservative treatment:** As union is seldom a problem in intertrochanteric and pertrochanteric fractures, they can be successfully treated by bed rest and traction. A Thomas splint may be used if desired for additional support. This form of treatment may be adopted if, for example, the patient is unfit for anaesthesia, or there are problems with other injuries; the risks must outweigh the advantages of early mobilisation.

**112. After care in pertrochanteric fractures:** In stable fractures (e.g. 1 & 2 in 266, 105) with high quality internal fixation, the patient may be mobilised early, with weight bearing at any stage. In less stable injuries the decision when to permit weight bearing is even more dependent on the rigidity of the form of fixation employed. In the very unstable fracture premature weight bearing may lead to mechanical failure of the internal fixation device, and it is often wise to advocate non-weight bearing with crutches until callous appears and is seen to be offering appreciable local reinforcing support.

*Complications:* The commonest complication is failure of fixation with drift into coxa vara (usually secondary to cutting out of the fixation device). If this occurs before much callous has appeared, it can usually be corrected by returning the patient to bed and applying skeletal traction of 5–7 kg. This is maintained till union is established. If coxa vara is discovered late, the position has usually to be accepted.

**113. Fractures of the femoral neck in children:** These uncommon injuries result from severe violence, and have been classified by Delbet into 4 types: Type I: Subcapital (or trans-epiphyseal)—these are fracture–dislocations with the capital epiphysis being extruded from the joint. Avascular necrosis is virtually inevitable. Type II transcervical—the commonest injury. If undisplaced (Illus.) avascular necrosis is uncommon, but if

displaced it is very high (60%). In Type III, cervico-trochanteric (basal) and Type IV, per-trochanteric fractures, the incidence of avascular necrosis is lower, but is also related to displacement. Coxa vara and non-union are two further complications of these serious injuries.

*Treatment:* (1) *All undisplaced fractures* should be treated with a hip spica maintained till union. Complications are low in this group. In displaced fractures (2), if the child is under 10 years, manipulative reduction should be tried, and if successful, the fracture secured with Knowles pins. Capsulotomy is sometimes advocated to reduce the incidence of avascular necrosis. (3) Open reduction is undertaken in Type I injuries. In the others, if reduction fails or if the child is over 10, primary subtrochanteric osteotomy with plaster fixation is advised to reduce the incidence of non-union and coxa vara. (4) Osteotomy may also be advised for non-union. The extent of avascular necrosis is variable and should be treated expectantly. Sometimes hip fusion may be required.

**114. Subtrochanteric fractures:** Fractures at this level are often pathological (e.g. from metastases). If the patient's general condition is very poor, pain relief may be obtained by traction in a Thomas splint (Illus.). In all other cases, internal fixation is advocated by, for example, a Russell–Taylor Reconstruction nail. Where there is a large osteolytic defect, acrylic cement packed into it will give much additional support to the internal fixation device, and immediate mobilisation may be possible.

**115. Trochanteric fractures:** Isolated fractures of the greater (Illus.) or lesser trochanters may result from sudden muscle contraction (avulsion of gluteus medius, or iliopsoas insertions). Fractures of the greater trochanter may also result from direct violence. Symptomatic treatment only is required, and the patient may be mobilised after a few days' bed rest.

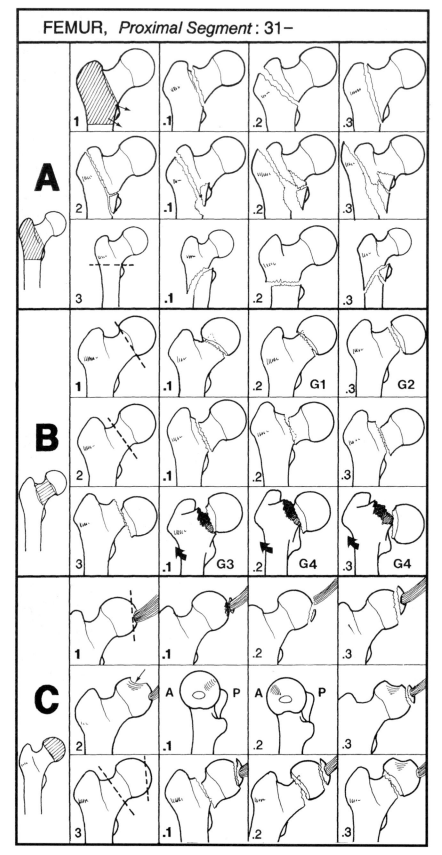

FEMUR, *Proximal Segment* : 31–

**116. AO Classification of Fractures of the Femur, Proximal Segment (31–):**

**Type A** fractures involve the trochanteric area (bounded by the intertrochanteric line and the line separating the diaphysis from the proximal segment, at the level of the distal limit of the lesser trochanter).

A1 = Simple fractures beginning anywhere in the region of the greater trochanter, and ending above or below the lesser trochanter: .1 the fracture runs along the intertrochanteric line; .2 it passes through the greater trochanter; .3 it passes below the lesser trochanter.

A2 = Multifragmentary fractures starting anywhere on the greater trochanter and running into the medial cortex which is broken at two levels: .1 with one intermediate fragment; .2 with several intermediate fragments; .3 with the medial border of the fracture extending more than 1 cm below the lesser trochanter.

A3 = The fracture line extends from below the greater trochanter to above the lesser trochanter: .1 simple oblique; .2 simple transverse; .3 multifragmentary.
[Note: Avulsion fractures of the greater and lesser trochanters cannot be classified with other Type A fractures, and have a separate classification, namely 31–D1.]

**Type B** fractures involve the femoral neck.
B1 = Minimally displaced subcapital fractures: .1 impacted with 15° or more valgus; .2 impacted with less than 15° of valgus; .3 non-impacted fractures.
B2 = Transcervical fractures: .1 basal; .2 adduction pattern; .3 shear pattern.
B3 = Displaced subcapital fractures: .1 moderate varus displacement with external rotation; .2 moderate displacement with shortening and external rotation; .3 marked displacement.

**Type C** fractures involve the femoral head; they are rare, and are generally seen as a complication of posterior dislocation of the hip.
C1 = Split fractures: .1 avulsion of the ligamentum teres; .2 with detachment of the ligamentum teres; .3 with a large fragment.
C2 = Depressed fracture of the head: .1 posterior superior; .2 anterior superior; .3 depression with a split fracture.
C3 = Fracture of the head and the neck: .1 split fracture with a transcervical fracture; .2 split fracture with a sub-capital fracture; .3 depressed fracture with a fracture of the neck.
*Note:* 1. The distinction between fractures in Type B is somewhat arbitrary as the great majority of fractures within this group are of a common pattern, the apparent radiological differences being due to differences in positioning or projection.
2. The AO Group observe the following approximate equivalents with the Garden Classification:
Garden 1 = 31–B1.2
Garden 2 = 31–B1.3
Garden 3 = 31–B3.1
Garden 4 = 31–B3.2 or 31–B3.3.

117. Following a head injury and a dislocation of the hip which was reduced by manipulation, this patient complained of persistent pain and stiffness in the hip. What is the cause of this?

118. Nine months after internal fixation of a femoral neck fracture by a tri-fin nail this patient complained of pain in his hip.
a. What is the source of his complaint?
b. What was the level of the fracture?
c. Has it united?
d. What deformity of the femoral neck existed before the injury?

119. This radiograph is of a young man who was complaining of severe pain in the hip and difficulty in weight bearing after a sudden sprint while playing football. What abnormality is present?

120. This radiograph is of a child who complained of pain in the hip and inability to weight bear after a fall from a tree. What injury is present, and what complications might ensue from this?

121. What does this radiograph show? How would you treat this?

122. What pathology is present, and how has it been dealt with?

123. What fracture has occurred here? What treatment has been carried out? What is the result?

124. What is this fracture? How has it been treated?

125. What injuries are present? How might this be treated?

126. What is this fracture? What complication may be present?

127. What injury is present?

128. What abnormality is present? Assuming this is the only injury, how would you treat it?

129. What class of pelvic fracture is showing in this radiograph?

130. What complication is present in this untreated intracapsular fracture of the femoral neck?

131. Describe this injury. How might it be treated?

132. What type of injury has been treated here? What complication has ensued? How might this be treated?

117. Myositis ossificans.

118. a. Avascular necrosis with bone collapse
    b. Subcapital.
    c. Yes.
    d. Coxa valga (secondary to poliomyelitis).

119. Avulsion fracture of the anterior inferior iliac spine (rectus femoris).

120. Type III (cervicotrochanteric or basal) fracture of the femoral neck with displacement. Possible complications include avascular necrosis, delayed or non-union, and coxa vara.

121. There is a multilocular cyst involving the femoral neck and proximal femoral shaft, with a fracture running across it. This is an undisplaced (as yet) extracapsular fracture of the femur in a case of fibrous dysplasia. The diagnosis would have to be confirmed by biopsy; normally the area would be curetted, packed with bone chips, and the fracture secured with a pin and large plate.

122. Slipped proximal femoral epiphysis. There is some persisting deformity. The position has been accepted (a lateral would be required to confirm the extent of the slip) and held with three pins.

123. This is an unstable pertrochanteric fracture which has been treated with a one-piece nail-plate device. This has broken (due to the severe stresses it has been subjected to), but the fracture has gone on to unite, albeit in coxa vara.

124. The fracture is uniting and the original fracture lines are hard to see. Nevertheless a spiral fracture of the proximal femur can be made out, with separation of part of the greater trochanter and involvement of the medial side of the femoral neck at its base. It has been treated by cerclage wiring and Enders nailing. (These intramedullary nails are introduced at the level of the medial femoral condyle under image intensifier control. There is an appreciable complication rate, and for this reason their use is becoming less frequent. A Russell–Taylor Reconstruction Nail would be one good alternative.)

125. There is an obvious dislocation of the hip. In addition there is a fracture of the floor of the acetabulum. Further radiographs and a CAT scan would be required to clarify the extent of the latter, but the impression is of a comparatively undisplaced transverse fracture through the acetabular floor.

Assuming this impression is confirmed, the dislocation would be reduced by manipulation; the acetabular fracture would then be re-assessed; if displacement of the fracture is minimal, then conservative management with traction and early hip movements would be advocated.

126. This is a quadripartite (butterfly) fracture of the pubic rami; there is risk of damage to the urethra or bladder.

127. This shows a posterior dislocation of the hip which was unstable due to an associated fracture of the acetabular rim; the fragment in question can be seen lying in proximity to the upper and outer quadrant of the femoral head. The hip was reduced, and to maintain the reduction, the rim fragment had to be exposed through a posterior approach and screwed back into position.

128. There is a symphyseal separation of just under 2.5 cm. This should be treated by bed rest until the pain settles. The separation should be monitored by repeated radiographs, and more active treatment pursued (e.g. with the use of an external fixator) should deterioration occur.

129. Examination of the symphysis shows a degree of overlap. The sacro-iliac joints appear intact, but there is a fracture involving the blade of the pelvis and the floor of the acetabulum on the right; the hemipelvis is displaced proximally. This is a Tile Type C3 injury.

130. Non-union.

131. There is an undisplaced crack fracture of the femoral neck in a child. This may be treated by the application of a hip spica.

132. There has been a fracture of the acetabular floor which has been reduced and held by two plates and a number of screws. The fracture has united, but there is loss of joint space and a degree of persisting protrusio. Should symptoms merit further treatment, a total hip replacement would have to be considered, but removal of the internal fixation materials would be required as a prior procedure.

# 12. Fractures of the femur and injuries about the knee

1. **Classification:** In the AO Classification system (see 289, 74 for full details) the femoral shaft is defined as in effect stretching between the inferior margin of the lesser trochanter (proximal segment) (1) and the upper border (2) of a square containing the distal end of the femur (the distal segment). For descriptive purposes the shaft (or diaphyseal segment) may in turn be divided into proximal (3), middle (4), and distal thirds (5). The proximal third is sometimes referred to as the subtrochanteric zone.

2. **Causes of fracture:** Considerable violence is usually required to fracture the femur, and the common causes include road traffic accidents, falls from a height, and crushing injuries. Pathological fractures may also occur: the commonest cause is senile osteoporosis but metastatic deposits, especially in the subtrochanteric region are frequently seen (1). Stress concentrations and bone erosions at the stem ends of prostheses may also be responsible (2).

3. **Fluid loss:** In a simple fracture, loss of ½–1 litre of blood into the tissues with accompanying shock is common. Fractures open from within out occur classically in the proximal third. Blood replacement is often required in closed fractures, and normally essential in open ones; grouping, cross-matching and setting up of an intravenous line should be done routinely (except in children). In the transport of patients to hospital, temporary splintage will help reduce local bleeding and shock.

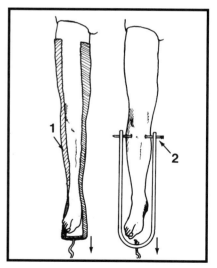

4. **Diagnosis:** This seldom presents any difficulty; weight bearing is impossible and there is abnormal mobility in the limb at the level of the fracture. The leg is often externally rotated, abducted at the hip, and shortened. Radiographs confirm the diagnosis. It is most important to exclude fracture of the patella, dislocation of the hip, and fracture of the pelvis of the central dislocation type.

5. **Conservative treatment:** Femoral shaft fractures are frequently treated conservatively, and the first principle to appreciate is that the large muscle masses of the quadriceps (1) and hamstrings (2) tend to produce displacement and shortening (3). Traction can overcome this, and is the basis of most conservative methods of treatment.

6. **Traction methods:** There are two methods of applying traction: **(1) Skin traction, using adhesive strapping:** This is used in children and young adults. There are occasional problems with skin sensitivity and pustular infections under the strapping. **(2) Skeletal traction**, using a Steinman pin through the tibial tuberosity. This is preferred in the older patient with inelastic skin and where heavy traction is required. There are occasional problems with pin track infections.

**7. Applying skin traction (1):** With the exercise of care and gentleness this can usually be done without an anaesthetic. (1) Begin by shaving the skin. (2) It is then traditional to swab or spray the skin with a mildly antiseptic solution of balsam of Peru in alcohol. This may facilitate the adhesion of the strapping.

**8. Applying skin traction (2):** Commercial traction sets use adhesive tapes which can stretch from side to side but not longitudinally. They come supplied with traction cords (1) and a spreader bar (2) with foam protection for the malleoli (3). Begin by applying the tape to the medial side of leg—do this by peeling off the protective backing with one hand (4) while pressing the tape down and advancing the other (5).

**9. Applying skin traction (3):** The leg is internally rotated and the tape applied to the outside of the leg, preferably a little more posterior than on the medial side. The tapes should extend up the leg as far as possible, irrespective of the site of the fracture. Now apply traction to the leg (1) and finally secure the tapes throughout their length with encircling crepe bandages (2).

**10. Applying skeletal traction (1):** The preferred site is the upper tibia a little under 2 cm (1″) posterior to the prominence of the tibial tuberosity (1). It is important to avoid the knee joint, and the growth plate in children: so begin by carefully identifying it by flexing the knee (2), noting its relationship to the tuberosity (3). If a general anaesthetic is not employed, infiltrate the skin and tissue down to periosteum with local anaesthetic (e.g. 2–3 ml of 1% lignocaine) (4).

**11. Skeletal traction (2):** Now make a small incision in the skin (1) enough to take the traction pin only; inset it until the point strikes bone. Drive the pin through the lateral tibial cortex by applying firm pressure and twisting the chuck handle (2). You should feel it penetrate the outer cortex and pass quickly with little resistance till it meets the medial cortex. Stop at this stage.

**12. Skeletal traction (3):** Infiltrate the skin down to periosteum on the medial side, using the lie of the pin to guide you to the expected exit area (3). Drive the pin through the medial cortex, and make a small incision over the tenting skin to allow it to come through. Protect the openings with gauze strips soaked in Nobecutane® or a similar sealant (4). Try to inset the pin at right angles to the leg.

13. **Traction systems (A): Skin traction in a Thomas splint (1):** The most important decision in selecting a Thomas splint is the ring size. To save time (e.g. before anaesthesia) the uninjured leg may be measured, and an allowance made for swelling, present and anticipated. It is nevertheless wise to have readily available a size above and below the estimate in case of inaccuracies.

14. **Thomas splint (2):** Applying traction with one hand on the spreader bar (1) the selected splint is pushed up the leg (2). It should reach the ischial tuberosity (or more likely the perineum) and it should be possible to pass one finger beneath the ring round its complete circumference. If the ring is too large or too small, maintain traction while the next size is tried.

15. **Thomas splint (3):** The choice of soft furnishings and their method of application is often made with a fanaticism that may amaze the uncommitted. Slings to bridge the side irons may be formed from strips of 15 cm (6″) wide calico bandage (1). It is traditional to secure these with large safety pins inserted from below, close to the outer iron (2). Sometimes spring clips are used. A double bandage thickness ensures greater rigidity (3).

16. **Thomas splint (4):** The sling placed directly beneath the fracture should preferably be unyielding, and one of canvas with web and buckle fastenings is often favoured in this situation. It is customary to apply the splint with the master sling in position; the other slings are then attached and adjusted to the contours of the limb. Less satisfactorily perhaps the splint is applied with all the slings already in position.

17. **Thomas splint (5):** Calico and canvas slings can drift, separate, or ruck, and many prefer the smoothness of an unbroken circular bandage, stretched in double thickness over the splint (e.g. Tubigrip®) (1). This has the disadvantage of 'waisting' the splint (2), being less than firm under the fracture and tending to drift distally (3). The last may be prevented by anchoring it to the ring with ribbon gauze or bandage (4).

18. **Thomas splint (6):** If separate slings are used, their tendency to separate may be minimised by pinning each to its neighbour (1). Nevertheless, a layer of wool should be placed between them and the limb to smooth out any unevenness (2) (not necessary with circular woven bandage). In all cases, a large pad (e.g. of gamgee) should be placed directly beneath the fracture to act as a fulcrum.

**19. Thomas splint (7):** In long oblique fractures and those with apposition no manipulation will be needed and the traction system may be completed by, for example, tying the cords to the end of the splint (1). The convention of passing the medial cord under the corresponding iron helps to control the tendency to lateral rotation (2). A Chinese windlass (of spatulae or a metal rod) may be used to take up slack (3).

**20. Thomas splint (8):** Where skeletal traction is being used a metal loop (1) (Tulloch–Brown loop) allows a direct pull to be made in the line of the limb. The loop may be tied to the end of the Thomas splint (2) and tensioned with a windlass as previously described (3). A stirrup may be employed to prevent springing of the loop (4). Protect the sharp ends of the pin with caps (5).

**21. Thomas splint (9): Manipulation:** With the exception of the young child, manipulation is advisable if there is loss of bony apposition. With the splint in position, but unattached, an assistant applies strong traction (1) while pressure is applied in the directions deduced from the radiographs (2). When the traction is eased off, the limb remains the same length if a hitch has been obtained (3) but telescopes if not (4).

**22. Thomas splint (10):** After the traction cords have been attached, the end of the splint can be raised temporarily on a pillow (1) while the limb is bandaged to the splint, using for example 15 cm (6″) crepe bandages (2). Note gamgee or wool padding behind the fracture to act as a fulcrum (3), behind the knee to keep it in slight flexion (4), and along the shin to avoid sores (5).

**23. Thomas splint (11):** The system described is normally referred to as fixed traction in a Thomas splint. The basic principles are straightforward, but it is important that they are thoroughly understood. Muscle tension (mainly quads and hams) tends to produce shortening (1); this can be overcome by traction, for example through a Steinman pin (2) aided by a loop and traction cord (3). If the traction cord is tied to a ringless Thomas splint, the reduction is maintained so long as a pull is kept on the cord (4); redisplacement occurs if the cord is released (5). This proximal migration is normally prevented by the ring (6) so that the reduction is maintained even when the traction cord is released (7). Note that muscle tone = tension in traction cord = ring pressure.

**24. Thomas splint (12):** This pressure of the ring of the Thomas splint tends to produce sores (1) (especially in the perineal, groin and ischial tuberosity regions) and must be relieved (3). This is done by applying traction (*c.* 3 kg/8 lb) to the anchored cords (4). If ring pressure is unrelieved, *increase the traction weights.*

**25. Thomas splint (13):** The traction weights have a tendency to pull the patient down towards the foot of the bed (1). This may continue till the splint comes to rest on the traction pulley (2). This may be countered if it becomes a problem by raising the foot of the bed (3), when the traction weight is balanced by the upward component of the patient's body weight (4).

**26. Thomas splint (14): Supporting the limb and the splint (1):** To allow the patient to move about the bed and prevent pressure on the heel, it is desirable to support the splint; this may be done most simply by tying a cord from the end of the splint to an overhead bar of the Balkan beam bed. The position of the suspension cord may be adjusted from near the midline to either side. (Illus.: lateral attachment to control external rotation.)

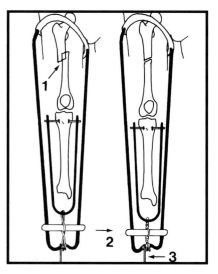

**27. Thomas splint (15): Supporting the splint (2):** Some prefer a lively system which can be achieved in various ways, e.g. by weights and a system of pulleys (1). The suspension cord may be arranged in Y-fashion to straddle both irons of the Thomas splint (2). Support for the proximal end of the splint (3) is less clearly an advantage although often pursued—it may cause extra pressure beneath the ring (4).

**28. Thomas splint (16): Supporting the splint (3):** Another form of lively splint support ('octopus') consists of elastic Bunjee cord (1), which can be adjusted with tensioners (2). The cords are attached to the splint with G-cramps (3) and to cross members of the Balkan beam (4) by means of a bar (5) along which a pulley (6) is free to move, allowing easy movement up and down the bed (7).

**29. Thomas splint (17):** Check radiographs should be taken after the application of a Thomas splint, after any major adjustment, and thereafter at fortnightly intervals till union.

**Corrections:** (a) If there is persistent shortening (1) tighten the windlass in a fixed traction system (2). This will inevitably increase ring pressure, and must be compensated by increasing the traction weight (3). (Soft tissue between the bone ends may nevertheless thwart reduction.)

**30. Thomas splint (18): Corrections:** (b) Where the proximal fragment is abducted (1) the position may be improved by increasing the traction (2) and abducting the leg (3). The position of the ring traction pulley and the splint supports will require corresponding adjustment. (c) If the proximal fragment is adducted (4) increase of traction alone (2) may lead to an improvement in the position. It may be helpful to apply side thrust with a pad (5) between the leg and the medial side iron. (d) Flexion and/or abduction of the proximal fragment (6) due to unresisted psoas and gluteal action is frequently a very painful complication. In the young patient, raising the splint (7) and/or abducting the leg and bandaging a local pad in position (8) may bring the fragments into alignment, but this manoeuvre is less certain in the older patient where internal fixation is frequently advisable for femoral fractures at this level and of this type. In any patient in whom this conservative technique is practised, care must be taken to avoid pressure in the region of the anterior superior iliac spine (9).

**31. Thomas splint (19): Corrections:** (e) Perhaps the commonest residual deformity requiring and amenable to correction is backward sag at the fracture site (9). If a continuous posterior support is used, the padding behind the fracture should be increased in thickness. If separate slings are used, the sling behind the fracture should be tightened and/or the padding behind the fracture increased (10).

**32. Thomas splint (20): After care (1):** During the first 72 hours following fracture, swelling of the thigh from haematoma and oedema may render the ring tight round its circumference. (Normally it should be easy to put a finger under the ring at any point.) To avoid changing the splint, split the ring with a hacksaw, ease the ends apart, and protect them with adhesive strapping.

**33. Thomas splint (21): After care (2):** The following items should be checked daily. Look for impending pressure sores (and take appropriate action). (a) *In the Achilles tendon region* if the slings stop at this level (1); (b) *Under the heel*, if the heel is included (2); If a circular woven support is used, a cruciate incision in it at heel level is prophylactic (3); (c) *Over the malleoli* (4).

**36. Thomas splint (24): After care (5):** In those cases where skeletal traction is employed, look for: (i) Loosening of the Steinman pin; this may require recentring; other treatment is seldom required, so that traction may be continued. (ii) Pin-track infection; a wound swab should be sent for bacteriological examination and the appropriate antibiotic administered. If infection is marked, the traction site may have to be abandoned. (iii) Shifting and digging-in of the loop; adjust with padding.

During the period a patient spends in bed he should practise quadriceps and general maintenance exercises. Splintage in children should be continued till union (6–12 weeks). In adults, mobilisation of the knee joint and/or the patient may be possible before union is complete.

**34. Thomas splint (22): After care (3):**
(d) *The ring area:* Good nursing care is vital to avoid skin breakdown. In addition for: (1) circumferential tightness—split the ring; (2) perineal pressure—increase the ring traction weight; (3) anterior spine pressure—lower the splint; (4) pressure behind the ring—decrease or remove any support weight and place a pillow above the ring (4); (e) pad the edge of the sling if needed (5).

**35. Thomas splint (23): After care (4):**
Check daily for weakness of ankle dorsiflexion (1) indicative of common peroneal nerve palsy and necessitating careful inspection of the neck of the fibula where the cause is generally felting of the wool padding, transmitting pressure from the side iron (2). Repad and fit a Sinclair foot support if the palsy is complete: expect recovery in 6 weeks.

**37. Early mobilisation techniques:** *(i)* Where there is abundant callus and the fracture cannot be sprung, splintage may be discarded and the knee mobilised till there is sufficient mature callus to allow weight bearing. *(ii) The Pearson knee-flexion piece:* this may be used as soon as some stabilising callus appears at the fracture site.

*Method:* The traction cord (1) is transferred to the Pearson attachment (2) which is fixed to the Thomas splint (3) and hinges at the level of the knee axis (4). An adjustable cord (5) may be used to gradually advance the range of permissable knee flexion. The end of the Thomas splint is raised (6) and supported (7) while a cord (8) may allow the patient to assist his knee extension manually.

**38. Early mobilisation techniques: (iii) Cast bracing (1):** After 4–8 weeks in a Thomas splint, cast bracing may be considered, especially in fractures of the distal half. Many techniques are practised. In a typical procedure the patient is sedated with diazepam, a sandbag placed under the buttocks, and a cast sock drawn over the knee (1). Circular woven bandages (stockingette) encase the limb in two sections (2) and are taped in position (3).

39. **Cast bracing (2):** A layer of wool roll is used to protect the bony prominences below the knee (4) and as a single layer of padding in the thigh (5). A below-knee plaster is then applied (6) and completed by turning back and incorporating the circular woven bandage (7). An appropriately sized bucket top of polythene is selected (8), trimmed as required and taped in position (9).

40. **Cast bracing (3):** Traction is applied to the leg (10), the bucket is pulled well into the groin (11), a plaster thigh piece applied, moulded in a quadrilateral fashion (to prevent rotation) (12) and completed (13). Maintaining traction in 10° flexion, polycentric hinges (14) are carefully positioned with a jig which is centred on the patella (15). The side-stays (16) are adjusted until the fixation plates (17) lie snugly against the upper and lower plaster components. Large encircling jubilee clips (18) may be used to hold the hinges in position while the jig is removed and flexion function checked. The hinges are plastered in position (19) and a rocker or boot applied (20). The hinges can be unlocked by removal of 2 set screws (21).

41. **Cast bracing (4):** The cast brace affords moderate support of the fracture, and mobilisation of the patient may be commenced at first using crutches and with the hinges locked. After 1–2 weeks or as progress determines, flexion can be permitted and the crutches gradually discarded. The brace is worn until union is complete.

A number of commercially produced cast-bracing kits are available using materials other than plaster of Paris (e.g. the bucket may be formed from pre-cut plastic sheet which can be temporarily softened by heating and moulded to shape: resin plaster bandages and polyethylene hinges can be employed). In many cases these render the technique comparatively simple, with the result that the so-called weight-relieving calliper, tubed into the patient's shoe, is now much less frequently employed for early mobilisation than in the past.

42. **Other methods of treating fractures of the femur: (1) Hamilton–Russell traction:** This is particularly applicable in the conservative treatment of bilateral fractures; it is a form of balanced traction where the pull on the limb (1) is countered by the body weight (2) through the bed being raised (3). The fracture and distal fragment are supported by a padded canvas sling (4), angled slightly towards the head (5) to counter a tendency to distal drift. The theory behind the classical arrangement is that the line of pull on the femur is the resultant (6) of a parallelogram of forces, where the horizontal component (7) is doubled because of the pulley arrangement (8). Friction losses spoil the theory, and many prefer direct control of all forces (9). This method of treatment, although often useful, gives restricted support to the fracture. Note that balanced traction can be carried out using a Thomas splint bandaged to the limb, but unattached to any of the traction cords.

**43. Gallows traction:** Children up to the age of 3 years (or 4 if light) are ideally treated by this method, which may sometimes be used at home if the circumstances are suitable. Traction tapes are applied to both legs and fixed to an overhead beam (1) so that the child's buttocks are just clear of the bed (2), making nursing easy. The body weight is responsible for the traction. Gallows traction should not be used in the older child as there is the risk of vascular spasm and peripheral gangrene.

prevented by horizontal screws; these are passed through openings in the intramedullary nail and engage cortical bone on either side. The use of interlocking nails is advocated in the presence of instability; this may be deduced from study of the radiographs, being by definition a feature of AO Type C fractures. Instability may also accompany certain Type B fractures, and may not become apparent until sometime during the course of surgery.

Nailing is usually carried out by a blind (closed) technique, with the fracture not being exposed unless reduction cannot otherwise be obtained. Plain nails may also be inserted using the retrograde technique. Reaming is contra-indicated in most Grade III open femoral fractures (but see 284, 55).

**44. (3) Hip spica:** Stable femoral shaft fractures may be supported by a plaster hip spica; this must include the injured leg to the toes, the other leg to above the knee, and extend to above the nipple line. A hip spica may be used for the fretful child where good nursing care is available at home (with fortnightly out-patient reviews) or for the badly infected compound injury in the adult.

**46. Intramedullary nailing (2):** 'Blind' nailing may also be carried out with the good leg flexed at the hip and externally rotated to give access for the image intensifier which is required to give views of the fracture site in two planes. Traction is applied in the line of the limb through a Steinman pin (1), with the perineal post offering counter-traction (2). The affected side is adducted at the hip to give room for the passage of guide wires and reamers down the femoral shaft. Somer surgeons prefer a lateral recumbent position

**45. Intramedullary nailing (1):** In many centres internal fixation by intramedullary nailing is considered the preferred treatment for femoral shaft fractures in the adult. The prime advantage is that it generally permits early mobilisation of the patient, lessening the risks of pulmonary, circulatory, renal, joint and other complications, while promoting muscle activity and functional recovery. It may also alleviate problems of bed occupancy (which is the historic reason for its introduction). Intramedullary nailing is of particular value in cases of multiple injuries, where its use is advocated if the patient's general condition will allow.

The main patterns of nail in common use include:
(i) plain intramedullary nails (Kuntscher, clover-leaf and other patterns) which are inserted without preliminary reaming, or with reaming limited to removal of any medullary tight spots which might interfere with their passage.
(ii) AO (or other intramedullary nails of similar pattern) which are inserted after a thorough reaming, which is carried out to ensure that the nail has a tight fit throughout the length of the medullary canal.
(iii) Interlocking nails (e.g. Grosse–Kempf, Russell–Taylor and others) where rotation of the upper, lower, or both bone fragments is

**47. Intramedullary nailing (3):** The greater trochanter is exposed through a direct lateral incision, and the medullary canal entered through the piriform fossa (1), using an awl (2). Alternatively a guide wire (3) held in the chuck of an introducer may be used; when the position has been confirmed the opening may be enlarged with a cannulated cutter (4). It may be necessary to slightly trim a medially overhanging trochanter using bone nibblers.

**48. Intramedullary nailing (4):** A reaming rod (1) with its tip angled in one plane is passed down the medullary canal, across the fracture site, and down to the distal metaphysis. It can be rotated (2) (by means of forceps applied to its proximal protruding end) to facilitate entering the distal fragment (3). The distal fragment itself may be manipulated by altering the amount and direction of traction or by the use of a threaded pin inserted percutaneously (4); if all else fails, the fracture may be exposed.

**49. Intramedullary nailing (5):** Cannulated flexible reamers (1) of increasing diameter are fed down the reaming rod (2) (after use of a front cutting reamer), removing just sufficient bone to ensure that ultimately there will be good contact between the nail and bone over a reasonable length of the shaft. The diameter and length of the nail to be used is determined by the final reamer size and the length or reaming rod protruding above the trochanter. A threaded conical bolt (3) is screwed into the chosen nail (4).

**50. Intramedullary nailing (6):** An insertion handle (1) is fixed to the conical bolt (2) with a locking nut (3). Interlocking holes (4) are aligned with the handle which engages with slots in the upper lip of the nail. The reaming rod is replaced with a guide wire (5), and the end of the nail slipped over it (6). A ram guide (7) is screwed into the free end of the conical bolt, and is steadied with a grip (8). A guide wire retainer (9) prevents the guide wire backing out as the nail is driven home with the ram (10).

**51. Intramedullary nailing (7):** A proximal interlocking screw (1) may be inserted after preliminary drilling of the bone using a guide (2) pushed through a hole in the insertion handle which acts as a jig. If the distal, circular, hole (3) in the nail is used, the locking is described as static. If the proximal *slot* (4) is used, then some axial (telescoping) movement (5) is possible (dynamic locking). Distal locking screws (6) may be inserted, using an image intensifier to locate the holes in the intramedullary nail.

**52. Intramedullary nailing (8):** Plain, clover-leaf pattern intramedullary nails may be inserted by the retrograde method. While now in less frequent use this technique has the advantage of being able to be performed where image intensification facilities are not available. The fracture is exposed (1) and the selected nail driven up the proximal fragment (2) until it presents at the buttock where it is delivered through a small incision (3). The fracture is reduced (4), and the nail driven back down (5) across the fracture site into the distal fragment.

**53. Other methods of fixation: External fixators:** Fractures of the femur are less easy to control with external fixators than those of the tibia, owing to the magnitude of the stresses at the fracture site from the weight of the limb; the technique is employed mainly in the management of highly contaminated open fractures.

*Plating:* Compression plating, with a heavy-duty six- to eight-hole plate, is sometimes employed in conjunction with bone grafting for non-union following intramedullary nailing but is not often used in other circumstances.

*After care:* After care is dependent on the quality of fixation. If a tight-fitting, large-diameter nail is used, and if torsion is well controlled by interdigitating fragments or cross-screws, no additional splintage is necessary. The knee may be mobilised and the patient allowed up on crutches. To avoid the risks of the nail bending or fatigue fracture many prefer to defer weight bearing until some callus appears.

If fixation is less sound, a period of a few weeks with the leg cradled in a Thomas splint may be thought desirable.

After union of the fracture, the nail is removed routinely in all but the very frail to reduce the risk of a comparatively minor injury causing a fracture of the femoral neck (from local stress concentrations at the end of the nail).

**54. Special situations: (1) Ipsilateral fracture of the femur and tibia:** The complication rate for these combined injuries is high, irrespective of treatment. To allow early mobilisation internal fixation (e.g. by intramedullary nailing) of both fractures is often preferred. Where conservative treatment is indicated (e.g. in children) a Steinman pin is inserted proximally (1), the tibia manipulated, and a below-knee cast applied incorporating the pin (2). A Thomas splint (3) with traction through the pin (4) controls the femoral fracture.

**55. Special situations *ctd:* (2) Fracture in the confused patient:** Where there is a head injury or a senile confusional state, a patient being treated conservatively may try to remove his own splint; it is possible to prevent this by encircling it with plaster bandages laid on top of the normal crepe bandages (Tobruk splint). This procedure may also be used to give extra security when a patient is in transit.
**(3) Metastatic fracture:** If death is not imminent, intramedullary nailing is advised to relieve pain. Acrylic cement packed round any defect may give sufficient support to allow the patient to bear weight.
**(4) Femoral shaft fracture with (acute) ischaemia of the foot:** Nearly all will respond to reduction of the fracture which should be carried out under circumstances which will permit exploration should reduction fail. If the femoral artery is in fact divided, intramedullary nailing will be required prior to vessel repair.
**(5) Femoral shaft fracture with nerve palsy:** The majority are lesions in continuity, the common peroneal element being most often affected. If there is reason to believe that there may be nerve *division*, exploration and internal fixation may have to be undertaken.
**(6) Fracture of the femoral neck and shaft:** If the shaft fracture is proximal, both fractures may be treated by a dynamic hip screw and long plate. In many cases a Russell–Taylor reconstruction nail may be suitable.

**(7) Femoral neck fracture with dislocation of the hip:** see 256, 64.
**(8) Fractures of the femoral shaft and patella:** Note the following important points: (a) Early mobilisation of the knee is essential for retention of function. (b) Avoid patellar excision when mobilisation of the knee is going to be delayed. (c) Avoid if possible exposure of the femoral fracture and the creation of tethering adhesions between the femur and quadriceps.

The ideal treatment of the femoral fracture is closed nailing; see 292, 81 for treatment of patellar fractures. If the femoral fracture must be treated conservatively, it is best to leave even badly displaced or comminuted patellar fractures to unite by fibrous union; mobilise the knee as early as possible; excision of the patella can then be carried out as a late secondary procedure when no further flexion can be gained.
**(9) Open fractures:** If internal fixation is indicated (especially with multiple injuries) the infection rate in Grade I and Grade II injuries is said to be no greater after a meticulous debridement and blind nailing than in closed fractures. Grade IIIA fractures with good skin cover and no medullary contamination can be nailed in reasonable safety if reaming is avoided. Grade III B&C open fractures are generally best treated conservatively or with an external fixator.

**56. Other fractures of the femur. (1) Fractures of the upper third:** It is often hard to control fractures at this level by conservative measures (but see 279, 30). Severe, prolonged pain is often a further problem, and is due to the psoas and glutei causing involuntary movement of the proximal fragment. In the adult internal fixation should certainly be considered (Illus.: nailed femur in Thomas splint). Some cases are suitable for fixation with a pin and long plate, aiming to get three screws at least distal to the fracture.

**57. (2) Fractures in hip replacements:** Four fracture types are described. *In Type 1* there is fragmentation of bone round the stem with inevitable loosening. All require surgery, and this is often highly demanding. Methods include (i) a long-stemmed prosthesis inserted after reduction of the fracture and placement of cerclage wires which are tightened before the cement sets (Illus); (ii) where there has been gross bone destruction or infection, excision of the proximal shaft and the use of a custom-made prosthesis.

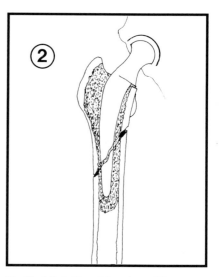

**58. (2 ctd):** *In Type 2* there is an oblique or spiral fracture round the stem. The stability of the fracture is maintained by the stem of the prosthesis. In treating these fractures it is important to obtain and maintain a good reduction, as in the majority the prosthesis eventually loosens and has to be replaced; mal-union, if it occurs, will cause difficulty. The initial treatment of these injuries may be *conservative* (e.g. by traction in a Thomas splint) or *surgical.*

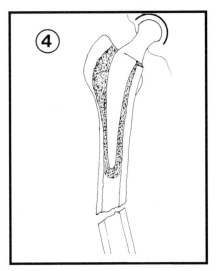

59. **(2 ctd)**: Type 2 injuries may be treated with Partridge nylon cerclage straps (1) used in conjunction with Partridge plates (2). The latter are also made of nylon, and contain slots for the straps. The plates have stand-off teeth, and the straps have recesses which reduce the area of bone contact, thereby lessening the risks of bone necrosis. These injuries may also be treated by plating (as described in 285, 60).

60. **(2 ctd)**: *In Type 3*, the commonest of these injuries, the fracture is at the tip of the prosthesis, and is unstable. Conservative treatment has a high complication rate (e.g. malunion, delayed union). If the prosthesis remains firm, consider (a) a long plate screwed to the trochanter, with additional screws passed in front of and behind the prosthesis (tapped into the cement mantle) and bone grafting; (b) a Mennen plate; (c) Partridge straps and plates. Avoid weight bearing until there are signs of union.

61. **(2 ctd)**: *In Type 4* the fracture lies entirely distal to the stem of the prosthesis. These carry a good prognosis, and may be treated equally effectively by conservative or surgical methods. *Conservatively* they may be treated by traction in a Thomas splint. *Surgically* they may dealt with by plates and screws (tapped into the cement if necessary), Mennen plating, or cerclage.

62. **(3) Supracondylar fractures (Type A fractures of the distal segment** — *see 290, 75 for full AO Classification)* **(1)**: In children, fractures in the distal third of the femur are frequently only minimally displaced, and may be successfully treated by the application of a cylinder plaster. Weight bearing should not be permitted till evidence of early union appears on the radiographs, but during this period the patient may be mobilised with crutches.

63. **Supracondylar fractures (2)**: In the adult especially, supracondylar fractures have a strong tendency for the distal fragment to rotate (1) under the continuous pull of the gastrocnemius (2) into a position of posterior angulation (anterior tilting) (3). If these injuries are being treated conservatively, this cannot be controlled by traction in the line of the limb (4). It is necessary to flex the knee and maintain the traction over a fulcrum (5).

64. **Supracondylar fractures (3)**: The necessary degree of knee flexion may be obtained using a Pearson knee flexion piece, or better still by bending the Thomas splint at the level of the fracture (Illus.). Mobilisation of the knee should be started as early as possible, as the risks of knee stiffness from the development of tethering adhesions (between the quadriceps muscle and the fracture) is high.

**65. Supracondylar fractures (4):** To allow early mobilisation of the knee and lessen the risks of stiffness many prefer internal fixation of these potentially difficult fractures. If the fracture is proximally situated, an interlocking intramedullary nail may be used (1). Otherwise good fixation may be achieved with a condylar blade-plate (2). These are available in a number of sizes, and are elbowed (3) so that they require little adjustment to fit the curve of the lateral femoral condyle.

**66. (4) Unicondylar fractures (Type B fractures) (1):** Where the displacement is slight (Illus.) these injuries may be treated successfully be conservative measures. A straight Thomas splint may be used for the first 1–2 weeks, but thereafter mobilisation should be started, either with a Pearson knee-flexion piece or with Hamilton–Russell traction.

**67. Unicondylar fractures (2):** Some prefer to treat all fractures of this pattern by internal fixation, and this is certainly indicated if displacement has seriously disturbed the contours of the articular surfaces. Where the bone is of good texture, use two cancellous screws (1), with washers (2) to prevent the heads sinking. A well-contoured buttress plate (3) and cancellous screws can be used if the bone is very soft, or where the fracture has occurred in the presence of a knee joint replacement.

**68. Unicondylar fractures (3):** Shearing fractures which are entirely intra-articular frequently fail to unite if treated conservatively, possibly due to dispersal of the fracture haematoma by the synovial fluid. Non-union may cause knee instability. These fractures may be held with two cancellous screws with their heads sunk below the level of the articular surface. Thereafter a 6 week period of non-weight bearing in a plaster cylinder is advised before vigorous mobilisation.

**69. (5) T- and Y-condylar fractures (Type C fractures) (1):** Undisplaced fractures may be treated conservatively or surgically. If the fracture is displaced without gross fragmentation a dynamic condylar screw may be used. The condyles are reduced first and the screw inserted. The plate is then attached and lined up and fixed to the shaft with cortical screws. The procedure requires an extensive exposure; it is seldom easy, often due to more fragmentation than suggested by the radiographs.

**70. T- and Y-condylar fractures (2):** Where there is a great deal of comminution, open reduction is likely to be unrewarding and the aim should be to restore the alignment of the knee and mobilise it as early as possible—e.g. by using Hamilton–Russell traction. Alternatively, in the elderly, primary joint replacement may be considered.

**71. (6) Displaced femoral epiphysis:**
This injury usually results from hyperextension, and there is risk of vascular complications; reduction should be carried out expeditiously by applying traction, flexing the knee to a right angle and pressing the epiphysis backwards into position. The knee should be kept in flexion for 3 weeks in a plaster slab, and for a further 3–5 weeks in a plaster cylinder in a more neutral position.

**72. (7) Segmental fractures:** These are uncommon in the femur, but are associated with a high incidence of non-union at one level. Fracture exposure may lose the tenuous blood supply to the intermediate segment. Although they may be treated conservatively (dealing with each complication as it arises), closed nailing, if reduction can be accomplished, is a more attractive alternative. A nail, locked at both ends, should be used. Static nailing may be converted at a later stage to dynamic nailing if union is delayed.

**73. COMPLICATIONS OF FRACTURES OF THE FEMUR**
Among the many complications which may accompany this fracture the following should be noted:

**1. Oligaemic shock:** (see p. 32).

**2. Fat embolism** (see p. 89).

**3. Slow or delayed union:** These are common complications, and if the fracture is being treated conservatively, may necessitate prolonged immobilisation of the knee, with risk of permanent stiffness. Where the fracture is being treated by an intramedullary locked nail, conversion from static to dynamic locking (by removal of the appropriate interlocking screws) may encourage union.

**4. Non-union:** In fractures being treated conservatively, this is generally dealt with as soon as it is confidently diagnosed, by intramedullary nailing and bone grafting.

If non-union occurs in a fracture which has been treated by intramedullary nailing, bone grafting will also usually be required. In addition, the quality of the fixation must be reviewed, and if this is found wanting, it must be dealt with. In some cases this will involve replacing the nail (after reaming the canal) with one of a larger diameter. Rotational instability must be controlled, and the use of interlocking screws is desirable. In some cases, in order to obtain compression of the fragments, the use of a dynamic compression plate may be considered to be a preferable method of treatment.

**5. Mal-union:** Persistent lateral angulation is the commonest deformity in shaft fractures, and if 25° or more then correction by osteotomy and intramedullary nailing should be considered. Angulation in the lateral plane seldom gives rise to much difficulty. Nearer the knee, angulation showing on the AP radiographs may give rise to instability, difficulty in walking and secondary osteo-arthritis in the knee. Each case must be assessed on its own merits, but again corrective osteotomy/osteoclasis should be considered.

**6. Limb shortening:** Shortening in the adult should be corrected by shoe alteration to within 1–2 cm (½″) of the limb discrepancy. In children, any difference in leg length usually corrects (or indeed overcorrects) spontaneously within 6–18 months of the injury, and alteration to the shoes is seldom required. Only rarely in epiphyseal injuries is there progressive shortening.

**7. Knee stiffness:** This is a common complication of femoral and tibial fractures, and of injuries to the extensor mechanism of the knee. Among the factors which are involved are the following:

*(a) Quadriceps tethering:* If the quadriceps becomes adherent to a femoral shaft fracture, it becomes unable to glide over the smooth distal shaft in the normal fashion, producing as a result fixation of the patella and restriction of movement in the knee. The closer the fracture is to the knee, the more important this effect. Surgical intervention tends to aggravate this tendency (unless it can be followed by rapid mobilisation).

*(b) Fractures involving the knee joint:* Fractures which involve the articular surfaces may give rise to intra-articular and peri-articular adhesions, or may form a mechanical block to movement. Early mobilisation is especially desirable where a fracture involves the joint.

*(c) Prolonged immobilisation:* Fixation of the knee for an undesirably long period, for example, by delay in union, may lead to stiffness, and this effect is particularly marked in the elderly.

**8. Infection:** Infection may sometimes supervene in femoral shaft fractures treated by intramedullary nailing. Sometimes the source is obvious (e.g. from a contaminated open wound where the initial debridement has been unsuccessful or insufficiently scrupulous), but often it may unaccountably follow a meticulously performed closed procedure. The course of treatment must be individually determined, but the following guide lines usually apply:

1. The causal organism should be isolated, and the appropriate antibiotic administered in effective doses for an adequate length of time.
2. If the infection has become established, it is unlikely to respond unless the fracture is firmly supported, and a most thorough debridement carried out under antibiotic cover.
3. If the fixation afforded by the nail remains good, the nail should be retained.
4. If the nail fixation is not good, and provided the debridement does not entail extensive bone removal, then consider using a larger diameter nail with locking screws.
5. If the fixation offered by the nail is poor, and much bone stock has to be removed, remove the nail and use an external fixator.

**TREATMENT**

**(a) Quadriceps exercises:** Stability in the knee and extension power are dependent on a good quadriceps. It is important that the muscle is not allowed to waste, and quadriceps exercises should be started as soon after injury as possible, and intensified on removal of any fixation. (Amongst the few exceptions are injuries to the extensor mechanism where quadriceps exercises are usually delayed for 2 weeks lest early contraction endanger a repair.)
**(b) Flexion exercises:** These should also be commenced as soon as possible, provided the means can be devised to support the fracture fully. Flexion should not be permitted unless

stress on the fracture can be reduced to a safe level or where healing can be more or less guaranteed (e.g. tibial table fractures).

**(c)  Discarding walking aids:** Walking without the support of sticks or crutches is frequently followed by an improvement in flexion, and such supportive measures should be discontinued as soon as the state of union and the patient's balance will allow.

**(d)  Physiotherapy:** Ideally quadriceps and flexion exercises should be supervised by a physiotherapist with access to aids and facilities such as weights, slings, local heat and hydrotherapy, but basically the patient should be instructed in quadriceps and flexion exercises, and the importance of performing these frequently should be stressed. Passive mobilisation of the patella in appropriate cases may also be helpful.

Physiotherapy should be continued until an acceptable functional range has been achieved (see below) or until a static position has been reached. For this it is necessary to record the range of movements in the knee with accuracy; this should be done initially at weekly and then at monthly intervals. A measurable gain in range, no matter how small, is an encouragement to the patient to further effort; and on the other hand the absence of any improvement should make it clear to him that to continue treatment is not justifiable.

## NOTES

**Acceptable functional range:** What is acceptable obviously varies considerably from case to case, being dependent on the gravity of the injury, the age of the patient, his occupation, athletic or outdoor pursuits, hobbies, etc., but the basic aim is a stable knee which places little restraint on normal everyday activities. The following factors are important:

**Lack of extension:** Loss of extension, both active and passive, may be found—e.g. in an angulated supracondylar fracture of the femur, or where there has been previous osteo-arthritis in the knee. Such losses are seldom severe enough to cause appreciable disability, usually being compensated at hip and ankle. If the knee can be passively but not actively extended, this is known as an *extension lag*. Extension lag frequently gives rise to 'giving way' of the knee. It is common to some degree after most cases of patellectomy, but usually recovers if quadriceps exercises are intensified.

Where extension lag is due to quadriceps tethering, quadriceps exercises should also be encouraged. The patient in most cases of persistent lag learns to compensate for the disability by using the hip extensors to keep the knee straight while standing.

**Lack of flexion:** Appreciable disability follows if flexion to 100° (i.e. 10° more than right-angle flexion) cannot be obtained, and 100° should be the aim. Flexion to 80–90° will permit sitting in inside seats (i.e. non-aisle seats) in public transport, cinemas, etc., but will not allow the patient to kneel. Less than 100° will cause difficulty with steps, deep tread and narrow stairs, and if both knees are affected, rising from armless chairs.

Where flexion has just become static at less than 100°, manipulation of the knee under general anaesthesia should be considered. This is best avoided, however, after patellectomy and quadriceps tendon and patellar ligament repairs because of the risks of secondary rupture. Gains in flexion by manipulation are seldom high, and late manipulations are usually very unrewarding.

Where 80° or less flexion is possible and the position static, the patient's functional disability and functional requirements should be carefully assessed. If there is a marked deficit, quadricepsplasty should be considered. In this procedure the vasti are divided close to the knee so that their tethering effect is eliminated; rectus femoris then becomes the sole extensor of the knee. This often gives a useful gain (often in the region of 40°) although sometimes this is at the expense of an extension lag, and always with some loss of power.

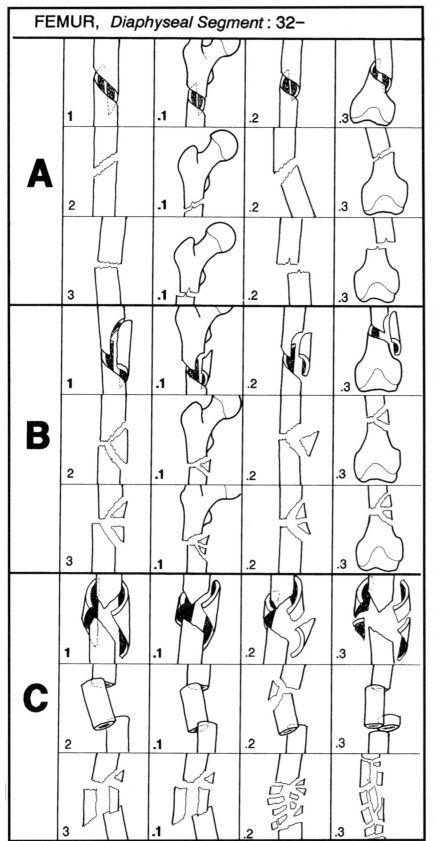

FEMUR, *Diaphyseal Segment* : 32–

**Type A** fractures are simple.
A1 = Spiral fractures: .1 subtrochanteric zone; .2 midshaft; .3 distal zone.
A2 = Oblique fracture (30° or more): .1 subtrochanteric; .2 midshaft; .3 distal zone.
A3 = Transverse fractures: .1 subtrochanteric; .2 midshaft; .3 distal zone.

**Type B** fractures are wedge fractures.
B1 = Spiral wedge fractures: .1 subtrochanteric; .2 midshaft; .3 distal zone.
B2 = Bending wedge fractures: .1 subtrochanteric; .2 midshaft; .3 distal segment.
B3 = Fragmented wedge fractures: .1 subtrochanteric; .2 midshaft; .3 distal segment.

**Type C** fractures are complex.
C1 = Spiral fractures: .1 with two intermediate fragments; .2 with three intermediate fragments; .3 with more than three intermediate fragments.
C2 = Segmental fractures: .1 with one intermediate segment; .2 with one intermediate segment and an additional wedge fracture; .3 with two intermediate segments.
C3 = Irregular fractures: .1 with two or three intermediate fragments; .2 with shattering limited to less than a 5 cm length of the bone; .3 with shattering over 5 cm or more of the bone.

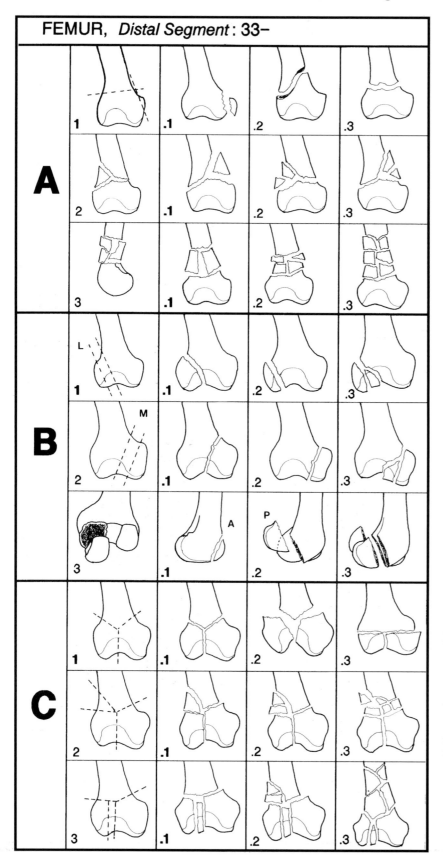

FEMUR, *Distal Segment* : 33–

**75. AO Classification of Fractures of the Femur, Distal Segment (33–):**

**Type A** fractures extra-articular.
A1 = Simple fractures: .1 avulsion fractures of the medial or lateral epicondyle; .2 fracture of the metaphysis, oblique or spiral; .3 fracture of the metaphysis, transverse.
A2 = Metaphyseal wedge fractures: .1 wedge intact; .2 lateral multifragmented wedge; .3 multifragmented medial wedge.
A3 = Complex metaphyseal fracture: .1 with a split intermediate segment; .2 irregular, but limited to the metaphysis; .3 irregular, and extending up into the diaphysis.

**Type B** fractures are partial articular.
B1 = Lateral condylar fractures in the sagittal plane: .1 simple through the intercondylar notch; .2 simple through the weight bearing surface; .3 multifragmentary.
B2 = Medial condylar fractures in the sagittal plane: .1 simple through the intercondylar notch; .2 simple through the weight bearing surface; .3 multifragmentary.
B3 = Frontal plane fractures: .1 flake fracture, anterior and lateral; .2 posterior unicondylar; .3 posterior bicondylar.

**Type C** fractures are complete articular.
C1 = Simple fractures of both the articular surface and the metaphysis: .1 slightly displaced T- or Y-fracture; .2 markedly displaced T- or Y-fracture; .3 distally situated T-fracture with the horizontal element involving the epiphysis.
C2 = Simple fracture of the articular surface, multifragmentary of the metaphysis: .1 with intact wedge; .2 multifragmented wedge; .3 complex.
C3 = Multifragmentary of the articular surface: .1 metaphyseal simple; .2 multifragmentary metaphysis; .3 multifragmentary of the metaphysis, extending into the shaft.

**76. Injuries of the patella and extensor mechanism of the knee: Mechanisms (1):** The *patella* may be fractured by direct violence, e.g. (a) In road traffic accidents in which the knee strikes the fascia (1). (Note the association between fracture of the patella, fracture of the femoral shaft and dislocation of the hip.) (b) By falls against a hard surface— e.g. the edge of a step (2). (c) By heavy objects falling across the knee (e.g. falling rock) (3).

**77. Mechanisms (2):** The patella may also be fractured by indirect violence, i.e. as a result of a sudden muscular contraction (1). This same mechanism may also cause: rupture of the quadriceps tendon (2), rupture of the patellar ligament (3), or avulsion of the tibial tubercle (4).

**78. Diagnosis (1):** Fracture of the patella should be suspected when there is a history of direct violence to the knee; fracture of the patella and other injuries to the extensor mechanism should be suspected when there is difficulty in standing after a sudden muscular effort (especially when there is a snapping sensation within the knee). In most cases *there is inability to extend the knee.*

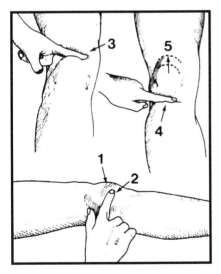

**79. Diagnosis (2):** Note clinically any of the following: bruising and abrasions (1); the presence and site of tenderness (2); any palpable gap above the patella (3) or beneath it (4); any obvious proximal displacement of the patella (5).

**80. Diagnosis (3):** In all cases, radiographs are essential to clarify the diagnosis. An AP projection and a lateral (preferably in extension) will generally suffice. In the acute case tangential projections cannot usually be obtained because of pain, but these views are often of value in the cases which present late. If there is doubt remaining, oblique projections may be helpful. Do not mistake a congenital bipartite patella (Illus.) for a fracture. This anomaly most frequently affects the *upper* and *outer* quadrant; it may be obvious in one view only. The edges are usually rounded, and this may help to differentiate it from a fracture. Other anomalies, such as tripartite patella, may also be distinguished by similar rounding and absence of local tenderness.

**81. Treatment (1): Vertical fractures:**
Fractures of this type are usually undisplaced and stable. They do not show in the lateral radiographs. In the AP view, the overlapping femoral shadow may make them difficult to detect, and in fact these fractures are frequently missed. Conservative treatment only is required.

**82. Treatment (2):** A 6-week period in a cylinder plaster (plaster cylinder, pipestem plaster) is usually advised.
*Method:* Apply a layer of stockingette (two pieces) from the hind foot to the groin (1). Protect the malleoli with a piece of felt (2), butt-joining the ends with adhesive tape (3). Note concavities for the Achilles tendon (4) and dorsum of the foot (5). Pad the leg with wool (6).

**83. Treatment (3):** The knee is normally kept in full extension (but not in recurvatum or hyperextension) while 20 cm (8″) plaster bandages are applied (7). A slab is not necessary. The edges of the stockingette are turned back before completion (8). Crutches are usually advised for the first 2 weeks, with a total of 6 weeks in plaster.

**84. Undisplaced horizontal fractures:**
Undisplaced horizontal fractures (even with some comminution) may be treated along similar lines with, however, radiographs at weekly intervals for the first 2–3 weeks to exclude late separation. After removal of the plaster at 6 weeks, physiotherapy will be required, and crutches may be needed again for the first few weeks till confidence is regained.

**85. Displaced horizontal fractures:** Fractures of this type should be explored so that (1) the exact nature of the pathology may be determined and (2) the appropriate treatment carried out.

Knee function after patellectomy is often excellent, but may fall a little short of perfect; although a full range of movements may be regained, there is often a feeling of instability while descending steep slopes, and there may be some weakness in rising from the squatting position. The patella should therefore be preserved, but only if the articular surface can be perfectly restored and maintained in that position until union occurs. In practice, this is only usually possible when there is no fragmentation, and although the radiographs (Illus.) may suggest that only two fragments are present, this can only be confirmed at exploration.

86. **Treatment (1):** If the joint surfaces can be restored, the fragments may be held in a number of ways. In *AO tension band wiring*, the fragments are reduced and then held in alignment with two hooked Kirschner wires (1) round which is looped a length of wire (2) which is tightened by twisting. A second wire in a figure of eight (3) may be used. The K wires are sunk home (4) and the distal ends trimmed (5). The strongest fixation is by *Pyrford wiring* employing a wire loop (6) and wire purse string (7).

87. **Treatment (2):** If the joint surfaces cannot be restored and held, or if, as illustrated, there is much fragmentation, a complete patellar excision should be carried out, with repair of the quadriceps insertion and lateral expansions. Note, however, that if the damage is confined to one pole of the patella, and the major part of the patella is spared, then good results can be obtained by *partial patellectomy*.

88. For exploration or excision, the patella may be exposed through a midline vertical incision (1) or a lazy S (2) with the raising of two flaps. The patellar fragments are carefully dissected free, taking care that every piece is removed (3). The insertion (4) along with the lateral expansions (5) are repaired with mattress sutures and a plaster cylinder applied. Crutches should be used for 4 weeks and mobilisation commenced at 6 weeks.

89. **Avulsion fractures of the tibial tubercle:** In the adult, or adolescent near skeletal maturity (Illus.) the displacement, if marked, should be reduced and the tubercle fixed with a screw. If displacement is slight, a 6-week period in a plaster cylinder should suffice. In children, surgery should be avoided if possible because of the risks of premature epiphyseal fusion but, if manipulative reduction fails, open reduction and fixing with a suture may become necessary.

90. **Rupture of the quadriceps tendon:** The diagnosis is essentially clinical, but sometimes may be confirmed by examination of the soft-tissue shadows on the radiographs (Illus.). The tendon must be re-attached surgically: it is often necessary to drill the patella to provide anchorage for the sutures. Thereafter a plaster cylinder is applied. Quadriceps exercises are commenced at 2 weeks, weight bearing at 4 weeks and knee flexion at 6 weeks.

91. **Rupture of the patellar ligament:** This is also a clinical diagnosis although proximal displacement of the patella (Illus.) may be suggestive. Treat these surgically like quadriceps tendon ruptures. When there is avulsion of the distal tip of the patella, the bony fragment should be removed. The patellar ligament may be re-attached using holes drilled through the patella for anchorage. Tension on the sutures may be relieved by a figure of eight wire between the quadriceps tendon and the tibial tuberosity.

**92. Osgood Schlatter's disease:** In children, sudden or repeated quadriceps contraction may be responsible for this condition, which is characterised by recurrent pain, tenderness, and swelling over the tibial tubial tubercle. It may be mistaken for an acute injury. While slow spontaneous resolution is the rule, an acute episode may be treated by 2 weeks in a plaster cylinder. Severe persistent symptoms occasionally merit excision of the detached fragment.

**93. Acute lateral dislocation of the patella (1):** In this condition the patella dislocates laterally, often as a result of sudden muscular contraction or a blow on its medial border. It may be reduced (unless of long standing) by applying firm pressure over its lateral aspect (anaesthesia is seldom required). If a first incident, a 6-week period of plaster fixation is advised; if not, apply a pressure bandage for 1–2 weeks.

**94. (2):** Lateral dislocation commonly occurs as first or subsequent incident in the course of recurrent dislocation of the patella, a condition seen most frequently in teenage girls. The presence on the tangential projection of the knee of a marginal osteochondral fracture is diagnostic, but may not be obvious until some weeks after a first incident (which may also be overlooked if spontaneous reduction occurs).

**95. (3):** Due to the femur meeting the tibia at an angle, the quadriceps (1) and patellar ligament (2) have a *lateral component* (3) during muscle contraction, and this is greater where there is genu valgum (5); it is resisted by the femoral gutter (4). An error in tracking, however, may cause the patella to dislocate. When this *starts in extension* (becoming more obvious as the knee flexes), patella alta (6) or an abnormal quadriceps insertion (8) may be additional factors. In these particular cases a re-alignment procedure may be required (e.g. Elmslie–Trillat, Hauser (Illus, 9) or Galeazzi; in the latter, more suitable in the adolescent, the divided semitendinosus tendon is threaded through a hole in the patella (10), and the stump sewn to semimembranosus (11)). Where the dislocation occurs *in flexion* there may be hypoplasia of the patella or lateral femoral condyle (7), with a shallow sulcus and tilting of the patella. Such cases may respond to a lateral tissue (vastus lateralis) release, with or without medial reefing, but sometimes they also require a re-alignment procedure. Where there is no tracking problem, ligament laxity is sometime blamed. Many of these latter cases respond to physiotherapy and the use of a knee brace during athletic activities.

**96. Dislocation of the knee (1):** This injury may surprisingly follow comparatively minor trauma. Most commonly the tibia is displaced anteriorly, but medial, lateral, posterior and rotational displacements are also found. There is inevitably major damage to the ligaments of the knee; all or most may be torn along with the joint capsule.

**97. Dislocation of the knee (2):**
Sometimes there is displacement of the menisci, fractures of the tibial spines, common peroneal nerve palsy, and most seriously, popliteal artery damage.

*Treatment:* Closed reduction appears to give better results in the majority of cases than attempts at operative repair. Reduction is generally easy by traction and the application of pressure over the displaced tibia. Thereafter the leg should be supported by light traction (2–3 kg/6 lb) in a Thomas splint for 3–4 weeks, followed by a further 4 weeks in a plaster cylinder before mobilisation is commenced. Surgery is indicated in the following circumstances: (1) if closed reduction fails (generally due to button-holing of the capsule by a femoral condyle), or (2) if there is persistent circulatory impairment in the limb after reduction, when popliteal artery exploration is indicated.

**98. Soft-tissue injuries of the knee:** When there has been trauma to the knee and the radiographs show little in the way of bony injury, a significant soft-tissue injury should be suspected. It would be unrealistic to say that injuries of this type are easy to diagnose; they sometimes are, but often cause much difficulty. There is the common clinical picture of pain in the knee, swelling, and difficulty in weight bearing shared by many lesions. Investigation of each case should aim to exclude: (1) damage to the extensor apparatus, (2) lateral dislocation of the patella with spontaneous reduction, (3) tears of the ligaments of the knee, (4) meniscus tears.

In some centres, when the injury is suspected of being more than trivial, further investigation is pursued in an aggressive fashion: any haemarthrosis is aspirated, and the soft-tissue elements examined directly by arthroscopy, or indirectly by MRI scan.

If there is no hard evidence to implicate any of the major soft tissue structures (and this is so in the *majority* of cases) a provisional (and rather unsatisfactory) diagnosis of 'knee sprain' or 'sprained ligaments with traumatic effusion' may be made, and the case treated appropriately (e.g. by the application of a crepe bandage support, Jones pressure bandage, or circular woven bandage (Tubigrip®)). The case should be re-assessed at weekly intervals thereafter until either the symptoms have settled completely, or a more accurate diagnosis can be established.

**99. Medial ligament injuries (1):** The commonest cause is a blow on the lateral side of the knee (1) which forces the joint into valgus (2). With slight force, there is partial tearing of the medial ligament (knee sprain) and the knee remains stable on clinical testing. With greater violence, the deep portion of the ligament ruptures (partial tear) (3); stressing the knee in 30° flexion with the foot internally rotated (F) causes more opening up of the joint than normal, but stressing the joint in extension (E) has no effect. There may be clinical evidence of rotatory instability. With greater violence, superficial *and* deep parts of the ligament rupture (4) and the tear rapidly spreads across the posterior ligament (5). The medial meniscus (6) may also tear. When the knee is stressed in extension (E) slight to moderate opening up will be noted, and if the edge of the ligament rolls over it may be felt subcutaneously (7). With severe violence, the cruciates (especially anterior cruciate) rupture (8) and the joint opens widely on stressing as at (E). Bruising on the lateral side (9) and medial tenderness (10) are suggestive of medial ligament damage. If there is remaining doubt regarding its integrity, repeat clinical tests after aspiration, or take stress radiographs, comparing one side with the other.

**100. Medial ligament injuries:**
**Treatment (1) Sprain:** Crepe bandages or a Jones pressure bandage should be applied and the patient given crutches to use until the acute symptoms have settled, when the knee may be fully mobilised.

**(2) Isolated tear**, with no evidence of 'rolling over' of the medial ligament: POP fixation *with the knee at 45° flexion* for 8 weeks, or the use of a limited motion knee brace.

**(3) Major tear:** If isolated and uncomplicated, conservative management should also be pursued, and a good result expected. If there is evidence of involvement of other structures, then operative repair should be carried out. If the anterior cruciate ligament has been detached or torn, an attempt should be made to re-attach or repair it. An associated meniscus injury should be carefully assessed and treated on its merits: the meniscus should be preserved if feasible, and in some cases it may be possible to re-attach it.

**Complications of medial ligament injury: (1) Late valgus instability:** It may be possible to improve stability by a reconstructive procedure; semitendinosus may be rerouted and used to reinforce a defective medial ligament, or a prosthetic ligament replacement may be carried out.

**(2) Persistent rotatory instability:** Improvement may follow a medial capsular repair and pes anserinus transposition, although the late results are often disappointing.

**101. Pelligrini–Stieda disease:** A valgus strain of the knee may produce partial avulsion of the medial ligament, with subsequent calcification in the subperiosteal haematoma. There is prolonged pain and local tenderness, with limitation of flexion, but no instability. In the acute phase, plaster, immobilisation for 2–3 weeks is advised, followed by mobilisation. Local hydrocortisone infiltrations are sometimes advocated for the chronic case.

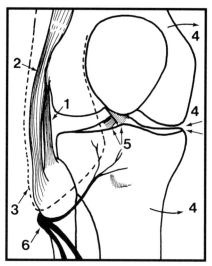

**102. Injuries to the lateral ligament (1):** The lateral ligament (1) is part of a complex which includes the biceps femoris tendon (2) and the fascia lata (3) attached to tibia, fibula and patella. All these structures may be damaged if the knee is subjected to a varus stress (4), and with severe violence the cruciates (5) will also be torn. The common peroneal nerve (6) may be stretched or torn.

**103. Lateral ligament (2):** Test the stability of the knee by applying a varus stress with the knee in extension (1), looking for opening-up of the joint on the lateral side (2). Test for common peroneal involvement by looking for weakness of dorsiflexion of the foot and toes (3), and/or sensory loss on the dorsum of the foot and side of the leg (4).

**104. Lateral ligament (3):** In some cases the radiographs may show tell-tale avulsion fractures of the fibular head or tibia. (Illus.: note a small undisplaced fracture of the head of the fibula, produced by the lateral ligament, and a large displaced fragment, indicated by a pointer, avulsed by the biceps.) *Treatment:* (a) If the knee is clinically stable, symptomatic treatment only is required (e.g. a crepe bandage and crutches).

**105. Lateral ligament (3)** *ctd: Treatment ctd:* (b) If there is instability, operative repair is indicated, unless there is a definite, undisplaced fracture which seems likely to go on to union; in such circumstances a plaster cylinder should be applied and retained for 6–8 weeks before mobilisation. (c) Common peroneal nerve palsy, if present, is likely to be due either to a lesion in continuity, or a complete disruption of the nerve over an extensive area. In neither case is exploration indicated for the neurological injury alone, although if the ligament is being repaired, the opportunity should be taken to inspect the nerve. In both cases treatment for drop foot should be started. With a lesion in continuity, recovery usually starts within 6 weeks, but a disruptive lesion carries a poor prognosis.

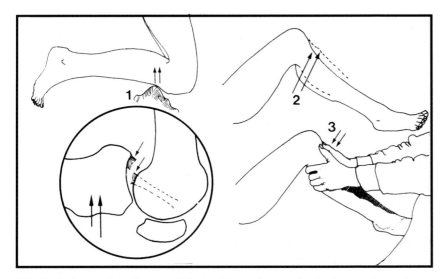

**106. Posterior cruciate ligament injuries:** The mechanism whereby the posterior cruciate ligament is damaged is usually either a fall, in which the tibia strikes a rock or some other object and is forced backwards (1) or from dashboard impact in road traffic accidents. There is often associated damage to the medial or lateral ligaments.

*Diagnosis:* (a) In most cases there is a striking alteration in the profile of the knee when placed in flexion: the tibia sags backwards (2) and this explains why the anterior drawer test (for the *anterior* cruciate ligament) often gives a false positive; the displaced tibia can be pulled forward to the normal position. (b) The posterior drawer sign may be positive (3). If there is remaining doubt, the knee should be aspirated and examined under anaesthetic.

**107. Posterior cruciate ligament injuries *ctd:* (c)** Radiographs may show avulsion fractures of the posterior cruciate ligament attachments.

*Treatment*: If untreated instability persists, disability is considerable, and osteo-arthritis often advances with great rapidity. (a) If there is an undisplaced fracture of the posterior tibial spine representing an avulsion of the posterior attachment of the ligament, the leg should be kept in a plaster cylinder for 6–8 weeks before mobilisation. (b) A displaced tibial spine fracture should be reduced and held with a screw. (c) A detached ligament should be re-attached to bone. As the majority of detachments are posterior, procedures (b) and (c) involve a posterior (popliteal) approach to the knee.

**108. Anterior cruciate ligament tears (1):** Isolated tears are uncommon (forced flexion or hyperextension injuries); tears of the medial ligament and/or medial meniscus may be associated.

*Diagnosis:* (1) Note variations in the anterior drawer sign: slight slip + internal rotation of the tibia (S + I) = isolated anterior cruciate tear; slight slip + external rotation (S + E) = medial ligament tear; marked slip without rotation (M) = tear anterior cruciate + medial ligament.

**109. Anterior cruciate ligament tears (2):** *Diagnosis:* (2) Carefully examine AP and lateral radiographs of the knee, looking for tell-tale avulsion fractures (Illus.: avulsion of the anterior attachment—the anterior tibial spine—indicated with pointer).
(3) Independently test the medial ligament, and look for evidence of meniscus injury. (4) Consider performing an arthroscopy to obtain unequivocal evidence of concurrent meniscal and cruciate ligament tears.

**110. Anterior cruciate ligament tears (3):** *Treatment:* (1) If the anterior tibial spine is undisplaced, treat with a 6–8 week period of fixation in a plaster cylinder. (2) If there is a substantial tibial spine fracture which is displaced, it should be carefully repositioned at open operation and fixed with a screw. (3) If the anterior attachment of the ligament is avulsed, it should be re-attached to bone at operation. (4) The results of surgical treatment of tears of the central portion of the anterior cruciate ligament are somewhat uncertain. In some cases, it may be possible to effect a direct repair, but generally the shredding and attenuation of the torn ends render this ineffective. An augmented repair (which seems to give the best results) or a secondary reconstruction may be possible, using for example: (a) a portion of the patellar ligament and part of the patella (used to anchor the end of the 'new' ligament); (b) part of iliotibial tract formed into a tube pedicle anchored with a block of bone; (c) a synthetic ligament replacement. (5) Associated tears of the medial meniscus and medial ligament take precedence in treatment. Any residual anteroposterior drift should be dealt with by intensive quadriceps building and the judicious use of a dynamic knee brace.

**111. Meniscus injuries:** In the young adult, the menisci are generally injured as a result of a rotational stress applied to the flexed, weight bearing knee (1). Injury can also result from rapid knee extension (anterior horn tears) and direct violence (cysts). The medial (M) and lateral (L) menisci are attached at their anterior and posterior horns to the tibia, and by coronary ligaments (C) to the femur and tibia. The majority of tears commence as vertical splits in the substance of the meniscus ('longitudinal tear') (2); the free edge may displace centrally, forming a bucket handle tear (3) or a racquet tear of the posterior (4) or anterior horns. The central edge may rupture forming a parrot-beak tear (5). In peripheral detachments the whole meniscus may displace centrally (6) or, more commonly, the posterior horn only of the lateral meniscus is affected (7). Congenital discoid menisci may also become detached (12) with ridging of their upper surfaces (11)—a common condition in children. Detachments of the anterior horn also occur, but are less common. A meniscus cyst (8) may result from a direct blow (such as a kick) and the lateral meniscus is most commonly affected. Cysts of the medial meniscus must be distinguished from pes anserinus ganglions. In middle age, horizontal tears may occur within the substance of the meniscus (9), sometimes without trauma, and may convert to tears with potential for displacement (10).

**112. Diagnosis of meniscus injuries: Note the following points:**

1. Acute tears in the young adult generally result from a clear-cut incident of weight-bearing stress, often while engaging in an athletic pursuit such as football. There is immediate pain in the knee and difficulty in weight bearing. Initial disability is usually marked, and if the patient has been playing football, he will be unable to continue. This important aspect of the history should be clarified.

2. Meniscus tears are very uncommon in women. Dislocation of the patella or chondromalacia patellae should always be eliminated before the diagnosis of a torn meniscus is contemplated in women.

3. Absence of knee swelling may be deceptive. After peripheral tears there is certainly usually a rapidly forming haemarthrosis but there may be no immediate swelling after longitudinal tears (the menisci are avascular). Any reactionary synovitis may appear quite late (e.g. several days) after the initial incident.

4. There is almost invariably joint-line tenderness, but as many minor lesions give this finding this is of little diagnostic value apart form localisation to either side of the joint.

5. A springy block to full extension is however almost diagnostic of a displaced, bucket-handle tear.

6. Some days after the first incident other signs may appear, such as quadriceps wasting and slight oedema in the joint line. When pain subsides, other confirmatory tests such as MacMurray's manoeuvre may give positive results.

7. Radiographs should always be taken to exclude other pathology.

8. In chronic lesions, positive physical signs are often lacking, and further investigation may be required (e.g. by arthroscopy, MRI scan, arthrography, provocative exercises).

**Treatment**

1. *Locked knee:* Admission at an early date for surgical treatment. Pending admission, a pressure bandage support, crutches, and analgesics may be prescribed. Attempts to unlock the knee are of questionable value.

2. *Case where the history and findings suggest a fresh meniscus tear:* Treat conservatively. Remember that peripheral detachments can unite, and that many joint injuries may mimic a torn meniscus yet recover completely. A pressure bandage should be applied, the patient given crutches and advised to practise quadriceps exercises. Analgesics may be required. If the knee fails to settle within 2 weeks, the usual practice is to perform a diagnostic arthroscopy followed by the procedure appropriate to the findings and available facilities. In general terms, the aim should be to preserve any part of the meniscus that can be made to make a contribution to the proper functioning of the knee (e.g. excision of the central portion only of a bucket handle tear, leaving an intact peripheral rim). In some circumstances re-attachment of a peripherally detached meniscus is feasible. In many cases it is possible to carry out the procedure required using the arthroscope and without opening the joint: this may make it possible to mobilise the patient at a very early stage, and may shorten the initial period of convalescence.

3. *Meniscus cysts:* Excise the cyst. In addition, many advocate removal of the associated meniscus which is not infrequently torn.

4. *Horizontal cleavage tears:* Symptoms may resolve with physiotherapy alone, and meniscectomy may frequently be avoided.

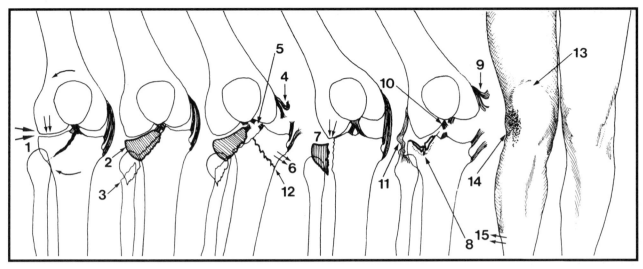

113. **Fractures of the lateral tibial table:**
These generally result from a severe valgus stress, and several patterns of injury are found.

(a) Impact of the mass of the lateral femoral condyle may be responsible for the 'sliding fracture' which passes downwards and laterally from the tibial spine region, the main articular surface remaining intact (1). With increasing violence the tibial fragment is depressed (2) and there may be an associated fracture of the fibular neck (3). In the severe cases there may be rupture of the medial ligament (4), rupture of the cruciates (5), and medial subluxation of the tibia (6). (b) The 'corner' of the lateral femoral condyle may cause a split fracture (7), or (c) a crush fracture (8) of the tibial table. In either of these cases there may be tearing of the medial ligament (9), or the cruciates (10), relative lengthening of the lateral ligament (11), or crushing of the lateral mensicus, (d) A second fracture line (12) may convert any of these injuries into a bicondylar fracture. (e) Fractures of the medial tibial table are uncommon, but do occur. They may be associated with lateral ligament ruptures and common peroneal nerve palsy. (Their treatment is along similiar lines to lateral tibial table injuries).

*Diagnosis:* (1) The clinical findings of lateral tibial table fracture include: haemarthrosis (13), lateral bruising and abrasions (14), valgus deformity of the knee (15).

114. **Diagnosis (2):** This is confirmed by radiographs, an AP view with a 15° tube tilt giving the most information. Measure the maximal depression of any fragment relative to neighbouring intact bone or a line projected from the (intact) medial table. If the medial ligament is suspect (e.g. local tenderness, etc.) stress films (preferably after aspiration and under GA) may be helpful. (Illus.: small split fracture with stress films showing medial ligament tear.) The tibial table may also be assessed by CAT scans.

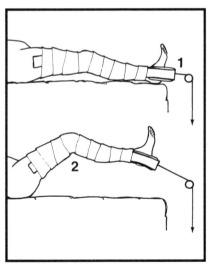

115. **Treatment (1):** *No ligament damage, no tibial subluxation, and a depression of less than 10 mm:* Apply skin traction of 3 kg (6–7 lb) (1); quadriceps exercises should be commenced immediately and flexion as soon as pain will permit (2). Traction may often be discontinued after 4 weeks; weight bearing may be permitted after 8 weeks. The late results are generally excellent.

116. **Treatment (2):** *Displaced unicondylar fractures (1):* These are included in Type B injuries of the proximal tibial segment: see 301, 123 for full details. If the displacement is more than 10 mm and is not reduced, there will be persistent valgus deformity of the knee, and often some residual instability leading to appreciable disability. Note in the illustration the large lateral fragment and the medial subluxation of the tibia of a degree suggesting medial ligament damage.

**117. Treatment (3):** These injuries should be treated by open reduction and internal fixation. When the fracture has been fixed, the medial ligament should be re-tested, and if found to be ruptured it should be repaired. It may also be possible to re-attach any displaced meniscus using absorbable sutures. (The radiograph shows the previous fracture after open reduction and internal fixation with a single cortical screw: it has gone on to union.)

**118. Treatment (4):** In some cases more stable fixation can be obtained using a cortical screw to lock the inferior margin of the lateral fragment (1), with one or more cancellous screws to obtain compression (2). If it is thought that the deforming forces are unlikely to be sufficiently countered by these measures, then a T- (3) or L-plate with the appropriate cortical and cancellous bone screws may be used.

**119. Treatment (5):** If the articular surface of the tibial plateau is depressed more than 10 mm, even in the absence of depression of the upper lateral tibial margin, the chances of obtaining a good result by conservative treatment becomes less likely. In assessing the indications for surgery, the extent and degree of depression of the lateral tibial plateau may be apparent on AP or lateral (Illus.) radiographic projections; further information on the bony disturbance may be obtained by CAT scans.

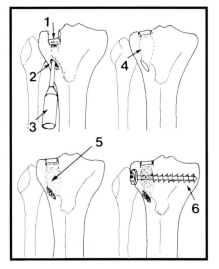

**120. Treatment (6):** It may be possible to elevate the bony depression (1) with its cartilaginous covering by making an opening (2) on the lateral tibial flare through which a narrow punch (3) may be inserted. Elevation of the depressed area inevitably leaves a defect (4) which should be tightly packed with bone grafts (5). It may be necessary to stabilise the elevated fragments with a cross screw (6). Thereafter the ligamentous structures should be tested and dealt with as required.

**121. Treatment (7):** Where there is depression of both the tibial margin (1) and the upper articular surface (2), reconstruction is technically more difficult. The steps in reconstruction that have been recommended are (i) reduction of the fracture and temporary fixation with Kirschner wires (3); (ii) packing the remaining defect (4) with bone grafts (5); (iii) supporting the fracture with a T- (6) or L-plate and the appropriate cancellous and cortical screws.

**122. Treatment (8): Bicondylar fractures (Type C):** If undisplaced, they may be treated conservatively by 6–8 weeks' traction (initially in a Thomas splint), mobilising as soon as the pain settles. If badly displaced (1), treat surgically along the lines indicated in the previous frame. Reduction may be greatly facilitated by the use of a distractor or external fixator (2), which may be retained (yet allow some movement) for 3–4 weeks if the quality of the fixation, even with plating, remains somewhat delicate.

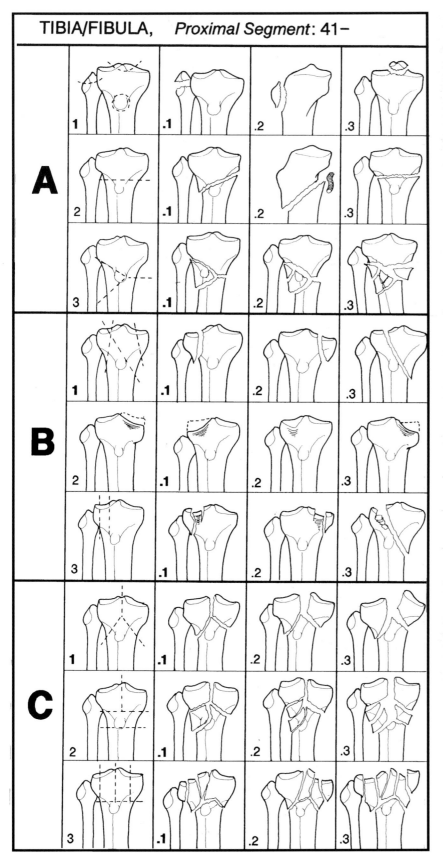

TIBIA/FIBULA,   *Proximal Segment*: 41–

### 123. AO Classification of Fractures of the Tibia/Fibula, Proximal Segment (41—):

**Type A** fractures are all extra-articular.

A1 = Avulsion fractures: .1 of the head of the fibula (lateral ligament); .2 of the tibial tuberosity (patellar ligament); .3 of the tibial spines (cruciate ligaments).

A2 = Simple metaphyseal fractures: .1 oblique from side to side; .2 oblique from posterior to anterior, often with vascular damage; .3 transverse.

A3 = Multifragmentary metaphyseal: .1 wedge intact; .2 fragmented wedge; .3 complex.

**Type B** fractures are partial articular.

B1 = Split fractures only: .1 lateral; .2 medial; .3 including the area of the tibial spines and one tibial table.

B2 = Depressed fractures only: .1 all of the lateral tibial table; .2 part only of the lateral tibial table; .3 part or all of the medial tibial table.

B3 = Combined split and depression: .1 lateral; .2 medial; .3 oblique, involving the tibial spines and one tibial table.

**Type C** fractures are complete articular.

C1 = Articular simple, metaphyseal simple: .1 minimal displacement; .2 one condyle displaced; .3 both condyles displaced.

C2 = Articular simple, metaphyseal multifragmentary: .1 intact wedge; .2 fragmented wedge; .3 complex.

C3 = Multifragmentary articular: .1 lateral; .2 medial; .3 both lateral and medial.

124. What is the level of fracture shown on these radiographs? How is it being treated? Is the position acceptable?

125. Describe the fracture and the method of treatment. Is the position acceptable?

126. (Above) Describe this fracture. What is the unusual feature about the deformity? How might it be treated conservatively?

127. (Right) What fractures are present? What treatment is obvious?

128. What does this radiograph show? How might this be dealt with?

129. What fracture is present? What treatment should be carried out?

130. What fracture is present? What treatment might be advised?

131. What fracture is shown on the radiograph? What complication has occurred, and what is its most likely cause? What would you advise?

132. What fracture is present? How has it been fixed?

133. What fracture is shown on the radiograph? How might this be treated?

134. Describe this fracture: how is it being treated? Assuming conservative treatment was being continued, would you make any correction?

135. What does the radiograph show? What structure is at serious risk?

136. What is this fracture? How has it been treated? What alternative treatment might have been carried out?

## Answers to self test

124. Proximal third fracture of the femur being treated in a Thomas splint. The proximal fragment is flexed so that there is no bony apposition, and probably soft tissue between the bone ends. The position is unacceptable (risk of non-union or mal-union) and internal fixation would be advocated. AO = 32–A3.1.

125. Oblique fracture of the midshaft of the femur (with shortening and angulation) in a child. It is being treated in a plaster hip spica. The position is acceptable: union is likely to be rapid; the shortening will almost certainly resolve spontaneously; any residual angulation is also likely to disappear with re-modelling. AO = 32–A2.2.

126. Supracondylar fracture of the femur. Angulation is slight, and is in the reverse direction from normal. Traction in a straight Thomas splint might be used and mobilisation commenced at an early date. Alternatively, this fracture might be dealt with by Hamilton–Russell traction and cast bracing or internal fixation with a blade plate, a dynamic condylar screw or an intramedullary nail with interlocking screws. AO = 33–A1.2.

127. There is a fracture of the midshaft of the femur and a supracondylar fracture, both held in alignment with an intramedullary nail. In addition, there is a fracture of the proximal third of the tibia. Such injuries are typical of high-velocity road traffic accidents. AO = 32–B1.2 + (33–A2.3 or 32–B2.3) + 41–A3.

128. Fracture of the femoral shaft at the level of the tip of a replacement arthroplasty prosthesis (Type 3 fracture). Treat by open reduction and internal fixation, e.g. with a plate screwed to the greater trochanter and shaft, or by a Mennen plate or Partridge plates and cerclage straps.

129. Displaced, intra-articular fracture of the medial femoral condyle. Treat by open reduction and internal fixation with counter-sunk cancellous bone screws; otherwise non-union is likely even if reduction is achieved. Avascular necrosis of the fragment is probable. AO = 33–B2.2.

130. Highly comminuted fracture of the distal third of the femur, with a fracture extending between the femoral condyles. Surgical reconstruction is likely to prove impossible due to the degree of comminution, and conservation management with traction and early mobilisation is likely to yield the best result. However, in the elderly patient primary joint replacement should be considered. AO = 33–C3.3.

131. Fracture of the midshaft of the femur, treated by intramedullary nailing. Union is incomplete and the nail has bent, with angulation of the femur because of premature weight bearing. The nail should be removed without delay, and a new nail substituted after reaming. Removal of the nail will obviously be difficult. It may be possible to straighten the

bend by forcible manipulation, but if this fails it may be necessary to expose the fracture, saw through the nail and extract the two fragments separately. AO = 32–A3.2.

132. Supracondylar fracture of the femur supported with a one-piece blade plate and screws. AO = 32–A3.3.

133. Highly comminuted fracture of the distal portion of the patella, with retraction of the main fragment. The proportion of the patellar surface involved and the degree of comminution militates against preservation, and excision, with repair of the ruptured lateral expansions would probably be the best procedure here.

134. Fracture of the femoral shaft at the junction between the middle and distal thirds. It is being treated in a Thomas splint. Traction should be increased, and further padding placed under the fracture to correct the angulation. AO = 32–A2.2.

135. Dislocation of the knee (posterior dislocation with 90° rotational deformity superimposed). The popliteal artery is in grave danger.

136. A transverse fracture has been anatomically reduced and held with a single cortical screw. This fracture could also have been held by tension band wiring (e.g. with Kirschner wires, or by Pyrford wiring).

# 13. Fractures of the tibia

1. **General principles (1): Mechanisms of injury:** The tibia is vulnerable to torsional stresses (1) (e.g. sporting injuries), to violence transmitted through the feet (2) (e.g. falls from a height, road traffic accidents), and from direct blows (3) (e.g. road traffic accidents, blows from falling rock, masonry, etc.).

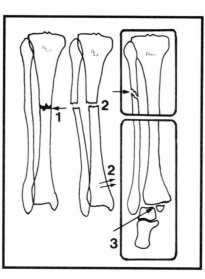

2. **General principles (2):** Isolated fractures of either the tibia or fibula may occur from direct violence (1) although this is comparatively uncommon. As in the case of the forearm bones, indirect violence leads to fracture of both tibia and fibula (2). Always obtain radiographs of the whole length of the limb to exclude a distal injury accompanying a proximal fracture (3).

3. **General principles (3):** Note that a third of the tibia is subcutaneous. There is little to resist the spiky end of a fractured tibia from penetrating the skin; again, any direct violence to the shin is uncushioned, and the skin is readily split; these factors account for the fact that tibial fractures are often open (either from within out or from without in).

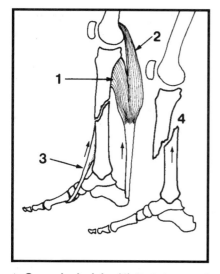

4. **General principles (4):** Partly because of its triangular shape, and partly because of the frequency of injury caused by torsional forces, oblique and spiral fractures of the tibia are common. Muscle tone in the soleus (1), gastrocnemius (2) and tibialis anterior (3) tends to produce shortening and displacement in fractures of this type (4).

5. **General principles (5):** The popliteal artery (1) is anchored as it passes under the origin of the soleus at the soleal line (2). It is susceptible to damage in upper tibial fractures (3) and may cause Volkmann's ischaemia of the calf with permanent flexion contracture of the ankle. Fractures of the tibia may be followed by ischaemia of the distal fragment (4) through interruption of the blood supply through the nutrient artery (5).

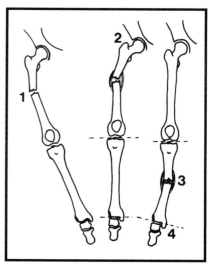

6. **General principles (6):** It is particularly important to correct angulation in fractures of this weight-bearing bone. Unlike angulation in femoral shaft fractures (1), which can be compensated at the hip (2), residual angulation in tibial fractures (3) will throw inevitable stress at the ankle (4) and/or the knee, perhaps leading to pain and secondary osteo-arthritis.

7. **Undisplaced fractures (1):** In children, owing to the thickness of the subcutaneous fat and periosteum, and the elasticity of the bones, fractures are often of greenstick pattern and simple. In many cases, too, the fractures are minimally displaced. (Illus.: Greenstick fracture distal tibia and fibula, betrayed by fibular kinking and tibial cortical buckling.)

8. **Undisplaced fractures (2):** When deformity is minimal, apply a long leg plaster immediately over a generous layer of wool (1) (mild sedation only may be required). A sandbag under the buttocks (2) may be helpful, while an assistant holds the toes (3) and supports the calf (4). The knee is slightly flexed (5) and the plaster may be applied in one stage with or without a slab (6).

9. **Undisplaced fractures (3):** Elevation of the leg and a regular, careful check of the circulation is essential, and admission for this is desirable. In a child, non-weight-bearing with crutches can usually be allowed as soon as there is no circulatory risk (say 2–3 days post injury).
Thereafter the child should be seen every 2–3 weeks (the casualty rate in children's plasters is high).

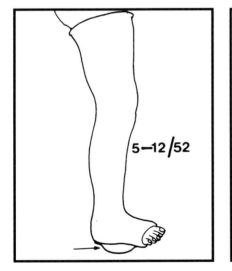

10. **Undisplaced fractures (4):** A walking heel can certainly be applied when there is evidence of early callus on the radiographs (e.g. after 3–4 weeks in a child of 9 years). Before that a heel may be applied if in your assessment there is no risk of displacement or problems from swelling. Any hesitation may sometimes be dispelled by the appearance of the sole of the plaster which often indicates premature successful weight bearing!

11. **Undisplaced fractures (5):** The fracture may be assessed for union after say 4–5 weeks in a child of 4 years, 8 weeks in a child of 8, and 8–12 weeks in a child of 12. On removal of the plaster no support for the limb is usually required, but confidence may be raised by a crepe bandage. Crutches for the first few days are advocated as the child often shows timidity in commencing weight bearing: and the parents may require reassurance.

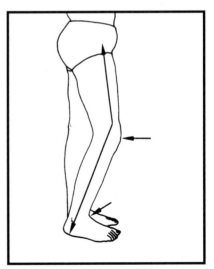

12. **Undisplaced fractures (6):** The child should be reviewed 2 weeks after removal of the plaster. In most cases he will be walking unsupported, the movements in the knee and ankle will have returned, and the limb lengths will be equal. The child may then be discharged. The parents should be reassured that any residual limp will resolve, and that athletic activities may be resumed say in a further 2 months.

**13. Angled fractures in children (1):**
These are reduced under general anaesthesia. One hand is placed over the fracture site (1) while the other, at the ankle (2), is used to correct the angulation. Although the AP plane only is illustrated, naturally any deformity in the lateral plane should be similarly corrected.

**14. Angled fractures (2):** The pressure of the hand at the ankle should be released, and any tendency for the deformity to recur noted (indicating springy intact periosteum). If this is found, particular care must be taken during the application of the plaster to maintain full correction; alternatively, complete tearing of the periosteum may be obtained by over correction of the deformity.

**15. Angled fractures (3):** If there is little tendency to recurrence of angulation, the plaster may be applied as follows: wool roll is wound round the limb from toes to groin (1); one assistant supports the fracture and the toes (2) while the second takes the weight of the thigh (3). The knee is flexed to 15° (4) and the ankle maintained at right angles (5). The supporting hands are moved during the application of the plaster (6). Use a sandbag under the buttocks.

**16. Angled fractures (4):** If there is a tendency to re-angulation, the plaster must be moulded while it sets. Except in the smallest of children it is difficult to apply a full length plaster and mould the fracture within the setting time. A two-stage technique may be used; *either* apply a below knee plaster (1), mould and complete the thigh (2), *or* apply the thigh cuff first (3), complete the plaster (4) and then mould.

**17. Displaced fractures of the tibia (1):**
An assistant applies strong traction in the line of the limb (1) while strong pressure is applied with the heels of the hands above (2) and below (3) the fracture to correct the displacement. The traction is then slackened off to allow the bone ends to engage.

**18. Displaced fractures of the tibia (2):**
Checking the reduction clinically can be difficult. Try palpating the fracture line along the subcutaneous border (1) or in the case of a transverse fracture confirm that a hitch is present by noting resistance to attempted telescoping (2).

**19. Displaced fractures of the tibia (3):**
If the reduction obtained by manipulation is somewhat precarious and it is feared that the fracture might slip during the application of plaster, place the limb on a firm plaster pillow (1), steady the leg by holding the toes (2) and apply a thick, anterior, plaster slab (3) tucking the edges well round the limb. When it has set, the leg can then be carefully bandaged into the slab.

**20. Wedging (1):** Ultimately, if necessitated by circumstance, displacement and even off-ending may be accepted in children. If, however, the radiographs indicate residual angulation, this should be corrected, and this may usually be done by wedging. Begin by marking the plaster circumferentially at the level of the fracture (1) using the radiographs as a guide (2).

**21. Wedging (2):** Now carefully work out where the plaster must hinge to correct the deformity. For example, where there is medial angulation (1) and the lateral projection is normal (2), the hinge should lie medially (3). Where there is lateral angulation (4) along with posterior angulation (5) the hinge should be positioned posterolaterally (6).

**22. Wedging (3):** Cut through 7/8 of the circumference of the plaster at the marked level, sparing the hinge; use a plaster saw or a hacksaw with a fine blade. Now spring the plaster 1–2 cm open; maintain the position temporarily by placing a suitably sized piece of previously prepared cork into the mouth of the wedge.

**23. Wedging (4):** Check radiographs should be taken, and any adjustment made on the result. If a satisfactory correction has been obtained, wool should be packed lightly into the gap on either side of the cork, and the plaster reconstituted locally with a 15 cm (6″) plaster bandage.

(Illus.: A badly angled fracture in the distal third of the tibia has been corrected by wedging. Although the level of the wedge is more distal than it should be, an almost anatomical position has been achieved.) General anaesthesia is not required for wedging, but mild sedation is desirable. After care should follow the lines described for undisplaced fractures (307, 9–12).

**24. Tibial fractures in the adult (1):** In the adult many tibial fractures may be treated conservatively, and where good results with few complications are the rule it is unwise to advocate surgery with its additional risks. Conservative treatment may with good reason always be advised for stress, isolated (Illus.) and undisplaced fractures, and for slightly displaced stable fractures.

**25. Minimally displaced fractures is the adult (2):** A long leg plaster is applied, check radiographs are taken, and the limb elevated (1) for 3–7 days until swelling subsides. The plaster is checked for slackness and changed if required. As soon as the patient has mastered crutches he may be allowed home (2). A walking heel is applied (3) usually after 3–6 weeks (depending on your assessment of stability) and the plaster retained till union.

**26. Sarmiento plaster (1):** Alternatively, at 4–6 weeks post injury, the long leg plaster is removed and a Sarmiento cast applied. The patient sits on the edge of the plaster table (1), the foot being steadied by the lap of the operator. Stockingette (2) and wool roll are applied, and the plaster extended over the knee (3). It is firmly moulded (before setting) round the patellar ligament (4).

**27. Sarmiento plaster (2):** The plaster is then trimmed from the upper pole of the patella (5) round to the upper part of the calf (6); check that knee movement is free before turning down the stockingette and finishing in the usual way. A rocker sole may then be applied (7) and weight bearing and knee flexion commenced. The plaster is retained until union is sound.

**28. Functional bracing with a gaiter:** In the later stages of fixation, or even as early as 4 weeks when instability is not a problem, a supporting gaiter may be used instead of plaster. The type illustrated may be fashioned from perforated Orthoplast® (Johnson & Johnson) thermoplastic sheet (1). For additional support a plastic heel seat (2) may be secured to the brace with polyethylene hinges (3) and a garter strap (4).

**29. After care:** (1) Intervals between hospital attendances should not exceed 4 weeks, and the fixation—plaster or brace—changed if it becomes unduly slack. (2) Tibial fractures take an average 16 weeks to unite, but union may be sought in 8—12 weeks in the case of a hairline crack, and after 12 weeks in a transverse fracture. Radiographs should be taken (Illus. advanced union in tibial fracture) preferably out of plaster.

30. **After care *ctd:*** (3) Apparent radiological union should be confirmed by clinical examination. (4) If union is judged sound a crepe bandage support is prescribed for the leg and knee, and full unsupported weight bearing commenced. Sticks or crutches may be required to give confidence over the first few weeks, but the patient should be encouraged to discard these as soon as possible (although the elderly patient may have difficulty in this respect). (5) The patient should be reviewed 2 weeks after plaster has been discarded. The following problems may be encountered:

(a) *The knee: pain or discomfort* in the knee at the beginning of mobilisation is normal. A small to moderate *effusion* is common. If the period of immobilisation is under 16 weeks, return of flexion is usually rapid.

Physiotherapy is nevertheless advisable in the majority of cases to encourage knee flexion, to develop the quadriceps and to help restore the gait to normal.

(b) *The ankle: Slight swelling and oedema* of the foot and ankle are usual for several months after tibial fractures. A crepe bandage or circular woven support is advised until this swelling subsides. Gross swelling with marked stiffness and pain in the foot and ankle should suggest Sudeck's atrophy. Swelling which is maximal over the fracture calls for re-assessment of union. Slight *restriction of ankle movements* is common after tibial fractures, but is seldom incapacitating.

(c) *Athletic activities:* Swimming may be permitted almost as soon as the plaster has been discarded, and should be encouraged. *Cycling* can be allowed as soon as knee flexion will allow (*c.* 110°). Golf may be allowed as soon as limb swelling is no longer a problem. *Rugby, football and gymnastics* should not be permitted until endosteal callus is sound, till knee flexion is nearly normal (say 130°) and muscle power is restored.

(d) *Return to work:* The patient should be encouraged to return to work as soon as possible, and in sedentary work the patient may do so while in plaster. Factors which may delay return are: (a) severe persistent oedema in jobs involving prolonged standing; (b) lack of knee flexion in work involving kneeling; (c) muscle and functional weakness in jobs involving work at heights.

31. **Displaced but potentially stable fractures in the adult:** Transverse fractures of the tibia in particular are potentially stable if good bony apposition can be obtained. While the tendency is to treat injuries of this pattern by closed intramedullary nailing, they may also be dealt with conservatively along the lines already described, reserving surgery for those cases where a satisfactory reduction cannot be achieved.

32. **Reduction techniques:** (a) The fracture may be manipulated as already described for the child (308, 17). (b) It is often helpful, especially if assistance is limited, to let gravity work to your advantage. The patient's knee is flexed over the end of the table (1). Use your own knees to steady or to apply traction to the foot (2). Both hands are free to manipulate the fracture (3).

33. **Reduction techniques *ctd:*** (c) Alternatively, it is sometimes possible to apply temporary traction using skin traction tapes (1). The traction may be controlled by the operator's foot on the spreader bar (2) and by elevating the table (3). After manipulation a padded plaster is applied over the tapes from the heel to the knee (4). The tapes are cut, and the foot of the plaster completed.

**34. Reduction techniques** *ctd:* Once the leg and foot have been encased in plaster in methods (b) and (c), the knee is gently extended to 15°, wool applied to the thigh, and the thigh cuff completed with 20 cm (8″) plaster bandages. Check radiographs are desirable on completion of the below-knee portion of the plaster, and after the thigh cuff has been added.

**35. Reduction techniques** *ctd:* If manipulation succeeds in bringing the bone ends into apposition, any residual angulation may be corrected within the first few weeks by wedging. (Illus.: Postmanipulation radiograph of the previous fracture (311, 31). There is an unacceptable degree of angulation although good apposition has been obtained. The angulation was easily corrected by wedging and union proceeded uneventfully.)

**36. Unstable fractures with minimal displacement:** Oblique and spiral fractures are potentially unstable. Although they may be managed conservatively along the lines indicated, meticulous supervision is necessary during the first 6 weeks. Slackness in the plaster must be promptly dealt with. Slight slipping of the fracture may be accepted, but if evidence of substantial displacement is found, internal fixation should be considered.

**37. Displaced unstable fractures: Closed intramedullary nailing (1):** Fractures which are unstable because of their pattern may be treated by manipulation to the best position that can be obtained, and by controlling angulation by wedging. Nevertheless this method of treatment requires much experienced supervision: shortening is inevitable, union may be delayed, and stiffness in the knee and ankle may become a problem. For the majority of fractures under normal circumstances closed intramedullary nailing (with interlocking nails) is the treatment of choice.

**Method (1):** The operation is performed as soon as the patient's condition will allow, and prophylactic antibiotic cover is frequently advocated. The fracture must be amenable to reduction by traction, but in practice this is seldom a problem. (If reduction cannot be achieved, the fracture must be exposed and openly reduced; thereafter it may be fixed by nailing or some other procedure.) Traction may be effected by a Steinman pin through the heel. (A plastic boot may be used instead, but its size will prevent the insertion of any distal locking screws.)

**38. Closed intramedullary nailing (2):** The leg must be positioned so that traction can be applied while providing surgical and image intensifier access. The knee should be flexed, and the other leg supported clear of the field (e.g. by lithotomy straps). Care must be taken to avoid undue pressure on the popliteal structures. All this may be achieved in a number of ways on an orthopaedic table, but the use of a Watson–Jones frame (Illus.) after removal of the table end-piece gives particularly good access.

39. **Closed nailing (3):** After checking the reduction, a 7.5 cm transverse incision is made between the level of the knee joint and the tibial tuberosity (1). An awl (2) is then used to locate and enter the medullary canal under the medial edge of the patellar ligament and 1 cm distal to the knee joint (which is not opened). A curved hand reamer may be used to open up the track in the proximal fragment before passing a reaming rod (3) across the fracture into the distal segment under intensifier control.

40. **Closed nailing (4):** The medullary canal may then be opened out with flexible powered reamers (1) of increasing size until the chosen nail will be a good fit in both main fragments. The reaming rod is then replaced with a guide wire (2) and the intramedullary nail inserted (3). (Grosse–Kempf (and other) tibial nails are angled (4) to accommodate the anterior access point. The length chosen should be 4 cm less than the distance between the tip of the medial malleolus and the joint line of the sound leg (5).)

41. **Closed nailing (5):** The nail should be driven well home to lessen the risks of persisting knee pain. The position for the insertion of proximal locking screws (1) may be determined by use of the insertion handle (2) which doubles as a jig. Due to the cumulative errors caused by nail flexibility and lost motion distal locating jigs are not very successful, and the holes in the nail for distal locking screws (3) are generally best located free-hand using the image intensifier.

42. **Closed nailing (6): After care:** Mobilisation of the knee and ankle may be commenced immediately, and as a result complete recovery of movements in these joints is the rule. As regards weight bearing, advice on when this should be permitted is dependent on the nature of the fracture and the quality of fixation. Absence of pain at the fracture site on weight bearing has been said to be a valuable guide as to when full unsupported weight may be taken through the limb. The fracture should be followed up until soundly united, when a decision, based on the usual criteria, should be made regarding removal of the fixation device. Return to work and athletic activities follows along the lines discussed in 311, 30. *Complications: Knee pain* occurs in about 40% of cases, and generally settles on removal of the nail. *Delayed union* may be treated by converting from static to dynamic fixation by removal of the appropriate locking screws, sometimes with an osteotomy of the fibula if it has united. *Hypertrophic non-union* may be dealt with by exchange nailing (removal of the existing nail, re-reaming to a greater diameter, and using a larger nail). *Infection* is uncommon, and should be dealt with along the usual lines, preferably retaining the nail until union has occurred. *Compartment syndromes* are also uncommon, but occasionally required decompression.

43. **Alternative methods of treatment (1):** Many tibial fractures are amenable to treatment by plating; a well-contoured dynamic compression plate can often provide a high quality of rigid internal fixation, and butterfly and other separate fragments may be secured with interfragmentary screws. Image intensification and the use of an orthopaedic table are of course not required. Plating may be used (with bone grafting) to deal with non-union in fractures which have been previously treated by conservative methods.

44. **Alternative methods of treatment (2):** External fixators are of particular value in open fractures. Good support is provided with 2–3 threaded cantilever pins on each side of the fracture, with a rigid connector which can give axial compression. The most rigid systems use a total of 12 pins, inserted in pairs at right angles to one another, with two linking bars. At the other end of the scale, tibial length may be preserved in conservatively treated fractures with two Steinman pins incorporated in the plaster.

**45. Special situations (1): Double (segmental) fractures:** Plaster fixation gives poor support, and the incidence of-non-union at one level in fractures treated this way is high. (Nevertheless, if this occurs, and if alignment is satisfactory, success may follow internal fixation and grafting.) The most useful primary treatment is *closed* intramedullary nailing with the insertion of proximal and distal locking screws. *Open reduction* and plating carries the risk of further devitalisation of the intermediate segment.

**46. Special situations (2): Gross fragmentation:** Where the bone is highly fragmented (as may occur in high energy dissipation situations) the multiplicity of small, detached avascular bone fragments will prevent any meaningful reduction. Alignment should be restored by manipulation; thereafter length and position may be maintained by Steinman pins incorporated in a plaster cast or by the use of an external fixator. Although generally undesirable, it may be necessary to bridge the knee (see 300, 122).

**47. Special situations (3): Fractures of the distal shaft:** Many of these fractures can be treated conservatively by reduction and plaster fixation, with or without a Steinman pin through the heel to help maintain alignment. Some permanent restriction of ankle joint movements is common. Alternatively, some can be internally fixed so that early movements can be permitted (e.g. by using a buttress plate with proximal cortical and distal cancellous screws).

**48. Special situations (4): Isolated fractures of the fibula:** The fibula may be fractured by direct violence; symptomatic treatment only is required (e.g. a below-knee walking plaster for 6 weeks). Always ensure, however, that the tibia is not fractured at another level, or that the fibular fracture represents part of a more complex injury to the ankle joint.

**49. Special situations (5): Open fractures:** The frequency with which fractures of the tibia are found to be open, and the reasons for this have been given at the beginning of this section. The AO and Gustilo classifications of open fractures, and the general principles of treatment are dealt with separately in Chapter 4.

It does no harm to restate that primary closure of the skin is generally to be avoided (although good results have been claimed in children where contamination has been minimal); in the absence of established infection, small wounds close spontaneously; larger wounds should only be dealt with by secondary suture if this can be performed without tension; and granulating surfaces may readily be covered by split skin grafts.

The importance of the thoroughness of initial and subsequent debridements has been stressed, along with the necessity of obtaining early soft-tissue cover of bone; a number of plastic surgical techniques to this end have been described.

There has been much controversy over the use of internal fixation in the treatment of open fractures, but in many cases the fears expressed of increasing the risks of infection have been shown to be unjustified. In open fractures of Types 1 & 2 (Gustilo) the infection rate following intramedullary nailing using the closed technique has been shown to be low and no greater than in closed injuries of a similar pattern.

In Grade 3 open fracture it has been suggested that reaming of the medullary cavity is undesirable, and for this reason the AO Group recommend the use in these circumstances of a solid intramedullary nail. This pattern of nail is angled and of sufficiently small profile to allow it to negotiate most tibiae without any reaming. Others have shown that in the majority of Grade 3 open fractures that the results of nailing (with the use of locking screws) after reaming are comparable in terms of infection with those obtained when external fixators have been employed; and that they are better in terms of joint stiffness, mal-union, access for plastic reconstructions, and patient preference. Nevertheless, where there has been gross tissue contamination, many would still prefer to use external fixation or where applicable, simple plaster cast support until the situation regarding wound infection has been resolved. Note the following:
1. If there is a pin track infection following the use of an external fixator reaming of the medullary canal is contraindicated; reaming carries the almost certain risk of disseminating infection throughout the bone.
2. If there is a bone defect involving more than 50% of the circumference of the bone, and more than 2 cm long, then bone grafting will ultimately be required in all cases; where the bone defect is smaller, healing may occur without grafting.

**50. AO Classification of Fractures of the Tibia/Fibula, Diaphyseal Segment (42–):**

**Type A** fractures are simple fractures.

A1 = Spiral: .1 fibula intact; .2 fibula fractured at another level; .3 fibula fractured at the same level.

A2 = Oblique fracture (30° or more): .1 fibula intact; .2 fibula fractured at another level; .3 fibula fractured at the same level.

A3 = Transverse fracture (less than 30° of obliquity): .1 fibula intact; .2 fibula fractured at another level; .3 fibula fractured at the same level.

**Type B** fractures are wedge fractures.

B1 = Spiral: .1 fibula intact; .2 fibula fractured at another level; .3 fibula fractured at the same level.

B2 = Bending wedge fracture: .1 fibula intact; .2 fibula fractured at another level; .3 fibula fractured at the same level.

B3 = Fragmented wedge: .1 fibula intact; fibula fractured at another level; .3 fibula fractured at the same level.

**Type C** fractures are complex fractures.

C1 = Spiral: .1 with two intermediate fragments; .2 with three intermediate fragments; .3 with more than three intermediate fragments.

C2 = Segmental: .1 with one intermediate segment; .2 with an intermediate segment and additional wedge; .3 with two intermediate segments.

C3 = Irregular: .1 with two or three intermediate fragments; .2 with shattering over a length.of less than 4 cm; .3 with shattering over a length of 4 cm or more.

51. What complication has occurred in this uniting fracture of the tibia in the distal third?

52. What pattern of fracture is present? How is it being treated?

53. What complication is present in this united tibial fracture? What effect will this have?

54. What type of fracture is present, and how has it been dealt with?

55. What complication is shown in this radiograph of a tibial fracture?

56. These radiographs were taken through plaster 10 weeks after injury. Describe the fracture. What further treatment would you advocate? What is the prognosis?

51. The radiograph shows the disturbance of bone trabeculation typical of Sudeck's atrophy.

52. This shows a spiral fracture of the tibia at the junction of the mid and distal thirds being treated in plaster. The position in this *single* view appears excellent. AO = 42–A1.1.

53. Mal-union of the fracture is present with lateral angulation. The plane of the ankle joint is affected, and degenerative arthritis in it is possible.

54. There are fractures of the shafts of both the tibia and fibula at the level of the junction of their middle and distal thirds; in each there is a separate wedge (or butterfly) fragment. The tibial fracture has been held in alignment with a plate (of Eggar pattern) and screws. AO = 42–B1.3.

55. Hypertrophic non-union is present. AO = 42–A3.1.

56. The radiographs are of an oblique fracture of the tibia in the middle third, with an associated fibular fracture at the junction of the middle and lower thirds. Both fractures are uniting, and bridging callus is well formed. The general alignment is good. No correction is required: the patient will require to continue with fixation for about another 4 weeks before plaster can be discarded (or a cast brace may be substituted). There will be approximately 1 cm of shortening, but the functional prognosis is excellent. AO = 42–A2.2.

# 14.  Injuries about the ankle

1. **Anatomical considerations (1):** The ankle joint is often fairly compared with the mortise and tenon joint of the woodworker. The talus (1) resembles the tenon (T), and is supported by the two malleoli and the articular surface of the tibia (the ankle mortise).

The lateral malleolus is firmly attached to the tibia by the strong anterior and posterior tibiofibular ligaments (2).

2. **Anatomical considerations (2):** The talus is held in the mortise on the medial side by the very strong deltoid ligament (1), and on the lateral side by the lateral (external) ligament (2).

The anterior part of the upper articular surface of the talus is wider than the posterior part (3). When the foot is dorsiflexed, the talus pushes the fibula laterally (4) and is more firmly gripped in the ankle mortise.

3. **Mechanics of injury (1):** The *function* of the ankle mortise is threatened if the malleoli are fractured or the tibiofibular ligaments are torn. The *stability* of the talus may also be reduced by rupture of the medial or lateral ligaments. The commonest injury is when the talus is rotated in the mortise, fracturing one or both malleoli.

4. **Mechanics of injury (2):** External rotation of the talus may be produced in two different ways: (a) The foot may act as a long lever; any rotational force applied to the inside of the foot is transferred to the talus with a mechanical advantage as in any system of levers. Even greater leverage may occur if, for example, the foot is attached to a ski.

5. **Mechanics of injury (3):** (b) The axis of movement of the subtalar joint is known to run obliquely in the direction of the crease on this paper model (1).

Inversion of the heel, represented by folding the paper, results in external rotation of the talus (2) (Rose's torque-converter principle). A common history is of the ankle 'coggling over' on uneven ground.

6. **Mechanics of injury (4):** The talus may be forced into relatively pure adduction as, for example, when the side of the inverted foot strikes the ground heavily. (The external rotation of the talus, produced by inversion of the calcaneus, being countered by the internal rotation of the strike, resulting in net adduction.)

**7. Mechanics of injury (5):** Similarly, if force is applied to the medial side of the heel and foot, the talus will tend to abduct in the ankle mortise.

**8. Mechanics of injury (6):** Many injuries occur during the course of walking or running. Under these circumstances there are additional forces transmitted to the posterior part of the inferior articular surface of the tibia (posterior malleolus).

**9. Mechanics of injury (7):** Compression injuries may be caused by: (1) falls from a height, forces being transmitted vertically from heel impact, or (2) following rapid deceleration in car accidents—sometimes aggravated by the pedals being driven into the front compartment and the ankle being forcibly dorsiflexed. Comminution is a feature of this type of injury.

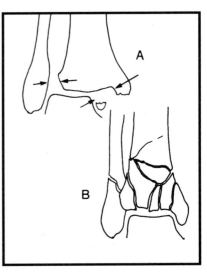

**10. Classification of ankle fractures (1):** There are several classifications of ankle fractures; for completeness (which none achieve) many are complex to a degree that makes commital to memory nigh impossible. Fractures involving the ankle joint are often loosely referred to as Pott's fractures; although the term is now somewhat archaic, there is some merit in its simplicity: in first degree Pott's fractures, one malleolus is fractured (1): in second degree Pott's fractures, two malleoli are fractured (bimalleolar fracture) (2).

**11. Classification of ankle fractures (2):** In third degree Pott's fracture (3) there is a bimalleolar fracture with in addition a fracture of the posterior part of the inferior articular surface of the tibia—often referred to as the third malleolus. These fractures may also be referred to as trimalleolar fractures.

**12. Classification of ankle fractures (3):** These fractures may be qualified by noting the presence of diastasis of the ankle or vertical compression.
(A) First degree Pott's fracture with diastasis.
(B) Second degree Pott's fracture with vertical compression.

**Classification of ankle fractures.** A fuller and widely accepted classification of ankle fractures is that of Lauge–Hansen which groups these fractures under double-barrelled headings. The first word in each group title refers to the position of the foot at the time of injury; the second refers to the direction in which the talus moves within the ankle mortise in response to the causal forces. There are five main groups; they have been arranged here in order of frequency and a common terminology of usage has been included.

| Order of frequency | Lauge–Hansen classification | Lauge–Hansen contraction | Position of foot | Direction of talar movement | **Common terminology** |
| --- | --- | --- | --- | --- | --- |
| 1 | Supination/lateral rotation | SL | Inversion | Lateral (external) rotation | External rotation injury without diastasis |
| 2 | Pronation/abduction | PA | Eversion | Abduction | Abduction injury |
| 3 | Pronation/lateral rotation | PL | Eversion | Lateral (external) rotation | External rotation injury with diastasis |
| 4 | Supination/adduction | SA | Inversion | Adduction | Adduction injury |
| 5 | Pronation/dorsiflexion | PD | Eversion | Dorsiflexion | Vertical compression injury |

*In the AO Classification* an initial distinction is made between fractures of the tibia/fibula, distal segment (43–) and fractures of tibia/fibula, malleolar segment (44–). On occasion there may be some difficulty in making a decision as to which of these two segments to assign a particular fracture. Note that the AO Classification of the malleolar segment does include complete tears of the lateral ligament of the ankle without any accompanying fracture. For full details of the AO Classification of both segments see the end of this section (339, 99 and 340, 100).

**13. Supination/lateral rotation injuries _(external rotation injury without diastasis)_ (1):** The foot inverts (1). Due to the torque-converter principle, the talus rotates laterally in the ankle mortise (2). The ankle joint structures are thrown under stress and fail in a regular sequence. As each structure fails, the next is stressed. The number of structures involved is dependent on the magnitude of the forces applied to the joint.

**14. Supination/lateral rotation injuries (2):** The rotating talus carries the fibula with it, leading first to rupture of the anterior (inferior) tibiofibular ligament (1). Alternatively, the ligament under stress may avulse its tibial attachment (T) (Tillaux fracture).

**15. Supination/lateral rotation injuries (3):** As external rotation continues, the fibula fractures in an oblique or spiral fashion (2). Note the direction of the spiral.

If displacement continues, the fibular fragment drags off the posterior malleolar fragment (3) to which it is attached by the posterior tibiofibular ligament (or the ligament tears).

**16. Supination/lateral rotation injuries (4):** If rotation continues, the fourth structure to fail is the medial ligament or its attachment (the medial malleolus) (4). Such injuries are potentially very unstable and should be carefully distinguished from Stage 1 and 2 lesions.

**17. Radiographs (1):** A spiral fracture of the fibula at the level shown is typical of an S/L injury: in the lateral radiograph the fracture runs downwards and forwards, and there was no evidence of a posterior malleolar fracture. Although there is very slight incongruity between the upper surfaces of the talus and the ankle mortise, absence of tenderness on the medial side of the ankle suggested this was a Stage 2 or 3 injury.

**18. Radiographs (2):** The avulsion fracture of the medial malleolus indicates that this is a stage 4 S/L injury. There is lateral shift of the talus in the ankle mortise but the main mass of the fibula maintains its relationship with the tibia, so there is no true diastasis. Nevertheless, this is a very unstable injury.

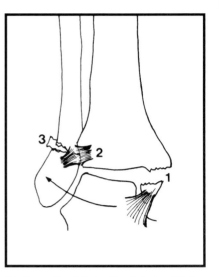

19. **Pronation/abduction injuries** *(abduction injuries)* **(1):** The foot everts and the talus swings into abduction. The first structures to be affected are on the medial side. Either (A) the deltoid ligament ruptures (rare) or there is an avulsion fracture of the medial malleolus. The fragment may be small (B) or large (C). In either case the fracture line runs horizontally.

20. **Pronation/abduction injuries (2):** In second stage injuries of this type, both the anterior and posterior tibiofibular ligaments rupture. In the case of the posterior tibiofibular ligament, its tibial attachment may be avulsed instead.

21. **Pronation/abduction injuries (3):** In the third stage the fibula fractures, often close to the level of the joint. Comminution may occur, sometimes with the formation of a triangular fragment of bone with its base directed laterally. The distal fibular fragment is tilted laterally (medial angulation). The fracture line is often horizontal.

22. **Radiographs (1):** In this example of a Stage 1 abduction fracture, note the small medial malleolar fragment, the intact fibula, and the undisplaced talus.

23. **Radiographs (2):** In this Stage 3 abduction fracture, note the direction of talar tilting, the avulsion fracture of the medial malleolus with a large fragment and the distally situated fibular fracture. The latter is not strictly horizontal, and its slightly spiral appearance suggests that there has been a rotational element.

24. **Pronation/lateral rotation** *(external rotation with diastasis)* **(1):** The talus is laterally rotated with the foot in the everted or neutral position (i.e. the foot does not invert). The rotating talus in the first stage produces an oblique fracture of the medial malleolus, or ruptures the deltoid ligament.

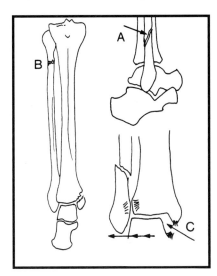

25. **Pronation/lateral rotation (2):** As the talus continues to twist, it impinges on the fibula. The anterior tibiofibular ligament is put under tension: in the second stage of P/L injuries, its tibial attachment is avulsed (Tillaux fracture) (2) or it ruptures.

26. **Pronation/lateral rotation (3):** In the third stage, the talus continues to rotate, producing a fracture of the fibula (3) that is spiral or oblique in pattern.

27. **Pronation/lateral rotation (4):** Note that in the lateral projection (A) the obliquity of the fibular fracture is in the opposite direction to that found in S/L injuries. The fibula may fracture proximally at the neck (B)—the Maisonneuve fracture. By Stage 3, the injury is unstable although stress films may be required to demonstrate diastasis (C).

28. **Pronation/lateral rotation (5):** If the talus continues to thrust laterally against the lateral malleolus, the posterior tibiofibular ligament now ruptures (A) or pulls off its bony attachment (B). The interosseous membrane rips and gross diastasis results (Dupuytren fracture—dislocation of the ankle: Stage 4).

29. **Radiograph:** Note in the lateral projection:
1. The line of the fibular fracture runs in the opposite direction to the fractures of the fibula found in supination/lateral rotation injuries.
2. The posterior subluxation of the talus.
Note in the anteroposterior projection:
1. The gross lateral displacement of the talus.
2. The obvious disruption which must have occurred in the interosseous membrane.
3. The avulsion of the attachment of the posterior tibiofibular ligament.

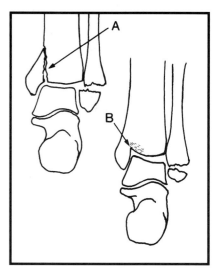

**30. Supination/adduction injuries:**
**(adduction injuries) (1):** The foot inverts,
but the tendency to external rotation of the
talus as a result of the torque convertor effect
is countered by the direction of forces applied
to the forefoot by the impact. The overall
effect is adduction of the talus in the mortise.
If the forces are slight, a partial tear of the
lateral ligament results (sprain of ankle).

**31. Supination/adduction injuries (2):**
With more severe violence there will be a
complete tear of all three bundles going to
form the lateral ligament (A) or there will be
an avulsion fracture of the lateral malleolus
(with a horizontally running fracture) (B).

**32. Supination/adduction injuries (3):**
In the second stage, the adducting talus strikes
the medial malleolus causing a *vertical* or *high
oblique fracture* (A). *Note:* (i) Instead of the
medial malleolus being pushed off, there may
be a compression fracture of the angle (B). (ii)
Occasionally the medial malleolus may be
broken off without damage first occurring to
the lateral ligament.

**33. Radiographs (1):** This radiograph
shows quite clearly an avulsion fracture of the
tip of the lateral malleolus, typical of a Stage 1
supination/adduction injury.

**34. Radiographs (2):** Note in a typical Stage
2 injury the fracture line tends to run almost
vertically from the medial corner of the ankle
mortise. There is some rotation in the
radiographic projection so that the fibular
shadow overlaps the tibia. The linear opacity
near the medial malleolus dates from a
previous Achilles tendon repair.

**35. Radiographs (3):** In this child's ankle
there is a greenstick-type fracture of the medial
malleolus with some compression of the angle
between the medial malleolus and the inferior
articular surface of the tibia.

**36. Pronation/dorsiflexion**
*(compression injuries)* **(1):** Commonly the foot is dorsiflexed at the ankle in association with an upward compression force—usually from a fall from a height or from a road traffic accident (A).

As the talus dorsiflexes, its wide anterior part is forced between the malleoli, shearing off the medial malleolus (B).

**37. Pronation/dorsiflexion injuries (2):** As violence continues, the anterior tibial margin (2) is fractured, to be followed by the lateral malleolus (3).

**38. Pronation/dorsiflexion injuries (3):** Fractures of the anterior tibial margin show quite clearly in lateral projections of the joint and help to identify quite clearly this class of fracture. The talus may sublux anteriorly, carrying the marginal fracture with it.

**39. Pronation/dorsiflexion injuries (4):** With still greater violence the tibia fractures in an irregular fashion, often with great comminution. There may be great irregularity of the inferior articular surface of the tibia. Note in the lateral radiograph the large anterior marginal fracture. In the anteroposterior view note the typical medial malleolar fracture, the gross comminution, and the disruption of the inferior articular surface of the tibia. In this case the fibula has remained intact.

**40. Other compression injuries:** If a fall occurs on to the plantar-flexed foot, the posterior articular surface of the tibia may be fractured. In addition, fractures of both malleoli (as in typical pronation/dorsiflexion injuries) may occur when the broad anterior portion of the talus is driven between them.

41. **Deformity:** Note the presence of any deformity. Look for: (1) External rotation of the foot relative to the leg. If the medial malleolus is fractured and laterally displaced, the distal end of the tibia may become quite prominent under the skin. (2) Posterior displacement of the foot, a common feature of posterior malleolar fractures.

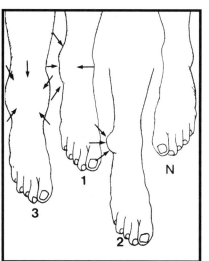

42. **Swelling:** Note the site and distribution of swelling and bruising, e.g. (1) Diffuse swelling in front of the lateral malleolus in many ankle injuries. (2) Egg-shaped swelling over the lateral malleolus shortly after complete lateral ligament tears or lateral malleolar fractures (McKenzie's sign). (3) Gross swelling and bruising in many trimalleolar and compression fractures.

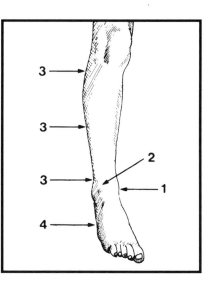

43. **Tenderness:** Try to localise tenderness if at all possible. In particular, check:
1. Medial malleolar area.
2. Anterior tibiofibular ligament area.
3. The whole length of the fibula.
4. The base of the fifth metatarsal. (Avulsion fractures following inversion injuries are often confused with ankle fractures.)

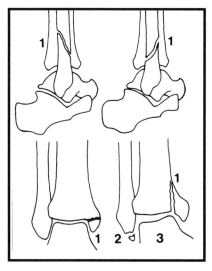

44. **Interpreting the radiographs (1):** In grouping and staging these injuries, note: (1) The site and slope of any fracture. (If in doubt, note the soft-tissue shadows, or examine an oblique (Cobb) projection.) (2) Small fragments suggesting avulsion injuries. (If in doubt about ligament integrity, stress films may be helpful.) (3) Talar tilting.

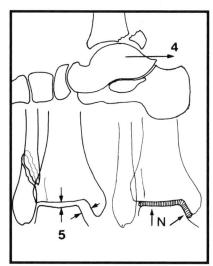

45. **Interpreting the radiographs (2):** Note also any shift of the talus relative to the tibia, e.g.: (4) Posterior subluxation, associated with a posterior malleolar fracture (5) lateral subluxation; note that the 'gap' above the talus should be the same as between the medial surface and the medial malleolus.

46. **Interpreting the radiographs (3):** Note the following possible appearances in the lateral: (1) Tibia and talus congruent: true lateral projection. (2) Tibia and talus congruent: slight rotation in lateral projection: two pairs of parallel articular shadows. (3) Tibia and talus not congruent.

### Principles of treatment of ankle injuries

The first considerations in treatment are:
1. The restoration and maintenance of the normal alignment of the talus with the tibia.
2. Ensuring good conditions for union or repair in the injured structures, so that there is no problem in the future with instability.
3. Ensuring optimum restoration of articulating surfaces to lessen the chances of osteo-arthritis in the joint.

Excellent results can be obtained by conservative methods in the majority of ankle fractures. Results are almost universally good in certain types—e.g. the stable lateral malleolar fracture—so that in these surgery would not normally be considered. The unstable bimalleolar or trimalleolar fracture, however, requires precision in reduction, great care in the techniques of plaster fixation, and above all skilled surveillance for many weeks following injury. Many surgeons prefer to avoid these uncertainties by accurate open reduction and internal fixation. In a number of fractures, especially where there has been soft-tissue interposition, reduction can only be achieved by open methods.

For the sake of simplicity, treatment has been divided into the following:

1. Fractures of one malleolus without talar shift.
2. Fractures of two or three malleoli (where there is actual or potential talar shift).
3. Injuries with diastasis and summary of postoperative care.
4. Compression fractures.
5. Lateral ligament injuries.
6. Epiphyseal and miscellaneous injuries.

**47. Fracture of one malleolus without talar shift:** (a) The commonest ankle fracture is the S/L (external rotation without diastasis) Stage 2 lesion, a stable injury (A). Associated tenderness over the medial aspect of the joint (B) is indicative of potential instability (S/L 4). Assuming that deformity has not occurred, the latter injury is usually treated by a below-knee plaster.

**48. Fracture of one malleolus with potential instability:** (b) The leg should then be elevated (1) and crutches used for 2–3 days till swelling has subsided. (2) A walking heel (or slip-on boot) may then be applied and the plaster retained for about 6 weeks. A circular woven bandage (3) or similar support may then be worn till any tendency to swelling settles. Physiotherapy is seldom required.

**49. Stable fracture of one malleolus:** If there is no medial tenderness (A) symptomatic treatment only is required; adhesive strapping, crepe bandaging or other support (B) may suffice, and should be retained till all swelling has subsided. In many stable injuries, however, symptoms can only be adequately controlled by plaster, and the regimen indicated in 330, 48 may be followed.

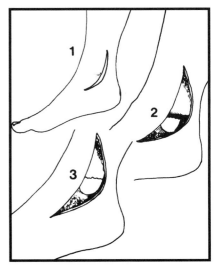

**50. Other fractures of one malleolus:** 1. Avulsion of the tip of the lateral malleolus (S/A Stage 1) may also be treated successfully by 6 weeks' plaster fixation. 2. Hair-line crack fractures of the medial malleolus (e.g. P/A Stage 1, P/L Stage 1) may be treated in a similar manner.

**51. Displaced medial malleolus (a):** Non-union of the medial malleolus is comparatively common and a frequent source of persisting pain and instability after ankle injuries. This is likely to occur if there is any persisting separation of the fragments (3). This is usually due to soft-tissue interposition (periosteum, extensor retinaculum, tibialis posterior tendon) and is an indication for open reduction and internal fixation.

**52. Displaced medial malleolus (b):** (1) A J-shaped incision is made under a tourniquet. (2) The medial malleolus is exposed, and any soft tissue between the fragments removed. (3) The fracture is then reduced under vision and held temporarily with a Charnley malleolar clamp or other device.

53. **Displaced medial malleolus (c):** The malleolus is then secured, with e.g.:
(1) one or two AO malleolar screws;
(2) one AO screw with an additional Kirschner wire to prevent rotation;
(3) a self-tapping screw penetrating the opposite cortex;
(4) a Zuelzer plate and self-tapping screws;
(5) Kirschner wires and tension band wiring;
(6) a dowel of biodegradable material (polyactide–glycolide copolymer).

54. **Displaced medial malleolus (d):** After closure of the wound, a padded below-knee plaster is applied, and the tourniquet released. The leg is elevated until swelling subsides (about 1 week). Non-weight bearing with crutches may then commence. The plaster is changed at about 2 weeks and the stitches removed. (The times indicate the approximate duration of each phase of treatment.)

55. **Displaced medial malleolus (e):** A walking heel may be applied at about 6 weeks, and this is retained until union is considered sound (usually at about 8 or 9 weeks). A circular woven bandage or crepe support is then worn until swelling subsides. Physiotherapy may be required.

56. **Posterior malleolar fractures (1):** Isolated fractures of the posterior malleolus are uncommon and do not fit neatly in the Lauge–Hansen classification. Assess on the basis of size and displacement: (A) If 25% or less of the articular surface, accept any displacement and treat as an S/L Stage 2 injury. (B) If more than 33%, and displaced, internal fixation is desirable.

57. **Posterior malleolar fractures (2):** (C) If 33% or more of the articular surface is involved and *undisplaced*, the injury may be treated conservatively by 8 weeks in a below-knee plaster. Nevertheless, there must be most careful surveillance, with radiographs being taken weekly in case there is some late slip (which would require internal fixation).

58. **Posterior malleolar fractures (3):** If a large posterior malleolar fragment is the sole injury, it may be exposed through a posterolateral approach. The patient is prone, with the ankle on a sandbag and the foot over the end of the table (1). The fracture is found between the Achilles tendon and flexor hallucis longus medially (2) and peroneus brevis laterally (3). It is fixed by one or two screws (4).

**Bimalleolar and trimalleolar fractures:** Bimalleolar fractures are unstable injuries and, where the posterior margin of the tibia is involved, instability is increased. Accurate reduction is essential for a good functional result. Conservatively treated cases must be most carefully supervised for the early detection of late displacement which may demand repeated manipulation or internal fixation.

Where internal fixation is employed, a decision must be made on its extent. Whatever procedure is contemplated, the medial malleolus should be fixed, for reasons already given. If the posterior malleolus is intact, fixation of the medial malleolus often restores very reasonable stability to the joint; this may be tested on the table. Nevertheless, any stability achieved remains dependent on the single screw usually employed for fixation; the additional support of a plaster is required until malleolar union is well advanced.

If both malleoli are adequately fixed, stability is guaranteed, and immediate plaster fixation is not required.

If the posterior malleolus is fractured and displaced, it frequently reduces if any accompanying fibular fracture is reduced and fixed. In spite of what would seem to be obvious, that anatomical restoration of the articular surface of the tibia would offer the best prospect of a good functional recovery, there is some doubt as to the value in practice of internal fixation of posterior malleolar fractures. Nevertheless many would still advocate accurate reduction and internal fixation of a large posterior malleolar fragment. If the fragment is small, and only two malleoli are fixed, immediate additional plaster support is desirable.

In women over the age of 50 years, conservative treatment gives on average as good or better results than surgery; this is due to the mechanical difficulty of securing small fragments of bone, which are often osteoporotic and subject to high levels of stress.

In men over the age of 50, operative treatment is often to be preferred. In both sexes, conservative treatment should also be considered if the patient is frail, a poor anaesthetic risk, or the skin and circulation poor. In the handling of ankle fractures it is important to be aware of the risks of delay. The complication rate soars eightfold for delays of 24 hours in initiating treatment. The presence of skin blistering or significant displacement double the complication rate.

**59. Posterior malleolar fractures (4):** In more extensive ankle injuries, advantage may be taken of medial and lateral malleolar exposures to visualise and reduce any posterior malleolar fragment. Where the fibula has been fractured, excellent access may be obtained by turning it downwards. The posterior malleolus may then be fixed by backwardly directed screws.

**60. Conservative treatment: manipulation (1):** Conservative treatment may be proposed if the patient is frail, a poor anaesthetic risk, or the skin and circulation poor. The patient is anaesthetised and the leg abducted over the edge of the table with a sandbag behind the thigh (1). The surgeon's stool (2) or the table should be adjusted until the toes can be steadied with the knee (3). A footstool may be helpful (4).

**61. Manipulation (2):** Carry out a reduction rehearsal. The malleoli generally preserve their relationship with the talus and the foot, so that in *essence it is a case of re-aligning the foot with the tibia*. In most cases, three elements require correction: (a) Begin by correcting any posterior subluxation by grasping the heel and lifting it anteriorly.

**62. Manipulation (3):** (b) Still grasping the hind foot, correct any external rotation. It should be noted that little force is required for these corrections, and in many cases re-alignment is completed by sensations similar to those experienced when reducing a dislocation.

63. **Manipulation (4):** (c) Finally correct any abduction deformity. *Note:* (1) The appearance of the ankle should be restored to normal. (2) Overcorrection is difficult or impossible. Repeat the procedure until you can remember the movements and force required for reduction.

64. **Manipulation (5):** Now apply wool roll to the limb making sure that the malleolar prominences are well covered (1). Without hurry follow this with two to three 15 cm (6″) plaster bandages from the level of the tibial tubercle to just above the ankle (2).

65. **Manipulation (6):** Smooth the plaster well down and then quickly apply two 15 cm (6″) plaster bandages to the foot and ankle. The toes may be steadied with your knee (3). On completion, you should be left with a plaster which is setting at the calf, but is quite soft and mouldable at the foot and ankle.

66. **Manipulation (7):** Now repeat the reduction manoeuvre and hold the limb in the reduced position until the plaster has set (4). Steady the forefoot with the knee (to keep the ankle at right angles) and ease the hands slightly upwards and downwards to prevent local indentation of the plaster. Extend it above the knee if the fracture is very unstable.

67. **Manipulation (8):** Check the position of the fracture with radiographs before the anaesthetic is discontinued, and if necessary, repeat the procedure (5).

Precautions should be taken over swelling— e.g. elevation, splitting of the plaster (6).

68. **Manipulation (9):** the plaster should be examined for slackness as swelling subsides. If it becomes slack, it must be changed with care to prevent slipping, and general anaesthesia may be necessary. Radiographs should be taken weekly; remanipulation under anaesthesia or internal fixation may have to be considered if there is any slip.

69. **After care (2):** A walking heel should not be applied before 6 weeks: prior to that the patient may be mobilised, non-weight bearing, with crutches. Plaster fixation should be maintained until union (usually 9–10 weeks). Confirm clinically and radiologically. Thereafter bandage supports should be worn till swelling subsides. Physiotherapy is often required.

70. **Internal fixation (a):** Indications for internal fixation and methods of fixing the medial and posterior malleoli have been discussed. Various techniques are used for the fibula. (1) In many cases an AO plate bent to fit the contours of the fibula and held with small fragment cortical and cancellous screws gives excellent fixation. (2) In some cases an oblique single Sherman or AO screw may give adequate support. (3) Intramedullary screws, although liked by some, are probably best avoided as they tend to tilt the fibula.

71. **Internal fixation (b):** If the fibular fragment is too small to take a screw without fragmenting, it may be successfully held with a well-contoured Zuelzer plate, which can usually be inserted with the minimum of local tissue dissection (4). Alternatively, a small fibular fragment may be held with tension band wiring, using two fine Kirschner wires (5). Accurate reduction and fixation of the fibula is regarded as one of the most important elements in the treatment of displaced ankle fractures.

72. **Internal fixation (c):** (6) High spiral fractures may be treated by cerclage, although a plate and screws (7) or cross-screwing (8) may be more surely followed by union. Especially where there is a tendency to diastasis, an oblique screw may be used: this should be inserted at the level of the joint and angled at 20° (a). *It should be removed as soon as union occurs.*

73. **Diastasis (1):** Wide separation of the tibia and fibula is a feature of P/L injuries (external rotation with diastasis) (1). In many other fractures the basic problem of talotibial misalignment may be present although there is no true diastasis (e.g. 2). In most cases diastasis is fully corrected if the malleolar components are fixed, and treatment should proceed along the lines detailed for malleolar fractures.

74. **Diastasis (2):** Persistence of diastasis may be due to (1) imperfect reduction of a Tillaux fracture or (2) an invaginated deltoid ligament. If attention is paid to these areas and diastasis still persists, cross-screwing as detailed above may be carried out. This must be done with the ankle in dorsiflexion, otherwise dorsiflexion may be permanently restricted.

**75. Postoperative treatment (1):** If all fragments are well held with screw fixation, a light pressure bandage may be applied, and immediate non-weight-bearing exercises commenced with the limb elevated. Crutches may be used after any swelling has subsided.

**76. Postoperative treatment (2):** After 2 weeks the stitches are removed and a close-fitting plaster is applied; assuming that swelling is not a problem, weight bearing can begin. Plaster is retained for about 6 weeks (after removal of the stitches) until there is evidence of union; thereafter a circular woven or crepe support is applied till any swelling subsides.

**77. Postoperative treatment (3):** If the medial malleolus only is fixed in a bimalleolar fracture (1) or the posterior malleolus not fixed in a trimalleolar fracture (2), plaster fixation is usually advised from the outset. Remove the sutures at 2 weeks, and apply a walking heel at 6 weeks. Union is usually sound after a further 4 weeks, when a crepe bandage or other support may be substituted, and physiotherapy commenced.

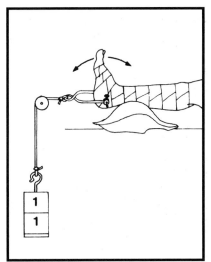

**78. Multifragmented compression (or pilon) fractures (1):** Surgery is technically difficult, but may be considered if there is at least one substantial intact articular fragment. The steps are (1) reduction and fixation of the fibula to obtain length and alignment; (2) reconstruction of the articular surface by placing the fragments over the talar dome and temporarily holding them with Kirschner wires; (3) packing defects with bone grafts; (4) fixing the main fragments with a buttress plate (and if required, cannulated screws).

**79. Compression fractures (2):** Where there is much fragmentation of the tibia, the reconstruction of the inferior articular surface of the tibia may be helped by the temporary use of a distractor (1). Where there is substantial skin and soft-tissue damage, an external fixator may be used (2). In all cases it is highly desirable to commence ankle joint movements as soon as the quality of fixation will allow. In some cases it is possible to achieve this by using a hinged external fixator (3) in the initial treatment.

**80. Compression fractures (3):** Conservative treatment may become necessary if the fragmentation of the distal tibia is so gross that no substantial articular fragment remains intact. Apply 2 kg of traction through a calcaneal pin to maintain alignment, and commence active exercises as soon as pain will permit. Weight bearing must be deferred until union is quite sound in order to avoid further compression. If secondary osteoarthritis becomes a problem ankle joint fusion may have to be considered.

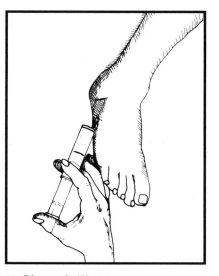

**81. Lateral ligament injuries: Diagnosis (1):** A soft tissue injury is diagnosed where there is a history of trauma and the radiographs are normal. A history of an inversion injury is obtainable in most lateral ligament injuries. In sprains, swelling and tenderness follow the fasciculi of the lateral ligament (1). In complete tears of the lateral ligament, swelling at first lies over the lateral malleolus (2).

**82. Diagnosis (2):** If the findings suggest a more substantial injury, grasp the foot and gently adduct the talus in the ankle mortise, feeling for any gap opening up at the outer corner of the joint. Compare with the other side. Excess movement of the talus on the injured side suggests a complete lateral ligament tear. (Note that the test is also positive in tears of the anterior tibiofibular ligament if the foot is not inverted in the *dorsiflexed* position.)

**83. Diagnosis (3):** If the manoeuvre cannot be performed adequately because of pain, infiltrate the fasciculi of the lateral ligament with local anaesthetic (e.g. 20 ml of 0.5% lignocaine) or administer a general anaesthetic. Repeat the manoeuvre, and for further confirmation, take AP radiographs under stress.

**84. Treatment (1):** Simple sprains resolve in a few days with local supportive measures (adhesive strapping, crepe bandaging, etc.) rest and elevation (1).

Complete lateral ligament tears should be treated either by surgical repair (of both anterior tibiofibular *and* calcaneofibular ligaments) or by plaster fixation for 6 weeks (2), followed by a lighter support till free from discomfort.

**85. Treatment (2):** If there is no obvious muscular or neurological problem, investigate chronic instability with plain and stress films (in two planes) and if indicated, arthroscopy. In many cases no abnormality can be found: these cases are labelled as functional instabilities, and thought to be due to disorders of muscle coordination or proprioception. Conservative treatment of instability involves physiotherapy to develop the evertors (1) and the use of lateral heel and sole wedges (2).

**86. Treatment (3):** Surgical reconstruction may be required if simple measures fail, and instability has been demonstrated. In the Watson–Jones reconstruction, the peroneus brevis tendon is threaded through holes drilled in the fibula and talus and sewn to itself. The upper stump is sewn to peroneus longus. The tendon replaces the torn ligament, and the success rate of the operation is high. Failure may indicate subtalar laxity.

**87. Epiphyseal injuries (1):** (a) Salter/ Harris Type 1 injuries are rare. (b) The commonest injury is sup./lateral rotation producing a Type 2 lesion. In many, displacement is minimal (1) and can be treated in a below-knee plaster for 4–6 weeks.

Where displacement is appreciable (2) the ankle should be manipulated as described for bimalleolar fractures.

**88. Epiphyseal injuries (2):** (c) A Salter/ Harris Type 3 injury may sometimes be reduced by applying firm local pressure under GA (1). If unsuccessful, cross-screwing may have to be considered, taking care to avoid damaging the epiphyseal plate (2). (d) Type 4 injuries (3) should be treated by open reduction. (e) In Type 5 Injuries (4) late corrective osteotomy may be needed (5).

**89. Sprain of inferior tibiofibular ligament:** Inversion injuries of the ankle may lead to a first stage sup./lateral rotational tearing of the inferior tibiofibular ligament. Pain may be quite severe, and tenderness well localised over the ligament. A 6-week period of plaster fixation is advised, although in cases of chronic disability hydrocortisone injections and even cross-screwing are advocated.

**90. Ankle dislocation without fracture:** Rarely the ankle may dislocate without fracture. Although rupture of both medial and lateral ligaments must take place, conservative management by closed manipulative reduction and plaster fixation may achieve a good result. Avascular necrosis of the talus is a minor risk in this situation.

**91. Recurrent dislocation of peroneal tendons:** This is a rare condition in which eversion causes painful clicking sensations as the peroneal tendons repeatedly snap over the lateral malleolus (1). The condition is associated with a defect in the superior peroneal retinaculum. A flap of bone and periosteum can be used to reconstruct the defective ligament (2).

**92. Footballers' ankle and osteochondritis tali:** Tibial and/or talar osteophytes (1) may arise in footballers from repeated anterior capsular tears, and limit dorsiflexion. Excision for this is seldom indicated. Pain may follow a fresh tear (treat symptomatically by POP fixation) or from early ankle joint osteo-arthritis.

(Osteochondritis tali (2)—see 349, 22.)

93. **Complications of ankle injuries:**
**Swelling:** Swelling persisting for weeks or
even months after fixation has been discarded
is so common as to be an almost normal
occurrence. Assuming that the fracture has
united a good position, local supportive
measures should be continued to resolution.
The patient should be reassured and advised
regarding elevation and activity.

94. **Sudeck's atrophy:** Where swelling is
gross, and especially if the toes are involved,
suspect Sudeck's atrophy. There may be
glazing of the skin and pain. Radiographs may
show typical porotic changes, and confirm
union of the fracture. Intensive physiotherapy
and continued use of supports will be required.
Convalescence may be expected to be slow
with occasionally some permanent functional
impairment.

95. **Stiffness, 'weakness' and
disturbance of gait:** Again, assuming sound
union, these symptoms generally respond
rapidly to appropriate physiotherapy and
occupational therapy. Progress may be
assessed by charting the range of ankle joint
movements. (The normal range is indicated,
but compare the sides.) Note also the range in
the subtalar joint.

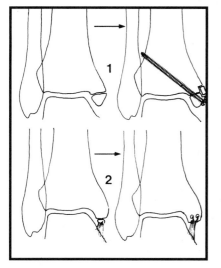

96. **Instability:** Instability due to lateral
ligament damage has been described;
instability may follow damage to the medial
structures.

   Non-union of a large medial malleolar
fragment should be treated by internal fixation:
additional grafting may be necessary (1).
When the tip only is involved, it may be
excised and the lateral ligament sutured to the
stump (2).

97. **Osteo-arthritis (1):** Considering the
incidence of ankle fractures, osteo-arthritis is
an uncommen complication. It is most likely to
follow compression fractures, and fractures
with residual diastasis or talotibial incongruity.
Note in this example of an old compression
fracture the central split in the tibial surface,
the broadening of the mortise and the
narrowed joint space.

98. **Osteo-arthritis (2):** If symptoms of
pain, swelling, stiffness and disturbance of gait
are troublesome, then fusion may be advised.
In the Crawford-Adams fusion, the articular
surfaces are cleared, the fibula is inlaid in the
talus and tibia and held in position with cross
screws. Late function is generally good due to
persistent midtarsal movement.

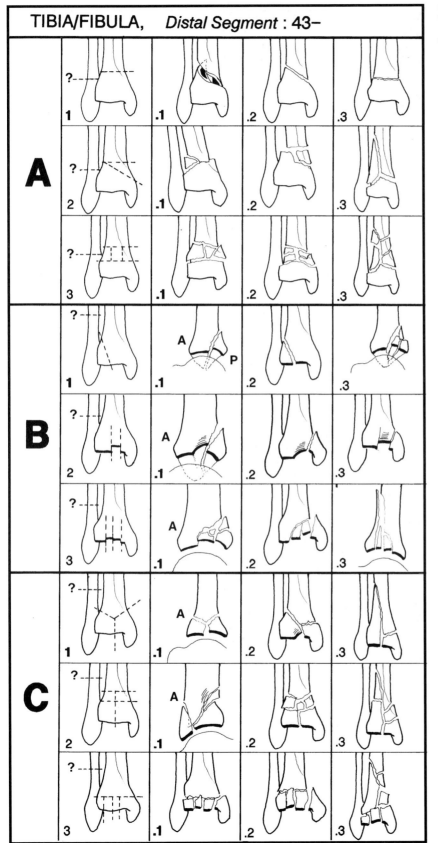

**TIBIA/FIBULA,** *Distal Segment* : 43–

**A**
1 · .1 · .2 · .3
2 · .1 · .2 · .3
3 · .1 · .2 · .3

**B**
1 · .1 · .2 · .3
2 · .1 · .2 · .3
3 · .1 · .2 · .3

**C**
1 · .1 · .2 · .3
2 · .1 · .2 · .3
3 · .1 · .2 · .3

**99. AO Classification of Fractures of the Tibia/Fibula, Distal Segment (43–):**

**Type A** fractures are extra-articular.
A1 = Metaphyseal simple, with or without an associated fibular fracture: .1 spiral; .2 oblique; .3 transverse.
A2 = Metaphyseal wedge fracture, with or without a fracture of the fibula: .1 with posterolateral impaction; .2 with an anteromedial wedge; .3 with the fracture extending proximally into the diaphysis.
A3 = Metaphyseal complex, with or without a fracture of the fibula: .1 with three intermediate fragments; .2 with more than three intermediate fragments; .3 with extension into the diaphysis.

**Type B** fractures are partial articular.
B1 = Pure split fracture with or without a fracture of the fibula: .1 frontal; .2 sagittal; .3 metaphyseal multifragmentary.
B2 = Split fracture with depression, with or without a fracture of the fibula: .1 frontal; .2 sagittal; .3 central.
B3 = Multifragmentary depressed fracture, with or without a fracture of the fibula: .1 frontal; .2 sagittal; .3 metaphyseal.

**Type C** fractures are complete articular.
C1 = Articular simple, metaphyseal simple, with or without a fracture of the fibula: .1 unimpacted; .2 with some depression of the articular surface; .3 with the fracture extending into the diaphysis.
C2 = Articular simple, metaphyseal multifragmentary, with or without a fracture of the fibula: .1 with uneven impaction; .2 without uneven impaction; .3 with the fracture extending into the diaphysis.
C3 = Multifragmentary, with or without a fracture of the fibula: .1 confined to the epiphysis; .2 confined to the epiphysis and metaphysis; .3 extending into the diaphysis.

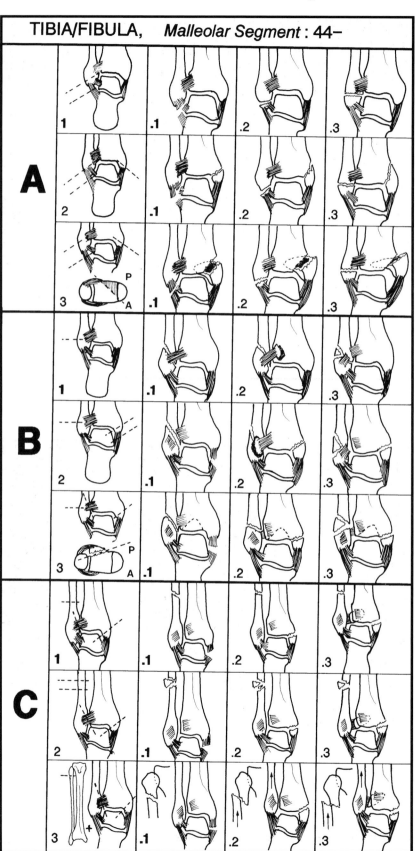

**TIBIA/FIBULA,** *Malleolar Segment : 44–*

## 100. AO Classification of Fractures of the Tibia/Fibula, Malleolar Segment (44—):

Note the following:

1. At this location the three Types (A, B, C) are selected by where the lateral lesion is placed in relation to the inferior tibio-fibular ligaments ('the syndesmotic ligaments').

2. In this exceptional situation, ligament lesions *without any accompanying fracture* have been included.

**Type A** lesions are infrasyndesmotic:

A1 = Isolated lesions of ligament or bone: .1 complete tear of the lateral ligament of the ankle; .2 avulsion fracture of the tip of the lateral malleolus; .3 transverse fracture of the lateral malleolus.

A2 = Bifocal lesions, with a fracture of the medial malleolus (which may be transverse, oblique or vertical) with: .1 a complete tear of the lateral ligament; .2 avulsion of the tip of the lateral malleolus; .3 transverse fracture of the lateral malleolus.

A3 = Bifocal lesions, with a medial malleolar fracture which extends posteriorly ('round the back') with: .1 a complete tear of the lateral ligament; .2 avulsion of the tip of the lateral malleolus; .3 transverse fracture of the the lateral malleolus.

**Type B** fractures of the fibula are trans-syndesmotic.

B1 = Where the lateral side of the joint only is involved: .1 simple; .2 with disruption of the anterior syndesmosis (anterior inferior tibio-fibular ligament tear or avulsion from the tibia (Tillaux fracture, Illus.) or from the fibula (le Fort fracture); .3 multifragmentary.

B2 = Fracture of the fibula with a medial lesion: .1 simple, with rupture of the medial (deltoid) ligament and disruption of the anterior syndesmosis; .2 simple, with fracture of the medial malleolus and disruption of the anterior syndesmosis (Illus.: le Fort); .3 multifragmentary lateral malleolar fracture with rupture of the medial ligament or a fracture of the medial malleolus.

B3 = Fracture of the fibula with both a medial lesion and a fracture of the postero-lateral rim (postero-lateral lip; fracture of the posterior malleolus): .1 simple fibula, ruptured medial ligament; .2 fibula simple, fracture of the medial malleolus; .3 multifragmentary fibula with fracture of the medial malleolus.

**Type C** are bifocal lesions with rupture of the anterior or both anterior and posterior inferior tibio-fibular ligaments. The fracture of the fibula is suprasyndesmotic (i.e. above the inferior tibio-fibular ligaments), and the medial lesion involves either the medial ligament or the medial malleolus.

C1 = Simple diaphyseal fracture of the fibula; .1 rupture of the medial ligament; .2 fracture of the medial malleolus; .3 with fracture of the medial malleolus and the posterior rim.

C2 = Multifragmentary diaphyseal fracture of the fibula: .1 with rupture of the medial ligament; .2 fracture of the medial malleolus; .3 fracture of the medial malleolus and the posterior rim.

C3 = Proximal fibular fracture (Maisonneuve fracture):. 1 without shortening; .2 with shortening; .3 with a posterior rim fracture.

101. This AP radiograph shows the position achieved by closed reduction of a Dupuytren fracture dislocation of the ankle (P/L (external rotation with diastasis) Stage 4 injury (AO = 44–C1.1)). Is reduction complete?

102. Classify this injury. Is the reduction satisfactory?

103. This radiograph was taken of a patient complaining of pain in the ankle after an inversion injury. Do you detect any abnormality?

104. On the information available on this lateral radiograph, classify this injury. Is the talus congruent with the tibia?

105. What is the most likely explanation for the broken screw showing on this radiograph?

106. What pattern of injury is shown in this lateral radiograph?

107. In this single lateral projection of the ankle, what are the most outstanding elements?

108. What treatment has been carried out for this ankle injury?

109. What is this injury? What atypical element is present?

110. What does this radiograph demonstrate?

111. What injury is present, and how has it been treated?

112. What is this injury? How has it been treated? What is the result?

101. No: there is persistent lateral talar shift (Note the gap between the talus and the medial malleolus) due to slight persistent diastasis. This position would be accepted by a number of surgeons, while others would prefer to correct this by cross-screwing.

102. The vertical fracture of the medial malleolus is typical of a supination/adduction Stage 2 injury (Adduction fracture) AO = 44–A3.1. Reduction is incomplete, and there is disturbance of the inferior articular surface of the tibia. Open reduction is indicated.

103. A small opacity is present distal to the tip of the lateral malleolus, and probably represents avulsion of the fibular attachment of the lateral ligament. The fragment is small, and clinical confirmation would be desirable. AO = 44–A1.2.

104. The direction of the spiral fracture of the fibula suggests that this is a P/L injury. The talus and tibia are not congruent (double talar shadow, single tibial shadow). AO = 44–C1.1.

105. The original pathology has been a fibular fracture or a diastasis treated by an oblique screw. Ankle movements have been permitted before removal of the screw. This has resulted in distortion of the inferior tibiofibular joint, and fracture of the screw, the lateral portion only of which has been accessible for removal.

106. This is an epiphyseal injury, in which there is slight backward displacement of the distal tibial epiphysis, along with a small fragment of metaphysis (juxta-epiphyseal fragment), i.e. a Salter–Harris Type 2 injury. There is some evidence on this lateral view of talotibial incongruity, and manipulation would be indicated.

107. There is a fracture of the posterior malleolus, with posterior subluxation of the talus. Half of the inferior articular surface of the tibia is involved. AO = 43–B1.3 or B2.1.

108. A small medial malleolar fragment has been reduced and held with a Zuelzer hook plate, and the limb placed in plaster.

109. This is a pronation/abduction injury with horizontal fractures of the medial and lateral malleoli and lateral displacement of the talus AO = 44–A2.3. There is an additional, atypical fracture of the fibula at a higher level.

110. Although comparison films of the other ankle should be taken, it is almost certain that a complete tear of the external ligament has been demonstrated in this inversion film. (Note the shadows of the lead gloves and the angle of talar tilting which has been marked on the radiograph.)

111. This is a pronation/lateral rotation (external rotation with diastasis) injury which has resulted in a fracture of the medial malleolus and a Tillaux fracture. The medial malleolar fracture has been held with a Sherman screw. With the fibula intact, this injury does not fit in to the normal AO Classification system.

112. There has been a bimalleolar fracture (supination/lateral rotation injury AO = 44–B2.2), and the lateral malleolus has been fixed with an oblique cross-screw. This has not been removed (as it should) so that there is virtually cross-union between the tibia and fibula. This has impaired ankle joint function, and osteo-arthritic changes are advancing. (Note the narrowing of the joint space between the tibia and the talus.)

# 15. Foot injuries

1. **Anatomical considerations (1):** The talus plays a key role in no less than 3 joints: (1) the ankle joint—articulating with the tibia and fibula; (2) the subtalar joint—articulating with the calcaneus. (3) the talonavicular joint: along with the calcaneocuboid joint, this forms the *midtarsal joint*. Secondary osteo-arthritic changes may occur following fractures which cause articular irregularity.

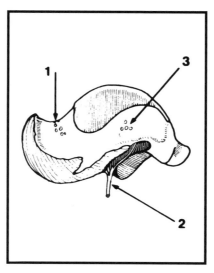

2. **Anatomical considerations (2):** Secondary osteo-arthritis may also follow avascular necrosis which occurs in half of all talar neck fractures. The blood supply of the talus enters at three sites: (1) the neck; (2) the sinus tarsi area; (3) the medial side of the body. The more sources are disturbed, the greater is the risk to the blood supply.

3. **Mechanisms of injury:** The commonest fracture is of the neck. This may occur in car accidents, when pedal impact (1) forces the talar neck against the tibial margin (2). (There is a long association between this injury and light aircraft crashes where the feet are violently dorsiflexed against the rudder pedals—'aviator's astragalus'.) The injury may also follow falls from a height in a crouching position.

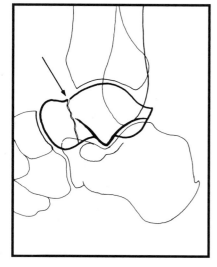

4. **Classification of talar neck fractures (1):** Talar neck fractures have been classified into four types of increasing severity. In *Type 1* the talar neck is fractured without displacement. Incomplete hair-line cracks are not uncommon. Only the blood supply through the neck is affected, and the incidence of avascular necrosis is under 10%.

5. **Classification (2):** In *Type 2* fractures there is an accompanying subtalar subluxation. The proximal portion of the talus adopts a position of plantar flexion (1). The *head* of the talus maintains its relationship with the navicular and calcaneus (and the rest of the foot) which sublux forwards (2).

6. **Classification (3):** Note in the radiographic example a more severe degree of plantar flexion of the proximal fragment, and greater subluxation. The blood supplies through the neck and sinus tarsi are both interrupted, and the incidence of avascular necrosis rises to 50% in fractures of this type.

7. **Classification (4):** *Type 3 injuries:* With further dorsiflexion and upward force (1) the tibia is driven between the two talar fragments. The posterior fragment is extruded backwards, while at the same time the convex posterior articular surface of the calcaneus (2) guides it medially. It comes to rest with its medial surface (3) caught on the sustentaculum tali (4).

8. **Classification (5):** In its final position (*ctd*) the main portion of the talus lies on the medial side of the ankle, with its fractured surface (5) pointing laterally. All three sources of blood supply are disturbed. The risks of avascular necrosis are high, rising to 85%.

9. **Classification (6):** In the rare *Type 4 injury,* the head of the talus dislocates from the navicular (1) in association with a Type 3 (2) or a Type 2 injury. The incidence of avascular necrosis here is also high.

10. **Diagnosis:** The diagnosis may be suspected from the history, but is made radiologically. Care must be taken to differentiate between Type 1 and Type 2 injuries. If doubt exists, two laterals, one in dorsiflexion (1) and one in plantar flexion (2) should be taken and compared. These will reveal any subluxation (Type 2 illustrated).

11. **Treatment of Type I injuries:** (1) Padded plaster with toe platform and elevation for about a week. (2) Non-weight bearing with crutches for 3 months. (3) The fracture is then assessed out of plaster for union and absence of avascular necrosis. (4) If there are no complications, weight bearing may commence with a light support. Physiotherapy will be required for ankle, subtalar joint and calf.

12. **Treatment of Type II injuries (1):** Reduction may be attempted by closed methods: (1) The foot is plantar flexed and everted. (2) A padded plaster is applied in this position and check radiographs taken. If a satisfactory reduction has been obtained, then conservative treatment may be continued.

13. **Treatment of Type II injuries (2):** (3) The limb is elevated for a week before (4) non-weight bearing is permitted. After 3–4 weeks the plaster is changed under intensifier control and the foot brought up to a right angle (5). Non-weight bearing is continued for a further 6 weeks. Thereafter, if the fracture is united and there is no evidence of avascular necrosis, weight bearing may be allowed with support (6). Physiotherapy will almost certainly be required.

14. **Treatment of Type II injuries (3):** If closed methods fail in obtaining a reduction, open reduction will be required. The fracture may be secured with a Kirschner wire passed backwards from the head of the talus into the body. The after care is as in 348, 13; the Kirschner wire may be removed at the change of plaster. These injuries may also be internally fixed as described in 348, 17 below.

15. **Treatment of Type III injuries (1):** The displaced portion of the talus is situated subcutaneously, and there should be no delay in reducing it as the overlying skin is tightly stretched over the bone and likely to slough. Facilities for open reduction should be available, but closed methods should be attempted first. (1) Begin by gripping the heel and applying traction to it (see 348, 16).

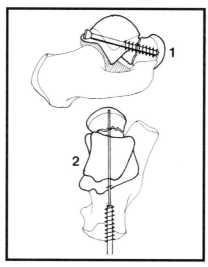

16. **Treatment of Type III injuries (2):** (2) Dorsiflex the foot with the knee. (3) Maintaining traction, pull the heel slightly forward and evert it to open up the space for the talus. (4) Apply strong pressure over the displaced body of the talus: press laterally, but also slightly anteriorly and downwards. (5) Plantar flex the foot. If purchase on the heel is poor, a Steinman pin through the heel and a calliper may be used.

17. **Treatment of Type III injuries (3):** (6) after reduction, proceed with elevation and gradual mobilisation as described in 348, 13 above. If closed reduction fails (as it often does), open reduction will be necessary. The condition of the skin and any planned internal fixation will dictate the incision(s). These

fractures may be fixed (best through a posterolateral incision) with one or two cortical or cancellous screws passed from behind through the body of the talus and into the head (1). Cannulated screws may also be used; these can be threaded over Kirschner wires which have been inserted temporarily to hold the reduction. (2) (The AO group, with an eye to rapid mobilisation, in fact recommend internal fixation along these lines for all talar neck fractures.) *Treatment of Type IV injuries:* These uncommon injuries are likely to require open reduction. All fragments should be retained, even if completely detached and obviously avascular. On no account should the talus be excised.

*Complications of talar neck fractures: (1) Skin necrosis:* The skin may become tightly stretched over a displaced talus and undergo necrosis with late sloughing. *Early reduction is imperative to avoid this complication. (2) Compound injuries:* Thorough debridement of the wound is essential, but again every effort must be made to retain the main fragments. Treatment should follow the usual lines established for the management of open fractures. If sepsis occurs *in conjunction with avascular necrosis,* healing may be obtained only after excision of the avascular fragments.

**18. Complications** *ctd:* **(3) Ankle fracture:** Rarely, malleolar fracture may be found complicating talar neck fractures. Closed reduction is here unreliable, and open reduction with internal fixation of the malleolar fracture is desirable. (Illus.: Type 3 fracture with fracture of the lateral malleolus.)

**19. Complications** *ctd:* **(4) Avascular necrosis:** The diagnosis is made from the radiographs. *Increased density* is often apparent by 6 and usually by 12 weeks, but do not be confused by the dense shadows cast by the overlying malleoli in the lateral. Revascularisation always occurs in closed injuries and is usually advanced by 8 months. (Check progress by monthly radiographs.) *Weight bearing before revascularisation is complete is likely to cause marked flattening of the talus (Illus.).* Local supports and physiotherapy will be required. Secondary osteo-arthritis is common and should be kept in mind. Because of its key position, avascular necrosis of the talus may lead to osteo-arthritis of the ankle, subtalar or midtarsal joints (or any combination of these).

**20. Complication** *ctd:* **(5) Osteo-arthritis:** This may occur secondary to avascular necrosis or mal-union. Determination of the joints involved is important, and this may be facilitated by the site of the pain and the clinical and radiological appearances. Local anaesthetic infiltration of suspected joints is occasionally helpful. Thereafter the appropriate fusion may be advised. (Where all three joints are involved, as here, all will require fusion.)

**21. Other talar lesions: (1) Dome fractures:** A portion of the upper articular surface of the talus may be detached as a result of a shearing injury: occasionally the fragment is inverted, effectively preventing union (1). If the fragment is substantial, it should be replaced and secured with, for example, Smillie pins (2); if the fragment is small, it may be excised. Thereafter, plaster fixation for 6 weeks is advisable.

**22. (2) Osteochondritis tali:** This may occur as a sequel to a non-displaced shearing fracture, although frequently there is no history of injury. (Note the lesion on the medial side of the upper articular surface.) Where there is appreciable pain and swelling, it is usual to place multiple drill holes through the base of the lesion in an attempt to encourage revascularisation.

23. **(3) Avulsion fractures:** Minor avulsion fractures of the talus may result from inversion, eversion, plantar flexion and rarely dorsiflexion strains of the ankle—when flakes of bone are pulled off by ligamentous or capsular attachments. These injuries require symptomatic treatment only (e.g. 2–4 weeks in a below-knee walking plaster).

24. **(4) Footballers' ankle:** Repeated forced plantar flexion may lead to avulsion of the anterior capsular attachments of the ankle with calcification developing in the haematomata. This produces exostoses of the tibia and talus and sometimes, as here, patchy areas of calcification in the anterior capsule (see also ankle, 337, 92).

25. **Fractures of the body of the talus:** (1) The upper articular surface of the talus may be fractured by the same mechanisms which produce compression fractures of the ankle. Vertical splits without significant disturbance of the ankle or subtalar joints (Illus.) may be treated as Type 1 talar neck fractures. (2) If displacement has occurred, accurate reduction and cross-screwing should be carried out. CT scans are useful in assessing dome fractures.

26. **Body fractures:** (3) Often there is a high degree of comminution. The convexity of the body may be flattened and the talus compressed as it is squeezed between the tibia and calcaneus. Such fractures may also involve the subtalar joint, and there is invariably extensive damage to the cartilaginous surfaces of the ankle joint. Surgical reconstruction is seldom possible.

27. **Treatment:** A typical conservative line of treatment might be: (1) Initial pressure bandaging and elevation. (2) Intensive active exercises as soon as pain and swelling will permit. (3) Avoidance of weight bearing until union is well advanced (about 8–10 weeks). Persistent pain and functional restriction would be indications for ankle fusion.

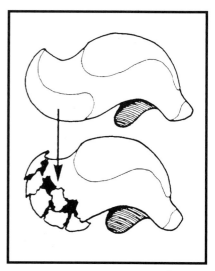

28. **(6) Compression fractures of the head of the talus:** These fractures are uncommon, but usually highly comminuted and unsuitable for attempts at reconstruction. Early mobilisation of the foot should be the aim, and a regimen similar to 350, 27 may be followed.

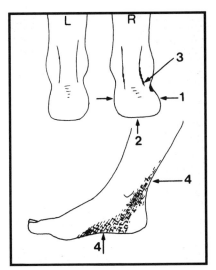

29. **Calcaneal fractures: mechanisms of injury (1):** The commonest cause of calcaneal fracture is a fall from a height on to the heels. Important factors include the height fallen, the nature of the ground, and the weight of the patient. The injury is common in slaters, window cleaners and construction workers. Rarely the injury may be produced by impact from below (e.g. a below-deck explosion on a ship).

30. **Mechanisms of injury (2):** Taking into account the commonest cause of injury, it is essential when examining a case of suspected calcaneal fracture that you do not overlook: (1) a similar fracture on the other side, (2) a wedge fracture of the spine. (Dorsolumbar junction fractures are present in 5% of calcaneal fractures.)

31. **Clinical appearance:** In major fractures, the heel when viewed from behind appears: (1) wider, (2) shorter and flatter, and (3) tilted laterally into valgus. There is often tense swelling of the heel, marked local tenderness, and later bruising (4), which may spread into the medial side of the sole and proximally to the calf. Weight bearing is usually, but not always, impossible.

32. **Radiographs (1):** The most important view is a well-centred and well-exposed lateral projection (1). An axial projection (2) is helpful in visualising the pillar of the heel (3), the sustentaculum tali (4), the anterior talocalcaneal joint (5) and the posterior talocalcaneal joint (6). This film is taken with the tube tilted at 40° from the vertical (7).

33. **Radiographs (2):** A line may be drawn from the anterior articular process of the calcaneus (1) through the posterior articular surface (2) to intersect with a second line touching the superior angle of the tuberosity (3). This *Bohler's salient angle* is normally about 40°. It is decreased (4) in fractures which flatten the heel profile.

34. **Radiographs (3):** An oblique projection may be helpful if doubt remains; note in this radiograph the split in the posterior articular surface of the calcaneus.

*Note that the key factor in assessing calcaneal fractures is whether or not there is involvement of the subtalar joint.* CAT scans close to the coronal plane are often of great value (see also 355, 54).

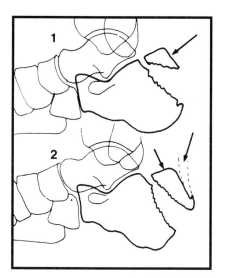

35. **Type of calcaneal fracture:** Seven common patterns of fracture have been described, and are arranged here roughly in order of increasing complexity. **I. Vertical fracture of the tuberosity:** The subtalar joint is not involved and the prognosis is excellent (1). Nevertheless, swelling may be severe, and should be controlled by firm bandaging over wool and elevation of the limb (2).

36. **Vertical fractures (2):** Weight bearing, whilst not harmful, will be painful or impossible, and crutches will be required for some weeks; they may be discarded when pain settles (3). A crepe bandage or similar support may be worn till swelling subsides. Any long-term heel pain may be controlled with a sorbo rubber heel cushion (4).

37. **II. Horizontal fractures (1):** These are of two types which must be distinguished. (1) The commoner injury involves the posterior superior angle of the calcaneus without disturbance of the Achilles tendon insertion; it is usually caused by local trauma (e.g. a kick). (2) The second is an avulsion fracture, produced by sudden muscle contraction.

38. **Horizontal fractures (2): Diagnosis:** Differentiate between the two main types of horizontal fracture by: (1) Noting the level of the fracture on the radiographs (Type 1 Illus.). (2) Studying the soft-tissue shadows on the radiograph, looking for upward (proximal) retraction of the Achilles tendon. (3) Feeling for a gap between the tendon insertion and the point of the heel.

39. **Treatment (1):** (1) If the fracture is of the avulsion type (or if there is continued doubt) it should be openly reduced and fixed with a screw. (2) To remove stress from the screw, a long leg plaster should be applied with the knee and ankle in flexion. (3) After 4 weeks a below-knee walking plaster may be substituted till union (about 8 weeks).

40. **Treatment (2):** (1) When the fracture is not of the avulsion type, it should be manipulated if severely displaced. Moderate residual displacement can usually be quite safely accepted. (2) Thereafter, a below-knee padded plaster may be applied, and crutches used for the first week or so. (3) A further 5 weeks in a below-knee walking plaster is then all that will be required.

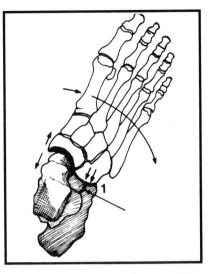

**41. III. Fractures of the sustentaculum tali (1):** These fractures result from eversion injuries (avulsion) (1). They are seen most clearly in axial projections, and indeed may be missed unless this view is taken and examined with care (2). Displacement is generally slight, and persisting disability is rare.

**42. Sustentaculum tali (2):** *Treatment:* Healing of the fracture is generally well advanced by 6 weeks. Prior to this the following treatments may be used: (a) A crepe bandage over wool pressure bandage and non-weight bearing with crutches for 6 weeks, or (b) a below-knee padded plaster with crutches initially and then a walking heel; after 6 weeks a circular woven support for a further 2 weeks or so.

**43. IV. Anterior calcaneal fractures (1):** This fracture affects the anterior part of the calcaneus which articulates with the cuboid. It may result from (1) Forced abduction of the forefoot in which the cuboid strikes the calcaneus. (2) Forced inversion injuries which have the same effect. (3) As part of a midtarsal dislocation.

**44. Anterior calcaneal fractures:** *Treatment:* (1) If there is no significant compression or shortening of the calcaneus (as in the vertical split illustrated) the injury may be treated conservatively along the lines already indicated for fractures of the sustentaculum tali (353, 42). (2) If there is evidence of midtarsal instability, treat as for midtarsal dislocation.

**45.** (3) If there is calcaneal shortening, the mechanisms of the midtarsal joint may be seriously disturbed, leading possibly to pain, restriction of movements in the foot and osteoarthritis. If the patient is elderly or has sustained multiple injuries, these risks may be accepted, and this injury also treated conservatively. In some other cases it may be possible by open operation and bone grafting to pack up the depressed articular fragments; this will improve function in the midtarsal joint and reduce the risks of secondary osteoarthritis.

**46. V. Fracture of the body of the calcaneus without involvement of the subtalar joint (1):** The fracture line passes just posterior to the posterior talocalcaneal joint. Frequently there is a decrease in the salient angle, and if this is the case (Illus.) then flattening of the heel profile may lead to troublesome localised and persistent heel pain.

47. **Body fractures (2):** Due to proximal displacement of the portion of the calcaneus carrying the Achilles tendon insertion, there is slackening of the calf muscles, so that there is weakness of plantar flexion at the ankle, and loss of spring in the step. This slackness is eventually taken up, but recovery is facilitated by *prolonged, intensive physiotherapy* in the form of calf resisting exercises.

48. **Body fractures (3): Treatment (1):** If displacement is slight, good results may be obtained by conservative treatment along the following lines: (a) Pressure bandaging, bed rest, elevation and analgesics for 2 weeks. (b) Crutches until graduated weight bearing can be commenced at about 6 weeks. (c) Calf resisting exercises as soon as pain will permit, and continued physiotherapy till maximal recovery.

49. **Body fracture (4): Treatment (2):** More severely displaced fractures may be treated along similar lines, or an attempt made to reduce the heel fragment. An open reduction may be performed through a lateral incision, with fixation of the fragments with screws or a reconstruction plate. Alternatively a Gissane spike may be driven into the heel which is then levered distally. The spike is incorporated in a plaster sabot which maintains the reduction while still permitting ankle movements.

50. **Body fractures (5): Treatment (3):** If a suitable spike is not available, a large diameter Steinman pin may be used. Image intensifier control is helpful. The pin should be inserted a little to the lateral side of the heel (1). The heel fragment is engaged (2) and brought down (3). The pin may if required be driven across the sinus tarsi into the head of the talus (following the axis of the subtalar joint) (4).

51. **Body fractures (6): Treatment (4):** The sabot and spike may be removed after 6 weeks and non-weight-bearing exercises continued for a further 2 weeks before full weight bearing. Pin-track infection is not uncommon, and at the first sign the pin should be removed and antibiotic treatment commenced. Because of this risk, this treatment should not be employed where there is any doubt about the peripheral circulation.

52. **VI. Calcaneal fractures with lateral displacement and involvement of the subtalar joint. (1):** Lateral displacement of the main fragment may cause: (1) calf impairment and local heel pain as previously described; (2) broadening of the heel, which may be unsightly and call for special footwear; (3) impingement symptoms from the lateral malleolus or squashed peroneal tendons.

**53. Subtalar joint involvement (2):** (4) Disruption of the subtalar joint is often most obvious in the tangential projection; there may be depression of the posterior joint on the lateral side, leading to fibrous adhesions and loss of inversion/eversion movements. (5) Secondary osteo-arthritis is extremely common, giving persistent pain and lack of confidence in walking. This plus an acquired fear of heights may lead to loss of work and alcoholism.

**54. Subtalar joint involvement (3):** CAT scans may be used to elucidate the extent of any subtalar joint involvement. Cuts made far back (left) show the tibia (T), fibula (F), talus (t) and the calcaneus (C). The illustration shows a displaced calcaneal fracture with involvement of the subtalar joint. More anteriorly placed cuts (right) may show the head of the talus and the navicular (N). (Illus.: fracture involving the sustentaculum tali and the anterior talonavicular joint.)

**55. Subtalar joint involvement (3): Treatment (1):** (a) Where deformity is not marked (Illus.) *or* where the peripheral circulation is poor *or* the patient elderly, the fracture should be treated along conservative lines as described in 354, 48. (b) In other cases, conservative treatment may also be employed. Although morbidity is high, the results of more active treatment are somewhat uncertain.

Nevertheless, the following alternative treatment may be considered: (1) Spike reduction of the major fragment (as in 354, 49 and 50). (2) *In addition* an attempt may be made to elevate any depressed lateral segment through a posterolateral incision. If necessary, the depressed articular surfaces may have to be packed up with bone grafts to maintain their position, and the fracture secured with screws and if required a reconstruction plate.

**Treatment after union:** (a) Physiotherapy and occupational therapy should be continued until nothing more can be gained.
(b) Pain under the heel should be treated by a sorbo pad.
(c) Broadening of the heel may require surgical footwear.
(d) Impingement symptoms with sharply localised pain and tenderness beneath the lateral malleolus may respond to local surgery (excision of any exostosis and freeing the peroneal tendons).
(e) Persistent pain and limp, due possibly to secondary subtalar osteo-arthritis, require careful assessment. Symptoms should be unremitting, persistent for 6–9 months *at least* after injury, and unresponsive to physiotherapy, before surgery is contemplated. Fresh radiographs should be compared with the original films to confirm subtalar joint involvement, and assess the calcaneocuboid joint.

If the subtalar joint only is involved, a subtalar fusion is advised. If there is any involvement of the calcaneocuboid joint, a full triple fusion will be necessary (fusion of the subtalar, calcaneocuboid and talonavicular joints).

**56. VII. Central crushing fractures:** In the most severe of calcaneal fractures, the talus drives like a wedge through the central part of the calcaneus, leading to comminution of a severe degree and disruption of the subtalar and calcaneocuboid joints. (In the united fracture illustrated note the changes in the calcaneocuboid and midtarsal joints.) Surgical reconstruction is generally impossible and complications are common. Nevertheless a number do well without requiring late fusion if treated wholly conservatively or by spike reduction.

**57. Peritalar dislocation: Pathology (1):**
Forcible inversion of the plantar flexed foot throws stress on the lateral ligament of the ankle and the talocalcaneal ligament. If the strong talocalcaneal ligament ruptures, the talus remains in the ankle mortise and a subtalar dislocation results.

**58. Pathology (2):** The forefoot remains with the calcaneus and the talonavicular joint dislocates: as the talus remains in position this injury is often described as a peritalar dislocation. It may be accompanied by fractures of the malleoli. The talus, freed from its attachments, goes into plantar flexion (and this is the position in which the foot must be placed during the initial stage of reduction).

**59. Diagnosis:** The diagnosis may be suspected clinically, but is always confirmed by radiographs. Note in the example how the talus has maintained its normal relationship with the tibia and fibula (somewhat concealed by the slight obliquity of the radiographic projection). Note that avascular necrosis of the talus does not occur, but late subtalar osteo-arthritis is common.

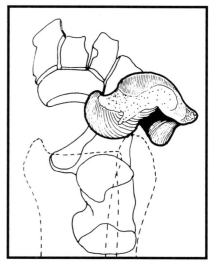

**60. Treatment (1):** Reduction is generally easy: under general anaesthesia (1) Plantar flex the foot. (2) Grasp the heel and the forefoot, apply a little traction, and swing the foot into eversion. Thereafter (3) Apply a padded below-knee plaster with the ankle at right angles and the foot in slight eversion (see 356, 61).

**61. Treatment (2):** (4) A walking plaster may be applied after a week and retained for a further 5 weeks.
  Open reduction is necessary if manipulation fails, and the talonavicular joint should be exposed first (5) as difficulty is usually due to button-holing of that joint. Instability may be controlled with Kirschner wire.

**62. Total dislocation of talus:**
**Pathology:** With greater violence than shown in 356, 57 there is complete rupture of all the other ligamentous attachments of the talus. The talus dislocates out of the ankle mortise and comes to lie subcutaneously in front of the ankle and on the lateral side of the foot. The head of the talus points medially and its calcaneal surface is directed posteriorly. (Very rarely eversion injuries may lead to medial dislocation of the talus.)

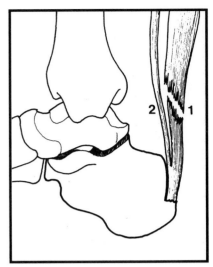

**63. Treatment (1):** Manipulative reduction should be attempted under general anaesthesia. It is imperative that delay is avoided, as there is always risk of skin sloughing where it is tightly stretched over the talus. The following technique may be employed: (1) Plantar flex the foot. (2) Invert the foot strongly. (3) The posterior part of the talus, lying laterally, should be pushed in a posteromedial direction.

**64. Treatment (2);** (4) When the talus starts to move into place, evert the foot.
If these measures fail, use a Steinman pin through the calcaneus to apply preliminary traction and control inversion. Occasionally open reduction may be required. (5) Thereafter apply a padded plaster. Avascular necrosis is almost inevitable. (Further care is as 349, 19.)

**65. Acute rupture of tendocalcaneus:** Rupture may follow sudden muscle activity (e.g. jumping or sprinting). It is especially common in the middle aged when degenerative changes are appearing in the tendon. It may be precipitated by local steroid injections. Usually the site is 4–8 cm above the insertion; rupture is complete (1) and the plantaris is spared (2). There is sudden pain with difficulty in walking and standing on the toes.

**66. Diagnosis:** The history and age of the patient may be suggestive. Clinically there may be: (1) a visible gap in the tendon, (2) weakness of plantar flexion against resistance, (3) lack of 'firmness' on side-to-side pressure at the site of the rupture, again when the foot is being plantar flexed against resistance. Soft-tissue radiographs or an MRI scan may show a defect in the continuity of the tendon in the lateral projection.

**67. Treatment:** Both conservative and surgical measures have their advocates, but neither guarantees freedom from complications, which include re-rupture, weakness of plantar flexion, stiffness of the ankle, poor wound healing (sometimes taking many months) and deep vein thrombosis.

*Conservative treatment:* This is often advocated for all cases seen within 48 hours, but is also particularly suitable for the elderly, frail or poor anaesthetic risk patient. The aim of treatment is to hold the foot in plantar flexion in order to approximate the tendon ends and to hold them there until healing is advanced. A long leg plaster is applied with the knee in about 45° of flexion and the ankle plantar flexed. This is retained for 4 weeks; a below-knee plaster is then substituted, with the ankle still a little in plantar flexion. After a further 4 weeks the plaster can be discarded, weight bearing permitted, and physiotherapy to improve the gait and calf strength commenced. To begin with, an inside shoe lift may be used to reduce dorsiflexion stresses on the healing tendon.

*Surgical treatment:* This gives the most satisfactory results where there is a delay of a week or more in making the diagnosis or initiating treatment. It is often also advocated for the young athletic patient. The tendon is approached through a vertical incision, a little to the side of the midline. A general anaesthetic, a tourniquet, and the prone position are advisable. The ends of the ruptured tendon will be found to come together when the foot is plantar flexed. It is held in that position during suturing. Absorbable, non-absorbable or Bunnell pull-out sutures may be inserted: all have their advocates and all are effective, but the frequency of wound breakdown is an added incentive for the use of absorbable sutures. Fascia lata may be used if there is much fraying of the tendon. After wound closure a long leg plaster cast is applied with the knee in flexion and the ankle plantar flexed. At 3 weeks the skin sutures may be removed and a below-knee plaster applied for a further 3 weeks with the ankle in a more neutral position. Discharging wounds are managed with patience along established lines, and only rarely require grafting.

**68. Midtarsal dislocations (1):**
Dislocation of the talonavicular portion of the midtarsal joint may accompany subtalar dislocations. The inversion mechanism has been described (see 356, 58). The subtalar joint may reduce (incompletely) spontaneously, so that the talonavicular dislocation is the main feature (Illus.).

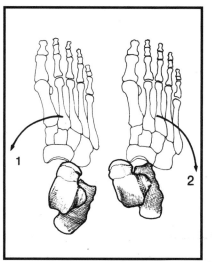

**69. Midtarsal dislocations (2):** The midtarsal joint lies between the talus and calcaneus posteriorly, and the navicular and cuboid anteriorly. *Both* elements of the joint may be disrupted as a result of (1) adduction (2) abduction forces applied to the forefoot.

**70. Midtarsal dislocations (3):** As in any other dislocation, abduction or adduction midtarsal dislocations are associated with ligament rupture or small avulsion fractures, but the talus, calcaneus, navicular and cuboid may escape significant fracture (Illus.: adduction midtarsal dislocation with small avulsion fracture of cuboid).

**71. Midtarsal dislocations (4):** On the other hand, a midtarsal dislocation may be associated with fracture of any of the components of the joint. The navicular is most frequently involved. (Illus.: an abduction type midtarsal dislocation with fractures of the navicular and cuboid.) When this is the case, reduction is more likely to be unstable, and secondary arthritic changes commoner.

**72. Treatment:** (1) Under general anaesthesia, traction is applied to the forefoot. (2) Maintaining traction, the forefoot is aligned with the hindfoot (abduction injury illus.). (3) If there is evidence of instability, the forefoot should be stabilised with percutaneous Kirschner wires. If manipulation fails, open reduction may be required; a large navicular fracture may sometimes merit screw fixation.

73. (4) A padded plaster is applied and split, and the limb elevated. (5) Non-weight bearing with crutches may commence after 1–2 weeks; any wires may be removed at 3–4 weeks. *Weekly* radiographs should be taken to detect late subluxation. (6) Plaster fixation may be discarded after 6–8 weeks and mobilisation commenced.

*Complications:* (1) Stiffness of the foot and ill-localised pain are common. This may be followed by (2) secondary osteo-arthritis. If this is confined to the calcaneocuboid joint, it may be treated by a local fusion: otherwise a full triple arthrodesis (arthrodesis of subtalar and midtarsal joints) may be required because of the functional interdependence of these joints. (3) Rarely medial plantar nerve palsy may be seen with intrinsic muscle wasting.

**74. Isolated fractures of the navicular:** (Do not mistake the common accessory centre of ossification for a fracture.) (1) The tuberosity may be fractured (illus.) by avulsion of the tibialis posterior; this and other undisplaced fractures may be treated conservatively (e.g. by 6 weeks in plaster). (2) Body fractures may be accompanied by dorsal extrusion of a large fragment which should be accurately reduced and fixed surgically.

**75. Tarsometatarsal dislocations (1):** Injuries to the tarsometatarsal region are infrequent and the mechanism of injury is not always clear. Dislocation of one or more metatarsals may result from the following: (A) A fall on the plantar flexed foot or a blow to the forefoot as in road traffic accidents. (B) A blow on the heel when in the kneeling position, e.g. when a horse falls on top of a thrown rider. (C) Run-over kerb-side accidents.

**76. Tarsometatarsal dislocations (2):** (D) Forced inversion, eversion or abduction of the forefoot as, for example, in a fall with the foot trapped. *Note:* (1) The dorsalis pedis/medial plantar anastomosis may be in jeopardy; (2) the metatarsal bases are keyed into the cuneiforms, and fracture of the second metatarsal base (3) will allow lateral drift (4). In eversion injuries, the first metatarsal may drift medially (5) and may be accompanied by the cuneiform (6).

**77. Treatment:** Reduction should be attempted promptly because of the risks of oedema and circulatory impairment. **(1)** If the deformity is a single, multiple, dorsal or plantar dislocation without fracture, reduction can often be achieved by applying traction in the line of the metatarsals and pressure over their bases. If stable, a padded plaster is used for 8 weeks before weight bearing and mobilisation.

**78. Treatment (2):** Where there is lateral drift of all the metatarsals, fracture of the second metatarsal base (not always obvious on a single projection as here) may make reduction difficult and unstable. Open reduction and Kirschner wire fixation are advisable, (carried out through a longitudinal incision lateral to the dorsalis pedis artery), and thereafter plaster fixation for 6 weeks.

**79. Treatment (3):** Where the first ray is displaced medially, this should be reduced first (by traction and inversion, or through a small medial incision. If unstable, the position should be held with longitudinal or transverse Kirschner wires. Thereafter, proceed as 359, 77 and 78. Anatomical reduction of all tarsometatarsal dislocations should be the aim for reasonable results in terms of pain, stiffness and freedom from limp.

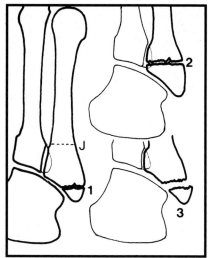

**80. Fractures of the fifth metatarsal base:** The commonest fracture of the lower limb is an avulsion fracture of the fifth metatarsal base: and it is often overlooked. It follows a sudden inversion strain (as, for example, from walking over uneven ground). In an effort to correct the progressive inversion of the foot, the peronei contract violently and the peroneus brevis avulses its bony attachment.

**81. Diagnosis (1):** Tenderness is marked and well localised over the fracture, so that diagnosis should be easy. As the fracture results from an inversion injury, the patient often complains of having sprained his ankle. If an adequate clinical examination is not carried out and radiographs taken of the ankle only, the *fracture line will not be visualised.* The diagnosis is confirmed by the correct radiographic projections.

**82. Diagnosis (2):** Note in the radiographs that the fracture line runs at right angles to the axis of the metatarsal shaft. The fracture involves the joint (1) with the cuboid, if the fragment is small and (2) with the fourth metatarsal, if the fragment is large. In the former case (3) separation of the fragments may occur. (Note that the classical (unrelated) Jones fracture (J) is situated distal to the intermetatarsal joint.)

**83. Diagnosis (3):** (4) Do not misinterpret the rounded shadows of accessory bones (e.g. the os peroneum in peroneus longus, the os Vesalianum in peroneus brevis). In children (5) the epiphysis lying *parallel* to the shaft may also be wrongly taken for fracture. Nevertheless (6) separation or (7) fracture of the epiphysis may occur.

**84. Treatment:** Most fractures are undisplaced (illus.) but even marked displacement does not merit reduction. If symptoms are slight, give a crepe or similar support for 2–3 weeks, and if marked a walking plaster for 5–7 weeks. Pain from the occasional non-union may be expected to resolve spontaneously, but Sudeck's atrophy is common and may require prolonged treatment.

**85. Jones fracture:** This fracture is not associated with inversion injuries, but tends to occur in athletes during training: it has some of the features of stress fractures. Non-union is common, and is most often associated with early weight bearing: because of this, treat with 7 weeks' fixation in a below-knee non-weight-bearing cast. In the professional athlete, internal fixation with an intramedullary AO cancellous bone screw may be considered. Treat delayed or non-union with medullary curettage and bone grafting.

**86. (1) Metatarsal shaft and neck fractures:** These frequently result from crushing accidents, and any associated soft-tissue injury will require careful surveillance (see 362, 96). Spiral fractures generally result from forced inversion or eversion of the forefoot. If the fracture is undisplaced (illus.: 2nd metatarsal fracture) without soft-tissue damage, treat symptomatically—viz. a crepe bandage support, or a walking plaster if pain is severe.

**87. (2) First metatarsal:** (1) AP and oblique projections illustrate a slightly displaced first metatarsal fracture. In this type of injury, damage to the peripheral circulation and post traumatic oedema may present problems. Admission for a short period of elevation and observation, with the limb supported in a well-padded split plaster is indicated. (Thereafter a below-knee walking plaster for 5-6 weeks.) (2) If there is marked displacement with off-ending, reduction should be carried out to avoid disturbance of the mechanics of the forefoot. Traction to the toe, with local pressure over the displaced metatarsal may suffice, but open reduction (and sometimes wire fixation) may be necessary (after care as above). (3) Hair-line fractures without soft-tissue crushing may be treated without preliminary elevation, while (4) compound injuries will require the appropriate wound treatment.

**88. (3) March fracture:** Fatigue fractures, usually of the second metatarsal neck or shaft, are not often seen until callus formation has occurred; reassurance, with at most a light support for 2–3 weeks, is all that is indicated. If seen at an early stage, severe pain will occasionally merit treatment in a below-knee walking plaster till union has taken place.

**89. (4) Multiple undisplaced fractures:** The radiograph shows fractures of the necks of the 2nd, 3rd and 4th metatarsals (the clue to the second metatarsal fracture is the kinking of the cortical shadow). Multiple fractures of this type without much displacement may be treated conservatively by plaster support (as 361, 87, 1 or 3).

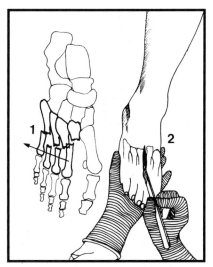

**90. (5) Multiple displaced fractures:** Fractures of the four lesser metatarsals is frequently accompanied by lateral drift, an unstable situation (1). Open reduction and internal fixation are advisable; frequently reduction and stabilisation of the second metatarsal will suffice as the intermetatarsal alignment is preserved. An approach (2) between the second and third metatarsals gives access to both and avoids the arterial anastomosis.

**91. Multiple displaced fractures (2):**
Stability may be preserved with an intramedullary wire and plaster fixation (after care as 361, 87, 1). *Displaced neck fractures* may be manipulated, but open reduction and Kirschner wire fixation are often required. A second incision may be needed to gain access to the 4th and 5th metatarsals. Mal-union may be treated by local trimming of any metatarsal head prominences in the sole.

**92. Freiberg's disease:** Osteochondritis of a metatarsal head (usually the second) may cause confusion in diagnosis. Although this condition may result from local trauma, symptoms are usually of gradual onset. An osteochondritic segment may be present, or more commonly there is narrowing of the MP joint and widening and flattening of the head. Persistent symptoms may require excision of the head.

**93. Phalangeal fractures:** Fractures of the terminal phalanx of the great toe are common in men and usually result from a heavy weight falling on the foot unprotected by industrial footwear. The fracture may involve the distal tuft only, but often runs into the IP joint. The fracture is often open.

**94. Treatment:** (1) All wounds should be cleaned and the edges loosely approximated. (2) The nail should be retained unless virtually separated. Some advocate evacuation of the subungual haematoma. (3) Thereafter the fracture may be supported by: (a) adhesive strapping to the adjacent toe, (b) a light dressing and the wearing of a stout shoe with, if necessary, a cut-out for the toe, or (c) a walking plaster with toe platform—all for 2–4 weeks. *Fractures of the terminal phalanges of the lesser toes* may be treated in a similar manner. *Fractures of the middle and proximal phalanges* should be treated by strapping to the adjacent toe for 3–4 weeks; but if there is marked displacement with obvious deformity of the toes, they should first be reduced by traction. *In the case of the great toe*, a walking plaster with toe platform for 4 weeks may give greater relief of symptoms. *Note: In all cases the circulation must be carefully assessed and additional precautions taken where necessary* (e.g. admission for elevation, etc.).

**95. Toe dislocations:** These should be reduced by traction. (Illus.: dislocations of the four lateral MP joints, with fractures of all proximal phalanges except the third.) If there is instability Kirschner wire fixation may be needed. Single dislocations may be reduced under local anaesthesia and supported by strapping to the adjacent toe: multiple dislocations will require general anaesthesia and a walking plaster with a toe platform for 4 weeks.

**96. Crushing injuries of the foot without fracture:** The foot is a resilient structure; it may be run over by a heavy vehicle or be severely crushed without sustaining any obvious fracture. If a history of this type of injury is obtained, admission is nevertheless advisable for: (1) light pressure bandaging by crepe bandage over several layers of wool, (2) elevation, (3) observation of circulation. Sloughing of the skin over a heart-shaped area on the dorsum is not uncommon, but the area requiring desloughing and skin grafting will be minimised by prompt early care.

Degloving injuries of the foot are potentially serious, especially when sole skin is involved, and require prompt plastic surgical attention.

97. What is this injury? What complication is likely to develop?

98. What abnormalities are shown on this radiograph?

99. What injury is present? What is the most likely late complaint? Why is the ultimate prognosis good?

100. Manipulation has failed to reduce this deformity: what is the injury and what treatment would be advised?

101. Describe this radiograph of a crushed foot. What would be the main principles of treatment?

97.  Type III fracture of the neck of the talus. The incidence of avascular necrosis in this type of injury approximates to 85%.

98.  There is an undisplaced fracture of the anterior process of the calcaneus as a result of recent trauma. In addition there is a small avulsion fracture of the dorsal aspect of the navicular, probably of long standing.

99.  Fracture of the tuberosity of the calcaneus. Local heel tenderness may persist for some time, but the ultimate prognosis is good because the subtalar joint is not involved in this class of fracture.

100.  Tarsometatarsal dislocation: if a recent injury, open reduction would be advised; if an old injury, surgical wedge correction with a tarsometatarsal fusion might be indicated.

101.  Comminuted fracture of the first metatarsal. Fractures of the shafts of the second and third metatarsals. Double fracture of the fourth metatarsal. Fracture of the neck of the fifth metatarsal. Lateral displacement. The injury is open (horizontal streaks of ingrained dirt can be seen). Treatment: if viable, (1) Debridement. (2) Reduction and Kirschner wire fixation of the first and then the second metatarsals. (3) Plaster back shell or split padded plaster, elevation, observation, infection prophylaxis (including antitetanus), etc.

# 16.  The fracture clinic

The organisation and running of fracture clinics varies from hospital to hospital. These differences are often dictated by the lay-out of the departments involved—records, appointments, secretarial, clinical, treatment, plaster, theatre and X-ray—and also by an established line of practice. A system which has worked for a number of years is difficult to change, as an apparently obvious improvement in one area may upset the smooth running of others—to the overall detriment; and change of any kind in an established system is unusual if it attracts universal acceptance. Those who work in fracture clinics have usually to do so within a framework imposed upon them, and it would be invidious to suggest a 'best way' of doing things. Nevertheless it might be helpful for the beginner who is confronted for the first time with a fracture clinic to offer a few guidelines on the handling of the actual consultation.

The newcomer to a fracture clinic is usually impressed by the number of cases dealt with in a short space of time. This speed often conceals the number of rather important decisions that are made about the patients' care. These decisions are of course determined by the basic principles of fracture treatment, but to ensure the smooth running of the clinic, the most professional and kindliest contact with the patient, and the avoidance of any error in management the use of a simple system, at least at the beginning, may be of some help.

Assuming that the usual courtesies of greeting have been made, each consultation should start with asking the two questions—'what' and 'when'—and end with asking 'when' and 'what'. In the middle there are a number of things to go through which can be conveniently dealt with under three headings, each starting with the letter A—'the three As'.

### i:  What:

Every decision that is made, and everything that is done, is directly dependent on the diagnosis. *This must be clearly stated at the beginning of the notes on the first fracture clinic attendance,* where they will serve as a guide to everyone who sees the patient subsequently. It is a never-ending source of astonishment how difficult it may be to find this information, the time taken often varying directly in proportion to the size of the records. If there is a problem, a glance at the initial radiographs (they alone are helpful to label) may give the answer. Time spent establishing the diagnosis is essential. Recording it will prevent the effort having to be repeated at the patient's next attendance.

### ii. When:

The point here is to establish the time that has passed since the patient's injury. While this can obviously be calculated on every occasion from the entries made on the day of injury and on the clinic visit, it is of greater practical value to give the elapsed time.

It is more professional to establish these primary facts before confronting the patient, rather than searching through the notes in his presence. When making the appropriate notes, where brevity should not compromise accuracy, the addition of a qualifier in the case of the diagnosis may be helpful: e.g. 'Undisplaced L Colles # 2/52 ago'; or '7/52: mid-shaft R femur, I-M locked nailing'.

On the solid basis of the knowledge of what you are dealing with, you can proceed to **Assessment, Action, and Advice.**

### iii. Assessment:

(a) The first step is to establish if the fracture to date has been treated *appropriately* and *adequately,* e.g. if a fracture has been manipulated, then it is necessary to consider whether this was the best method of treatment in the circumstances; the desirability of internal fixation or other methods of dealing with the condition should be reviewed. Then the check radiographs should be studied to assess the quality of the reduction, and an overall assessment made.

(b) If a plaster cast has been applied, it should be seen to be appropriate to the injury. It should be checked for tightness, slackness or other inadequacy, and if it is only a backslab, a decision should be made as to whether it needs completion. The presence of swelling, the quality of the circulation, and any impairment of nerve supply in the limb should be noted.

(c) If the fracture has been treated surgically, the need for inspection of the wound or removal of sutures should be assessed. If the fracture has been internally fixed, the quality of the fixation should be reviewed so that a decision may be made regarding the degree of mobilisation that may be permitted without the fracture coming adrift.

(d) If some time has elapsed since the injury, an assessment should be made as to whether a greater degree of freedom may be permitted, e.g. whether a supporting sling may be discarded or whether a cast may be removed to allow joint mobilisation, or whether a walking heel may be applied to a leg plaster.

(e) A decision when to remove all external splintage is not usually required until an appropriate length of time has elapsed since the injury, and in making the decision, radiographs may be required to check the state of union, and/or the cast may be removed so that a clinical assessment of the fracture may be made.

### iv. Action:

Having assessed the fracture, the appropriate action should be taken. What should be done generally follows in a clear cut fashion from the assessment: e.g. if a plaster is too tight it should be split, or if there is complaint of local pressure the plaster should be windowed or trimmed.

The only difficulties that are likely to arise are those associated with the assessment of the treatment that has been carried out. This tends to present less of a problem as experience grows, although with the variety and vagaries of chance and changing opinion the need for the critical analysis of every case is one of the continuing delights of fracture clinics and one which prevents them ever becoming dull. *The point which is imperative to note is that if there is any doubt regarding the treatment or progress of a fracture, a more senior opinion should be sought without delay.* Procrastination narrows the available treatment options, and will attract the criticism of why an earlier opinion was not sought. It is generally easy and a pleasure for a senior colleague to give timely advice on the treatment of a case, and gives him confidence in the reliability and common sense of his junior. Delay or failure in seeking advice may lead to an undesirable or even tragic outcome.

### v. Advice:

The patient should be given clear and appropriate advice. Some of the areas which might be considered include the following:
(a) He should be told or preferably shown what exercises he should do to encourage or preserve movements in the joints related to his fracture.
(b) If he has been given an arm sling he should be advised when and if he may discard it, and how the limb may be exercised with and without it. If he has a leg in plaster he should be given clear advice on how much weight if any he should be allowed to transmit through the limb.
(c) If appropriate he should be given advice on his fitness to drive or return to work.
(d) If he is being referred for physiotherapy he should be advised on what he should do between visits to reinforce the treatment that he will receive.

It is important to explain to the patient, with repetition if necessary, the nature of his injury. It is equally important to keep him informed of his progress and to give, wherever possible, assurance regarding the position of a fracture, and what stage of healing it is at. He should be given some idea of when he can reasonably expect to reach the landmarks in his planned line of treatment, e.g. when he can hope to come out of a cast, when he might be able to weight bear, when he might be able to return to work.

If a complication arises, this should not be concealed. The proposed line of treatment should be clearly explained, and what result might be hoped for.

Frankness at all stages lessens the chances of misunderstanding, and may avert litigation which in many cases is embarked upon when a patient's anger at a less than perfect result is vented on an imagined lapse in management rather than the seriousness of an injury which has not been clearly explained to him.

### vi. When:

The date and time of the next appointment is given, unless the patient is being discharged. In that event it is usually necessary to give a prognosis and advice regarding, for example, return to work or the procedure to follow should any complication arise. It may be necessary to give a recommendation about removal of an implant. It is usual to reinforce these points with the appropriate discharge letter to the patient's own doctor. Do not decide when to see a patient again by guesswork: instead, choose a date when you expect to have to make a further decision about the management of the case, e.g. whether a plaster will have to be changed or when union in a fracture might have to be assessed.

### vii.  What:

The purpose of the patient's next visit should be clearly stated so that the time and trouble that you have spent on assessing and treating the case can be pursued on the next attendance without any waste of precious time—of the patient or the clinic staff. For example it may be helpful to indicate that on the next visit the patient should have his plaster removed, and an X-ray taken to assess union, as soon as he arrives at the clinic. Depending of course on how the clinic is organised this may save valuable time by avoiding the patient having to wait and be seen twice.

### Patients' notes:

The smooth running of a clinic is dependent on the clinical notes, but these lose much of their value if they can only be read by the originator; and they become largely pointless if, as is not infrequent, even the writer has difficulty in interpreting them. If there is no facility for having *all* the notes typewritten, it is nevertheless strongly advised the notes should be typed on the first fracture clinic attendance *and* if there is any significant change in the line of treatment. Otherwise contractions in common usage, printed in upper case letters, may provide oases of understanding appreciated by every reader.

The following examples of two of the commonest conditions seen at fracture clinics are given to illustrate these points:

**I.  A wrist fracture:** A patient has had a Colles fracture which was only slightly displaced. The wrist was put in a plaster back shell without manipulation and the arm supported in a sling. Her plaster and the swelling and circulation were checked at a review clinic the following day. She is now attending her first fracture clinic 4 days later.

The post-fracture swelling has subsided and it would seem that the plaster backshell can be safely completed. Review of the initial radiographs indicate that the fracture was only slightly displaced, and the original decision not to manipulate the fracture seems quite correct. No radiographs have been taken to check the fracture, and while the chances of it having slipped are thought to be comparatively slight, it is desirable to have the position confirmed; for if the fracture has slipped and the position is not acceptable, it could be readily manipulated at this stage.

If check films are taken before the plaster is completed, there is the possibility that the position may alter during the course of that procedure. The action taken is therefore to complete the plaster and have check radiographs taken afterwards. These in fact show that the original position has been maintained, and it is thought that the risks of late slipping may now be judged to be slight.

The patient is assured that her fractured wrist is in good position, and that it is planned to see if it has joined in 5 weeks' time. She is warned that when she comes out of plaster that her wrist will be rather stiff, but that it is anticipated that eventually she will regain a good range of movements and have little handicap. Her sling is removed, and she is advised (for what is hoped to be the second time) how she may exercise her shoulder and her fingers.

She is asked to return in 2 weeks' time. The main purpose of that visit is to check her plaster.

Notes to cover this might be made along the following lines:

**R Colles # 4/7 ago. Circn OK, POP completed. Check X-ray satis. Discard sling. See 2/52 for POP check.**

When this next appointment is kept, no search has to be made (because of the content of the note above) for what is wrong or what would normally be expected at this visit. The plaster is checked and not found to be slack. It is decided on the basis of the original radiographs of this impacted fracture that if any slipping of the fracture has occurred that this is likely to be minimal and not requiring correction; so there is no call for further radiographs. There has been some discomfort because of pressure in the region of the metacarpal of the little finger and the plaster is trimmed in this region. The fingers and shoulders are found to have a full range of movements, and the patient is encouraged to continue with the exercises she has been shown. She is told that her plaster will be removed on her next visit to see whether her fracture has joined; she is warned that if it transpires that union is not sufficiently far advanced that she may have to go back into plaster for perhaps a further 2 weeks, although this is not particularly likely.

The note might read:

**2/52+. POP trimmed. See 3/52, POP off on arrival.**

On removal of her plaster 3 weeks later, no tenderness is found at the fracture site, and her fracture involving cancellous bone can be safely judged to have united. (Check radiographs are superfluous, and would not be indicated unless any complication were suspected.) There is no swelling, and the use of a Tubigrip or crepe bandage support is not considered necessary. She is advised to continue with her finger exercises, and shown what to do to mobilise her wrist. Her good progress is re-affirmed, and she is advised to return for review in 2 weeks' time when a decision will be made as to whether she needs to have any physiotherapy.

**Note: 5/52+. POP off. No tenderness. Mobilise. See 2/52 ? physio.**

Her next visit is her last as she had no complaints of pain, and has regained an excellent if not complete range of movements. She is told that as she has recovered such a good range of movements at this early stage that physiotherapy is not necessary. She is advised that it is expected that she will regain almost full movements in the wrist, and that she will recover excellent if not quite complete strength, perhaps over the course of the next year. Should she develop any problems with pain, swelling or tingling sensations in the thumb or fingers (anticipating Sudeck's atrophy or carpal tunnel syndrome

—now rather unlikely) she should make a review appointment. She should be told how this can be done.

A discharge letter would normally be written to her own doctor incorporating the diagnosis, her present state, and expected progress. The clinical note may be simply 'See discharge letter' or along the following lines:

**7/52+. Lacks 20° dorsiflexion and 15° supination. Full finger movements, good grip. Discharge.**

**II.  An ankle fracture:** A 25-year-old man has sustained an undisplaced fracture of the lateral malleolus and this has been treated by the application of a below-knee non-weight-bearing plaster cast. The notes record that at the time of his initial attendance on the day of the injury 4 days ago that he had tenderness over both malleoli. The injury has been judged as being potentially unstable, and the decision to treat it conservatively by use of a cast would appear to be correct. A check radiograph taken after application of the plaster shows the fracture in anatomical position, and there is no talar shift.

The notes record that he was seen the day following the injury and the circulation was thought to be satisfactory.

On his present attendance the toes are noted to be a little swollen, and he is complaining of pain in the little toe which is concealed by the cast which extends over it.

This area must be inspected, and the excess plaster is trimmed back exposing the toe. Although the toe is red, it is judged that the relief of local pressure will allow a rapid return to normal. The degree of swelling of the toes suggests that it might be unwise to permit weight bearing at this stage.

The patient is told that although his fracture is in excellent position, that as is commonly the case he has too much swelling to allow him to take weight as yet through his plaster. He is advised to continue using his crutches, and to elevate the limb whenever possible. He is encouraged to exercise the toes.

His job is found to be that of a representative, and involves a mixture of driving, walking and sitting. He is advised that he will have to remain in a plaster cast for 6–8 weeks, and that while in his plaster he should not attempt to drive. Considering the nature of his job which cannot be adjusted to suit his circumstances, he must expect to be absent for at least 2 months. His actual time off will depend on his progress after coming out of plaster, but that there is a good chance of his being able to get back to his particular job within 3 months of the injury.

His notes might read:

**4/7 since # R lat. mall. POP trimmed. See 2/52 ? heel.**

At his second fracture clinic appointment the toe swelling has subsided. The plaster is checked for slackness, and considered to be still offering adequate support. It is noted that the sole of the plaster is a little soft as a result of some weight having been put on it. The upper end of the cast at the back is a little high and is restricting knee flexion. The sole is reinforced, the calf of the plaster trimmed, and a walking heel or boot applied.

The patient is told that he may now start taking full weight through the limb; but that to begin with he should use his crutches until he has gained confidence, when he may or may not feel the need to use a single walking stick. He is asked to return in 4 weeks when it will be decided whether he can come out of plaster, or whether a short further period of plaster fixation will be needed. He is also advised to return in the interim if he has any problem with his plaster.

The note may read:

**2/52. Sole reinforced. Heel. See 4/52 POP off and X-ray ankle on arrival.**

On his third attendance the limb is inspected out of plaster. There is no swelling, and no tenderness in the region of the fracture. A check radiograph (which some would regard as being optional) shows some early callus formation in the region of the fracture whose position has been maintained. Movements of the ankle are restricted to 5° dorsiflexion and 10° plantar flexion.

Union of the fracture is assessed as being sufficient for the patient to remain out of plaster. It is anticipated that as he mobilises the ankle there will be some swelling, and he is given a Tubigrip or crepe bandage support. It is thought that he will rapidly regain most of his ankle and foot movements, and that although the need for physiotherapy will have to be kept in mind, this will probably not be required. He is shown how to exercise the foot and ankle on his own.

The patient is told that his fracture is progressing very well, but that he is likely to develop some rather persistent swelling of his ankle. The support he has been given to counteract this should be removed when in bed at night. He is advised to return in 2 weeks' time when he will be assessed regarding the need for further treatment or when he can return to work.

The note may read:

**6/52. POP off. # uniting. Tubigrip. See 2/52 ? physio. ?discharge.**

On his fourth visit a trace of swelling is noted, but he has recovered all but the last 5° of plantar flexion in the ankle, and foot movements are full. He has no complaint of pain and says he is anxious to return to work which he now thinks he will be able to manage. He wonders when he might return to playing golf and squash.

As he has no pain in the ankle and has recovered a good range of movements, no physiotherapy is necessary and it should be safe for him to drive and try going back to work. He is advised to continue wearing his support until any tendency to swelling has disappeared.

The presence of some swelling suggests that it would be wise not to overdo his weight bearing activities. A reasonable approach might be to recommend that after a further 2 weeks he might try a half round of golf, and be guided by any subsequent discomfort and swelling. As far as squash is concerned, where stress on the ankles is particularly high, it would be advisable to defer this until a full 3 months from the time of the original injury, and until all swelling of the ankle has subsided.

He should be told that at this stage, in view of his progress and the anticipation of a full recovery, that there is no immediate need for him to re-attend. Should however he become unhappy about his progress then he should make a review appointment. It should be mentioned that his doctor will be written with a summary of the history, present findings and recommendations.

The final note then need only be **'See discharge letter'.**

The discharge letter itself need not be long, but should cover the main points in the history, the diagnosis, the treatment, and the prognosis. Such a letter might read:

**'Mr . . . attended the Casualty Department on . . . with an undisplaced fracture of the right lateral malleolus sustained in a fall down some steps. It was treated by 6 weeks' fixation in POP and it has united in good position. He has regained a good range of movements in the ankle, but he has still a little swelling. He can now return to work, but should avoid contact sports for a further month at least. He has been discharged today, but I have advised him to return should he have any problem.'**

Enjoy your clinics!

# Index